OSCILLATIONS IN NEURAL SYSTEMS

THE INTERNATIONAL NEURAL NETWORKS SOCIETY SERIES

Harold Szu, Editor

Alspector/Goodman/Brown • *Proceedings of the International Workshop on Applications of Neural Networks to Telecommunications* (1993)

Alspector/Goodman/Brown • *Proceedings of the International Workshop on Applications of Neural Networks to Telecommunications, Vol. 2* (1993)

Freeman • *Societies of Brains: A Study in the Neuroscience of Love and Hate* (1995)

King/Pribram • *Scale in Conscious Experience: Is the Brain too Important to be Left to Specialists to Study?* (1995)

Lenaris/Grossberg/Kosko • *World Congress on Neural Networks: Proceedings of the 1993 INNS Annual Meeting*

Levine/Brown/Shirey • *Oscillations in Neural Systems* (2000)

Levine/Elsberry • *Optimality in Biological and Artificial Networks?* (1977)

Pribram • *Rethinking Neural Networks: Quantum Fields and Biological Data* (1993)

Pribram • *Origins: Brain and Self-Organization* (1994)

Pribram/King • *Learning as Self-Organization* (1996)

Sobajic • *Neural Network Computing for the Electric Power Industry* (1993)

OSCILLATIONS IN NEURAL SYSTEMS

Edited by

DANIEL S. LEVINE
University of Texas at Arlington

VINCENT R. BROWN
Clarkson University

V. TIMOTHY SHIREY
Metroplex Institute for Neural Dynamics

LEA
2000

LAWRENCE ERLBAUM ASSOCIATES, PUBLISHERS
Mahwah, New Jersey London

Lawrence Erlbaum Associates, Inc., Publishers
10 Industrial Avenue
Mahwah, New Jersey 07430

Cover design by Kathryn Houghtaling Lacey

Library of Congress Cataloging-in-Publication Data

Oscillations in neural systems / edited by Daniel S. Levine, Vincent R. Brown, V. Timothy Shirey
p. cm.
Includes bibliographical references
ISBN 0-8058-2066-3 (cloth : alk. paper)
1. Neural computers. 2. Neural networks (Computer science)
I. Levine, Daniel S. II. Brown, Vincent R. III. Shirey, V. Timothy
QA76.87.083 1999 99-39666
006.3'2--dc21 CIP

Books published by Lawrence Erlbaum Associates are printed on acid-free paper, and their bindings are chosen for strength and durability.

Printed in the United States of America
10 9 8 7 6 5 4 3 2 1

Contents

List of Contributors

Bill Baird, Department of Mathematics, University of California, Berkeley CA 94720 (baird@math.berkeley.edu)

Douglas A. Baxter, Department of Neurobiology and Anatomy, University of Texas Medical School, Houston TX 77030 (dbaxter@nba19.med.uth.tmc.edu)

Galina Borisyuk, Institute of Mathematical Problems in Biology, Russian Academy of Sciences, Pushchino, Moscow Region, 142292, Russia (borisyuk@impb.psn.ru)

Roman Borisyuk, School of Computing, University of Plymouth, Drake Circus, Plymouth, PL4 8AA, United Kingdom (borisyuk@soc.plym.ac.uk)

Anthony G. Brown, Room E502, DERA (Malvern), St. Andrews Road, Malvern, WORCS WR14 3PS, United Kingdom (abrown@signal.dera.gov.uk)

Vincent R. Brown (Editor), Department of Psychology, Clarkson University, Potsdam, NY 13699-5825 (brownv@clarkson.edu)

Robert J. Butera, Jr., Mathematical Research Branch, NIDDK, NIH, 9190 Wisconsin Ave., Suite 350, Bethesda MD 20184 (butera@helix.nih.gov)

John H. Byrne, Department of Neurobiology and Anatomy, University of Texas Medical School, Houston TX 77030 (jbyrne@nba19.med.uth.tmc.edu)

Carmen C. Canavier, Department of Psychology, University of New Orleans, New Orleans LA 70148 (cccps@uno.edu)

Larry J. Cauller, School of Human Development, Box 830688, University of Texas at Dallas, Richardson TX 75083 (lcauller@utdallas.edu)

John W. Clark, Jr., Department of Electrical and Computer Engineering, Rice University, Houston TX 77251 (jwc@rice.edu)

Steve Collins, Department of Engineering Science, University of Oxford, Parks Road, Oxford OX1 3PJ, United Kingdom (steve.collins@eng.ox.ac.uk)

Anthony A. DeFranceschi, Department of Electrical and Computer Engineering, Rice University, Houston TX 77251

David DeMaris, 1514 West 9th, Austin TX 78703 (demaris@ece.texas.edu)

John P. Edstrom, Oregon State University, The Mark O. Hatfield Marine Science Center, 2030 South Marine Science Drive, Newport, OR 97365 (edstrom@slugo.hmsc.orst.edu)

Frank Eeckman, Lawrence Berkeley National Lab, 1 Cyclotron Road, Mailstop 46A-1123, Berkelely CA 94720 (FHEeckman@lbl.gov)

Paul S. Fisher, Department of Computer Science, University of North Texas, P.O. Box 13886, Denton TX 76203-2989 (fisher@infinop.com)

Guenter Gross, Department of Biological Sciences, Center for Network Neuroscience, P.O. Box 305220, University of North Texas, Denton, TX 76203 (gross@morticia.cnns.unt.edu)

Stephen Grossberg, Department of Cognitive and Neural Systems, Boston University, 677 Beacon Street, Boston, MA 02215 (steve@cns.bu.edu)

Alexander Grunewald, Division of Biology, California Institute of Technology, Mail Code 216-76, Pasadena, CA 91125 (alex@vis.caltech.edu)

David Horn, School of Physics and Astronomy, Tel Aviv University, Tel Aviv 69978, Israel (horn@neuron.tau.ac.il, http://neuron.tau.ac.il/~horn)

Arun Jagota, Department of Computer Science, University of California at Santa Cruz, Santa Cruz, CA 95064 (jagota@cse.ucsc.edu)

Mark E. Jackson, Department of Neurobiology and Behavior, SUNY — Stony Brook, Life Science Building, Stony Brook, NY 11794-6661 (mjackson@utdallas.edu)

Yakov Kazanovich, Institute of Mathematical Problems in Biology, Russian Academy of Sciences, Pushchino, Moscow Region, 142292, Russia (kazanovich@impb.psn.ru)

Christof Koch, Computation and Neural Systems, 139-74, California Institute of Technology, Pasadena CA 91125 (koch@klab.caltech.edu)

Jacek M. Kowalski, Department of Physics, P.O. Box 305370, UNT Station, University of North Texas, Denton, TX 76203 (jmkow@worldnet.att.net)

Hilde A. Lechner, Department of Neurobiology and Anatomy, University of Texas Medical School, Houston TX 77030 (hlechner@nba19.med.uth.tmc.edu)

Daniel S. Levine (Editor), Department of Psychology, University of Texas at Arlington, Arlington, TX 76019-0528 (levine@uta.edu)

George E. Mobus, Department of Computer Science, MS 9062, Western Washington University, Bellingham, WA 98226 (mobus@cs.wwu.edu, http://www.cs.wwu.edu/faculty/mobus/)

George J. Mpitsos, Oregon State University, The Mark O. Hatfield Marine Science Center, 2030 South Marine Science Drive, Newport, OR 97365 (gmpitsos@slugo.hmsc.orst.edu)

Irit Opher, School of Physics and Astronomy, Tel Aviv University, Tel Aviv 69978, Israel (irito@post.tau.ac.il)

Nam Seog Park, Information Technology Laboratory, GE Corporate Research & Development, One Research Circle, Niskayuna, NY 12309 (parkns@crd.ge.com)

Barry K. Rhoades, Department of Biology, Wesleyan College, Macon, GA 31210 (brhoades@post.wesleyan-college.edu)

Dave Robertson, Department of Artificial Intelligence, University of Edinburgh, 80 South Bridge, Edinburgh EH1 1HN, United Kingdom (dr@dai.ed.ac.uk)

V. Timothy Shirey (Editor), 2706 Sam Houston Drive, Garland, TX 75044 (shirey@dal.asp.ti.com)

Ivan Soltesz, Department of Anatomy and Neurobiology, University of California, Irvine CA 92717-1250 (isoltesz@uci.edu)

Martin Stemmler, Innovationskolleg Theoretische Biologie, Humboldt-Universitaet zu Berlin, Invalidenstrasse 43, D-10115 Berlin, Germany (stemmler@pauling.biologie.hu-berlin.de)

Keith Stenning, The Human Communication Research Centre, University of Edinburgh, 2 Buccleuch Place, Edinburgh EH8 9LW, United Kingdom (keith@cogsci.ed.ac.uk)

Gary Strong, National Science Foundation, Suite 1500, 4201 Wilson Boulevard, Arlington, VA 22230(gstrong@nsf.gov)

David C. Tam, Department of Biological Sciences, University of North Texas, Denton, TX 76203-5220 (dtam@unt.edu, www.biol.unt.edu/~tam)

Elizabeth Thomas, Institute Leon Fredericq, University of Liège, Place del Cours 17, 4000 Liège, Belgium (ethomas@ulg.ac.be)

Todd Troyer, Department of Physiology, Box 0444, University of California, San Francisco CA 94143 (todd@phy.ucsf.edu)

Marius Usher, Department of Psychology, The University of Kent, Canterbury, Kent CT2 7NP, United Kingdom (M.Usher@ukc.ac.uk)

Xin Wang, 3005 Shrine Pl. #8, Los Angeles, CA 90007 (xwang@rcf.usc)

Seth Wolpert, W-256K Olmsted Bldg., Department of Electrical Engineering,Penn State-Harrisburg,777 W. Harrisburg Pike, Middletown, PA 17057-4898 (sxw33@ psu.edu)

David Young, 645 Sunset Boulevard, Baton Rouge, LA 70808-5082 (dyoung@ ee.lsu.edu)

Geoffrey L. Yuen, Morningstar Inc., 225 West Wacker Drive, Chicago IL 60606 (gyuen @ mstar.com)

Preface

This book is the fourth of a series of books based on conferences sponsored by the Metroplex Institute for Neural Dynamics (M.I.N.D.), an interdisciplinary organization of Dallas-Fort Worth area neural network professionals in both academia and industry. M.I.N.D. sponsors a conference every few years on some topic within neural networks. The topics are chosen (a) to be of broad interest both to those interested in designing machines to perform intelligent functions and those interested in studying how these functions are actually performed by living organisms, and (b) to generate discussion of basic and controversial issues in the study of mind. The subjects are chosen for depth and fascination of the problems covered, rather than for the availability of airtight conclusions; hence, well-thought-out speculation is encouraged at these conferences. Thus far, the topics have been as follows:

May 1988 — Motivation, Emotion, and Goal Direction in Neural Networks
June 1989 — Neural Networks for Adaptive Sensory-Motor Control
October 1990 — Neural Networks for Knowledge Representation and Inference
February 1992 — Optimality in Biological and Artificial Networks?
May 1994 — Oscillations in Neural Systems
May 1995 — Neural Networks for High-Order Rule Formation

Lawrence Erlbaum Associates, Inc., has published books based on the 1988 conference (in 1992), the 1990 conference (in 1994), the 1992 conference (in 1997), and now this one on the 1994 conference.

The topic of neural oscillations was chosen because of the increasing interest by neuroscientists and psychologists in both rhythmic and chaotic activity patterns observed in the nervous system. As for rhythmic activity patterns, Milner (1974) speculated that they could play a role in binding parts of a perceptual pattern into observed whole objects from the environment, and segmenting the temporal windows of different perceptual patterns. This speculation was confirmed by some observations of activity patterns in the cerebral cortex due to Gray and Singer (1989), and has been developed further in numerous models of perceptual binding (Grunewald & Grossberg, chap. 12, this volume; Horn & Opher, chap. 11, this volume; Singer, 1994; Stemmler, Usher, & Koch, chap. 4, this volume). This type of perceptual binding has been proposed to play strong roles in the generation of perceptual consciousness (Crick & Koch, 1990) and in various types of linguistic inference (Hummel & Holyoak, 1997; Shastri & Ajjanagadde, 1993). In addition, other neuroscientists have applied this notion of rhythmic pattern generation to the motor domain (see, e.g., Houk, 1987; Yuen, chap. 10, this volume).

Chaotic aspects of neural activity have been generally thought to play a somewhat different set of functional roles. Skarda and Freeman (1987), based on years of results on the olfactory cortex from Freeman's laboratory, proposed that chaos is important for flexibility of nervous system responses, enabling the dynamical system represented in the cortex to change the attractor it approaches based on changes in incoming stimuli or in internal motivational states. A similar role for chaotic patterns has been noted in invertebrate motion generation by Mpitsos and others (see Mpitsos & Edstrom, chap. 5, this volume). In a similar vein, chaos has been suggested to play a role in increasing the information processing capacity of the brain, particularly the cerebral cortex (Jackson & Cauller, chap. 8, this volume). This can also be a mechanism for switching between different interpretations of an ambiguous percept (e.g., DeMaris, chap. 13, this volume). This role of chaos has also been studied mathematically and applied to optimization problems (e.g., Jagota & Wang, chap. 19, this volume).

Yet neither the mathematical structure of neural oscillations nor their functional significance is precisely understood. There are a great many open problems in both the structure and function of neural oscillations, whether rhythmic, chaotic, or a combination of the two, and many of these problems are dealt with in different chapters of this book.

First of all, the nature of intrinsic oscillations of firing patterns in small groups of neurons is still under investigation. Several laboratories have cultured isolated neuron groups in an attempt to illuminate these patterns (Gross, Kowalski, & Rhoades, chap. 1, this volume). Other investigators have reproduced electrical patterns of neuronal groups in electronic chips (e.g., Wolpert, chap. 20, this volume). At the same time, there is still mathematical investigation both of the sequence of firings (*spike trains*) of individual neurons and of the interrelationships, including synchrony and correlation, between the spike trains of related neurons (Perkel, Gerstein, & Moore, 1967a, 1967b; Tam, chap. 2, this volume).

These investigations have raised questions about what is the source of a given oscillatory pattern, particularly when a rhythmic or synchronous pattern is observed at some location in the nervous system, such as the hippocampus (see Soltesz, chap. 6, this volume) or thalamocortical system (see Thomas, chap. 7, this volume). Is it single cells generating the pattern or is it a property of a larger neural system? Is it intrinsic to the area or group of cells where it is observed, or is it the results of outside inputs from another area? These questions are being investigated, both experimentally and in theoretical models, by adding various neuromodulators or transmitter agonists and antagonists and observing how these substances change the oscillatory pattern. Answers to these questions bear in turn on questions about the functions of the observed oscillations (e.g., in the case of the hippocampus, the theta rhythm observed in that region has been suggested to be related to short-term memory capacity; see Lisman & Idiart, 1995).

The synchronous patterns observed in nervous systems have a wide range of frequencies, from a few up to several hundred Hertz (or cycles per second). This range has led some investigators to propose that different frequencies might have different roles. For example, Borisyuk, Borisyuk, Kazanovich, and Strong (chap. 14, this volume) have proposed that low frequencies might be associated with preattentive processes, such as occur in visual feature binding, and high frequencies with attention and central executive processes that determine which features to attend to. Baird, Troyer, and Eeckman (chap. 15, this volume) discuss the attentional processes further, including a model of how signals from one region might control the frequencies expressed in another region.

As engineers and computer scientists have developed machines for sophisticated and complex applications, they have incorporated most of the major recent insights developed by neuroscientists and neural network theorists. The insights about oscillations in neural systems are no exception. Hence, oscillatory systems have played roles in devices for many applications including inference (e.g., Park, Robertson, & Stenning, chap. 18, this volume); associative memory (e.g., Brown & Collins, chap. 17, this volume); and robotics (e.g., Mobus & Fisher, chap. 16, this volume).

The different levels of analysis involved in studying neural oscillations has led us to group the chapters in this book as follows:

PART I: Oscillations in Single Neurons and Local Networks

Guenter Gross, Jacek Kowalski, and Barry Rhoades
David Tam
Douglas Baxter, Hilde Lechner, Carmen Canavier, Robert Butera, Anthony DeFranceschi, John Clark, and John Byrne
Martin Stemmler, Marius Usher, and Christof Koch
George Mpitsos and John Edstrom

PART II: Oscillations in Cortical and Cortical/Subcortical Systems

Ivan Soltesz
Elizabeth Thomas
Mark Jackson and Larry Cauller
David Young
Geoffrey Yuen

PART III: Oscillatory Models in Perception, Memory, and Cognition

David Horn and Irit Opher
Alexander Grunewald and Stephen Grossberg
David DeMaris
Galina Borisyuk, Roman Borisyuk, Yakov Kazanovich, and Gary Strong
Bill Baird, Todd Troyer, and Frank Eeckman

PART IV: Applications of Synchronized and Chaotic Oscillations

George Mobus and Paul Fisher
Anthony Brown and Steve Collins
Nam Seog Park, Dave Robertson, and Keith Stenning
Arun Jagota and Xin Wang
Seth Wolpert

We are pleased to acknowledge the assistance of various individuals who helped make this book possible. Lane Akers and Sondra Guideman, our editors at Lawrence Erlbaum Associates, Inc. (LEA) at different stages, were very helpful in seeing this book through and patient with the slow progress of collecting chapters. Arthur Lizza, Vice-President in charge of production at LEA, was helpful in making sure that the camera ready copy fit specifications.

The other members of the Metroplex Institute for Neural Dynamics (M.I.N.D.) gave great support, emotional and financial, to the running of the 1994 conference on which the book is based. In particular, several students then involved with M.I.N.D. — Raju Bapi, Jaynee Beach, Sriram Govindarajan, Paul Havig, and Nilendu Jani — provided indispensable assistance with the logistics of the meeting organization. The meeting was also supported by several departments at the University of Texas at Arlington: the main library, who provided the facilities at nominal cost; the College of Science and its Dean, Peter Rosen, the Department of Psychology and its Chair, Roger Mellgren, and the Department of Mathematics and its Chair, George Fix, all of whom gave financial assistance to M.I.N.D. for the conference.

Several distinguished scientists gave talks that contributed to the vitality of the conference but for various reasons were unable to contribute chapters to this book. These speakers were Adi Bulsara, Shien-Fong Lin, Alianna Maren, Andrew Penz, Mark Steyvers, Roger Traub, and Robert Wong. Also, we acknowledge the assistance of Dr. Rodney Carver in reviewing the original manuscripts of several of the chapters for clarity and mutual coherence.

Finally, we acknowledge the personal and emotional support of Lorraine P. Levine and Lynne D. Shirey.

Daniel S. Levine
Arlington, TX

Vincent R. Brown
Potsdam, NY

V. Timothy Shirey
Garland, TX

References

Crick, F., & Koch, C. (1990). Towards a neurobiological theory of consciousness. *Seminars in Neuroscience, 2*, 263-275.

Gray, C. M., & Singer, W. (1989). Stimulus-specific neuronal oscillations in orientation columns of cat visual cortex. *Proceedings of National Academy of Sciences of the USA, 86*, 1698-1702.

Houk, J. (1987). Model of the cerebellum as an array of adjustable pattern generators. In M. Glickstein, C. Yeo, & J. Stein (Eds.), *Cerebellum and Neural Plasticity* (pp. 249-260). New York: Plenum.

Hummel, J. E., & Holyoak, K. J. (1997). Distributed representations of structure: A theory of analogical access and mapping. *Psychological Review, 104*, 427-466.

Lisman, J. E., & Idiart, M. A. (1995). Storage of 7 +/- 2 short-term memories in oscillatory subcycles. *Science, 267*, 1512-1515.

Milner, P. M. (1974). A model for visual shape recognition. *Psychological Review, 81*, 521-535.

Perkel, D. H., Gerstein, G. L., & Moore, G. P. (1967a). Neuronal spike trains and stochastic point process. I. The single spike train. *Biophysical Journal, 7*, 391-418.

Perkel, D. H., Gerstein, G. L., & Moore, G. P. (1967b). Neuronal spike trains and stochastic point process. II. Simultaneous spike trains. *Biophysics Journal, 7*, 419-440.

Shastri, L., & Ajjanagadde, V. (1993). From simple associations to systematic reasoning: A connectionist representation of rules, variables and dynamic bindings using temporal synchrony. *Behavioral and Brain Sciences*, *16*, 417-494.

Singer, W. (1994). Putative functions of temporal correlations in neocortical processing. In C. Koch & J. Davis (Eds.), *Large-Scale Neuronal Theories of the Brain* (pp. 201-237). Cambridge, MA: MIT Press.

Skarda, C., & Freeman, W. J. (1987). How brains make chaos to make sense of the world. *The Behavioral and Brain Sciences*, *10*, 161-195.

I

Oscillations in Single Neurons and Local Networks

1

Spontaneous and Evoked Oscillations in Cultured Mammalian Neuronal Networks

Guenter Gross and Jacek M. Kowalski
University of North Texas

Barry K. Rhoades
Wesleyan College, Macon, GA

ABSTRACT

In monolayer networks derived from dissociated embryonic mouse spinal cord tissue and maintained in culture for up to 9 months, near-oscillatory activity states are common and represent the most reproducible of all network behaviors. The oscillations, which are normally coordinated among many of the electrodes, can be generated in all spontaneously active cultures. Extensive observations of self-organized oscillatory activity have demonstrated that such network states represent a generic feature of randomized networks in culture and suggest that possibly all neuronal networks may have a strong tendency to oscillate. Whereas oscillatory states in normal culture medium are highly transient, system disinhibition produced by blocking inhibitory glycine or $GABA_A$ receptors generates long-lasting oscillatory states that survive for hours with minimal changes in burst variables. Electrical stimulation at a single electrode can generate driven periodic states and repeated stimulus trains have been observed to induce episodes of coherent bursting lasting beyond the termination of the stimulus pattern. Such responses appear "epileptiform" and might be considered a cultured network parallel to electrical induction of an epileptic seizure *in vivo*. These experimental observations suggest that oscillation, and not quiescence, is a natural state of neural tissue and challenge theoretical efforts to focus on oscillations as the basic "engine" of spontaneous activity.

1. INTRODUCTION

1.1 Ubiquity of Synchronized, Oscillatory Bursting

Many investigators have reported complex oscillatory neural activity as part of normal central nervous system (CNS) function and it even has been suggested that the integration of distributed processes in the CNS may be accomplished by neuronal rhythms (Gray, 1994; Gray, König, Engel, & Singer, 1989; Malsburg, 1981; Milner, 1974; Singer, 1990; Sporns, Tononi, & Edelman, 1991). The ubiquity of oscillation implies that this phenomenon is a fundamental property of neural tissue and that it may underlie mechanisms of information processing in the CNS. Clearly, a better understanding of oscillatory activity should provide insight into the dynamics of neuronal ensembles and the roles played by oscillatory states in brain function and behavior. However, because of the complexity of neural systems, accelerated progress in this area will require great care in describing data, improved computational methods and theoretical models, as well as a focus on simple experimental dynamical systems in which oscillatory mechanisms can be investigated under highly controlled conditions and for long periods of time.

Among numerous examples, oscillatory EEG patterns have been observed in the thalamus of drowsy cats (spindle oscillations 7 to 14 Hz) and sleeping cats (delta waves 0.5 to 4 Hz); (Steriade, Curro Dossi, & Nuñez, 1991). In the human thalamus (VL nucleus), spontaneous burst frequencies of 3 to 6 Hz with burst durations of 10 to 30 ms were reported (Raeva, 1990). Oscillatory burst patterns were found in both the epileptic and normal human gyrus hippocampi, but with higher burst pattern frequencies detected on the focal side (Babb & Crandall, 1976). In the rat medial septal area (which projects to the hippocampus), about 40% of the neurons revealed rhythmic bursting (Jobert, Bassant, & Lamour, 1989). This was also shown by Stewart and Fox (1989) who demonstrated that this activity did not depend on feedback from the hippocampus. The suprachiasmatic nucleus of the hypothalamus maintains a circadian (spiking) rhythm of 7 to 10 Hz and 3 to 5 Hz during the light and dark phases, respectively (Hatton, 1984). In addition, phasic bursting, approximating slow oscillations at 2 to 3 bursts per minute, was seen in the paraventricular nucleus. Here, the vasopressin-containing neurons established electrotonic coupling under conditions of dehydration, resulting in massive phasic bursting that was inferred to be a population response (Hatton, 1984).

Investigations of thalamic slices (Jahnsen & Llinas, 1984a, 1984b; McCormick & Pape, 1990) showed extensive two-mode operations for neurons: stimulus-elicited spiking and synchronized bursting. Bursting could be promoted by disinhibition of thalamic interneurons and it was postulated that the oscillatory bursting mode corresponded to states of reduced attentiveness. Bursting states were shown insensitive to incoming stimuli (McCormick & Feeser, 1990), which confirmed a postulated "filtering" role for such states (Sporns et al., 1989). Unique insight has also been gained into oscillatory activity within the olfactory bulb where spatial patterns of phase, frequency, and amplitude of the induced field potential waves revealed no changes until odors were presented to the experimental animals in a behaviorally significant context (Freeman, 1978; Freeman & Schneider, 1982).

It is well established that oscillatory responses can be elicited in practically any region of the brain or spinal cord by disinhibiting agents (Alger, 1984; Gloor, Quesney, & Zumstein, 1977; Gutnick & Friedman, 1986). Under the influence of 30 to 120 μM (micromolar) NMDA, rhythmic burst patterns (200 to 800 ms in length) were seen in brainstem slices (Tell & Jean, 1990). Massive correlated bursting with oscillatory components also play an important role in embryonic development. It has long been thought that embryonic limb movement depends partially on endogenous oscillatory processes (Brown, 1914). Electrophysiological evidence has now confirmed that embryonic motility is spontaneous and patterned by spinal circuitry without any requirement for afferent impulses (Grillner, Buchanan, Wallen, & Brodin, 1988; Hamburger & Balaban, 1963; Provine, 1971). In developing chick embryos, massive polyneuronal burst discharges were identified within the ventral cord region at 4.5 days (Ripley & Provine, 1972). These experiments point to an inherent pattern-generation capability within spinal tissue of various species.

In light of the numerous *in vivo* observations of oscillatory bursting, it is significant that simple mouse monolayer cultures consisting of 200 to 800 neurons display spontaneous, coordinated burst patterns. These patterns are seen approximately two weeks after seeding and remain active for more than 9 months *in vitro* (Gross, 1994). Hence, after dissociation of embryonic CNS tissue into its cellular constituents, the self-assembly of networks in culture forms circuits that are, at least in this specific dynamic response, histiotypic (i.e., similar to the parent tissue). Transient oscillatory bursting also is commonly observed. If such networks are disinhibited with blocking agents of the inhibitory glycine and GABA circuits, highly regular oscillatory activity is induced. Such modes of activity are often stable for many hours, and are associated with a clear regularization of burst duration, burst period, and spike frequency within the bursts. The induced oscillatory response is one of the most reproducible of all *in vitro* network behaviors (Droge, Gross, Hightower, & Czisny, 1986; Gopal & Gross, 1996a, 1996b; Gross, 1994; Gross & Kowalski, 1991; Gross, Rhoades, Reust, & Schwalm, 1993; Hightower, 1988; Jordan, 1992; Maeda, Robinson, & Kawana, 1995; Rhoades & Gross, 1991a).

All simplified experimental systems have limitations that prevent direct extrapolation of data to living organisms. Cultured networks have a reduced synaptic density, seemingly random architecture, reduced glia cell number, and lack of sensory input. Questions of whether, or under what conditions, cultured networks duplicate the functions of *in situ* circuitry are pertinent. However, the presence of structural and dynamic fluctuations in these monolayer cultures should not prohibit statistical descriptions focusing on highly probable, gross behavioral features of a large family of similar cultures (with identical origin, similar neuronal densities, and environmental parameters). It is desirable to develop reference networks for which all functions and mechanisms can be well documented. The advantages of such *in vitro* preparations grown on microelectrode arrays are (1) a yield of spatial and temporal statistical data, with multiple chances to select high signal-to noise-ratio samples of representative spike activity; (2) application of flexible schemes of multielectrode recording and stimulation; (3) reproducible pharmacological manipulation; and (4) long-term (days to weeks) optical, photometric, and electrophysiological monitoring with stable cell-electrode coupling. In addition, such systems are amenable to experimental morphological alterations or developmental constraints that can be correlated with specific changes in network dynamics. As a consequence, they are becoming *generic platforms* for the study of the internal dynamics that underlie such key network phenomena as pattern generation, pattern recognition, pattern storage, and fault tolerance.

This chapter focuses on spontaneous and induced oscillatory activity patterns on the burst level of spike organization. Although it may still be possible to question whether minor changes in spike patterns are of significance or should be considered "noise," bursts are high frequency spike packets that have major influences on postsynaptic voltages and, therefore, will have functional consequences. Our opinions and conclusions are based on the evaluation of multichannel data from 64 channel recording arrays on which spinal cord and cortical networks were grown. This approach allows the monitoring of population responses without losing the important dynamic individualities of neurons contributing, through synergetic and antagonistic interactions, to transiently expressed and often synchronized oscillatory population patterns.

1.2. Summary of Experimental Methods

Nerve cells are grown in cell culture on transparent, photoetched microelectrode arrays featuring 64 electrodes in a 1-mm^2 area. Most data are collected from isolated networks centered on the recording matrix. The diameter of the monolayer networks usually ranges from 1 to 4 mm containing, respectively, 100 to 1,500 neurons. The cultures form stable cell-electrode coupling for long-term monitoring of spike traffic within a monolayer network (Gross, 1994; Gross & Kowalski, 1991; Gross, Wen, & Lin, 1985). Most networks show initial spiking activity at one week and generate complex, often coordinated burst patterns at three weeks. This chapter restricts itself to data derived from murine embryonic spinal cord, dissociated at 14 to 15 days gestation and seeded at a total concentration (neurons and glia) of approximately $5x10^5$ cells/ml (cf. Gross, 1994). Some spinal monolayers survived for more than 9 months in culture and routinely showed vigorous electrical activity at all ages above two weeks. Similar methods have recently led to an initial multi-channel exploration of auditory cortex in culture (Gopal & Gross, 1996a, 1996b).

The nerve cell culture is situated inside its recording and life-support chamber on the stage of an inverted microscope. Two VLSI preamplifier banks (CAR 2000, Department of Electrical Engineering at Southern Methodist University) containing 32 amplifiers each, are located to either side of the chamber and attached via edge connectors and zebra strips. This component is also able to select any combination of channels for stimulation with a maximum of four separate stimulation signals (Abuzaid et al., 1991). The pH of the bicarbonate-buffered medium is controlled by an Aalborg gas mixture controller (Dakota Institute, Monsey, NY) which passes a 10% CO_2/air mixture to a gas wash bottle (not shown) to increase the humidity before entering either a medium supply flask (closed recording chamber) or the cap of an open recording chamber at a flow rate of about 1 ml/min (Gross & Schwalm, 1994). Preamplified signals are fed to a second-stage computer-controlled amplifier and data processing system consisting of 16 digital signal processors that allow spike recognition and selection from a total set of 64 amplifiers. A maximum of 32 channels can be computer-selected for output to the patch panel, 14 to the analog tape recorder, and 4 to oscilloscopes. A subset of these channels can also be selected for digital processing and manipulation with a variety of statistical packages (Spectrum Scientific, Dallas). Signals from the patch panel are electronically integrated (time constant 700 ms) and available for display on a 12-channel chart recorder.

Typical multichannel data is shown in Fig. 1.1 with an 8-channel simultaneous recording of activity in the native state (i.e., spontaneous spiking and bursting from a culture in a recording chamber under the same medium as in the incubator, at pH 7.4 and 37°C). This panel shows a spontaneous transition from spiking on channels one and five to correlated bursting on all channels. It can also be seen that, after a damped oscillatory transient, the network enters a nearly periodic coordinated bursting mode. For native activity, such modes are almost always of short duration with approximate periodic oscillations that often are disrupted by aperiodic patterns. The lower part of Fig. 1.1 shows the equivalent integrated patterns for each channel, respectively. Integration is a convenient method of feature extraction that eliminates slow spiking and emphasizes bursts consisting of high frequency spike clusters. Although the figure represents digitized data, the program simulates analog electronic integration (time constant 700 ms) which is used extensively at several workstations in our laboratory.

1.3. Pattern Identification

There is no single, generally accepted terminology for describing spatiotemporal patterns because of the great variability in such patterns. In our approach, we assign temporal patterns to six general *activity modes* in order of increasing spike activity: (1) no spiking; (2) low frequency spiking; (3) patterned spiking with weak bursting; (4) patterned bursting; (5) periodic bursting; (6) burst fusion leading to continual high frequency spiking (Gross et al, 1993). Each category can be expanded to include a "fine structure" for incorporation of more complex patterns. At present, it allows a limited visual evaluation of the temporal evolution of activity modes of a single channel during experiments. For the description of spatial data provided by the simultaneous recording of many channels, we use the notions of coordination, synchronization, and coupling. Coordination implies a relationship between bursts on different channels and includes alternating activity. Synchronization is a special case of coordination when there are no phase differences between bursts. However, such cases are rare and the term synchronization has been broadened (by many) to include "nearly simultaneous events" without concern for small phase differences. This has been called "coarse-grain synchronization" or "approximate synchronization." We suggest that synchronization be used broadly and that cases of zero phase differences be termed "true" synchronization.

Statistical measures of activity states and activity modes can be attained in the burst regime with state-space cluster plots. The graphs represent a two parameter state space derived from a single random burst pattern variable (such as period, duration, duty cycle, integrated area, and integrated amplitude). Figure 1.2 shows the construction of such plots schematically for the burst period variable. A short data or time segment (10 to 20 bursts) is used to calculate a mean period and the concomitant standard deviation. The mean is then plotted against the normalized standard deviation (coefficient of variation), resulting in one data point that we define as a "channel state." If the channel

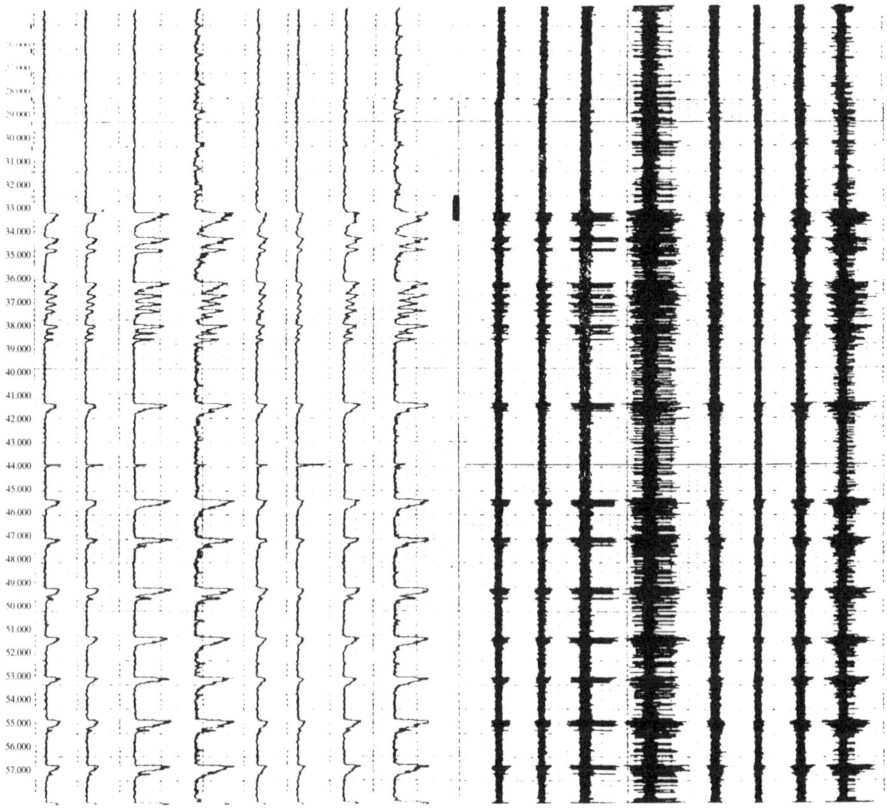

Fig. 1.1. Coordinated (approximately synchronized) activity. Bottom: Equivalent integrated patterns for each channel, respectively (time constant 700 ms; bar = 10 sec).

reports only one active unit, or if the units are separated by an appropriate spike recognition method, the channel state becomes a unit state representing one neuron. Our definition of "state" is not an instantaneous configuration of the network as suggested by Getting (1989) but rather a short data segment from which a mean and standard deviation (SD) can be calculated (Gross, 1994). A continuation of this process generates a state space cluster in which increasing periods (or duration) shift the data to the right and greater burst pattern irregularity shifts the data points away from the x-axis. The cluster, or primary domain of the cluster, is defined as a "channel (or unit) activity mode."

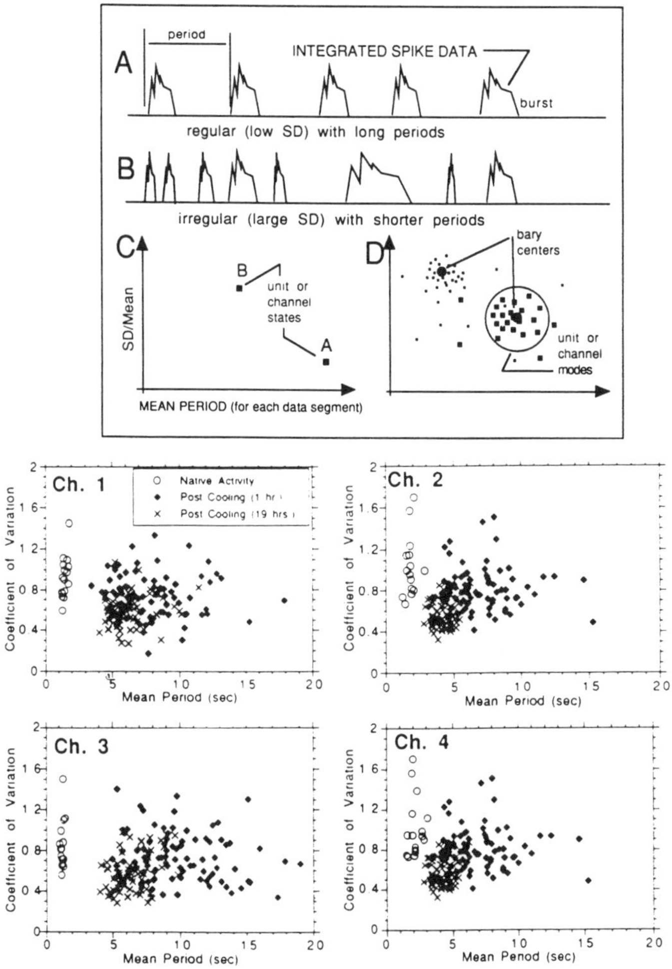

Fig. 1.2. Top: Construction of a two parameter state-space cluster plot derived from a single random burst variable. Variables such as period, duration, duty cycle, integrated area, and integrated amplitude can be represented in this manner. Unit or channel states represent short data segments from which a mean and standard deviation can be calculated. Activity modes are clusters of such states from which a barycenter can be determined. Clusters of barycenters approximate network activity modes. Bottom: Cluster plots for four channels over the same time period using the burst period as variable. The network was cooled to 10°C for one hour, returned to 37°C, monitored one hour after rewarming, and again 19 hours after rewarming. A native mode of short but variable periods changes to longer, irregular periods with some reorganization by 19 hours.

This procedure does not represent the network unless all units are truly synchronized (no phase differences) with identical burst variables, which is never the case. However, by calculating barycenters (arithmetic centers, or centers of gravity with mass 1), it is possible to determine a "mean activity mode" that, if plotted with the respective barycenters from other channels, now begins to approximate a "network activity mode." It is also possible to introduce one additional variable to give better emphasis to the larger bursts. In a center-of-gravity calculation using, for example, burst duration as the primary variable, burst amplitude or area can be entered to determine a "weighted" barycenter (not shown). The bottom panel of Fig. 1.4 shows actual data from an experiment investigating the effects of low temperature on burst pattern generation (Lucas et al., 1994). The network was cooled to 10°C for one hour, returned to 37°C, monitored one hour after rewarming, and monitored again 19 hours after rewarming. Cluster plots from four channels show a native mode of short but variable periods that changes to longer, irregular periods after exposure to low temperature. Some burst pattern reorganization can be seen by 19 hours. Channels 2 and 4 show almost periodic oscillatory activity at 19 hours.

2. NATIVE OSCILLATORY STATES

The spontaneous activity of cultured networks is complex and seems to reflect rapid transitions between short, stationary patterns as well as possible superposition of such patterns. Although bursting is often synchronized among channels, the degree of synchronization (number of channels synchronized) and the strength of synchronization (intensity of overlapping bursts on different channels) can vary greatly with time. Native oscillatory states in cultured networks are usually short-lived and typically damped in period. However some experiments have also shown long episodes of native oscillations, usually when the cultures are left undisturbed for long periods of time. The latter behavior has not yet been correlated with any obvious variable such as age, pH, cell density, or even culture stress. When long periods of spontaneous oscillations occur, the bursting is always approximately synchronized.

Figure 1.3 shows examples of complex (A) and simple (B) spatiotemporal activity. Panel A shows a coexistence of at least four different patterns. The problems of recognizing and classifying such activity is obvious. The temporal pattern shown is clearly irregular although, on a longer time scale, there could be repetition. The spatial pattern consists of subsets of synchronized channels with no overall (obvious) coordination. This activity may be identified as regionally synchronized, globally uncoordinated, and temporally irregular bursting. By comparison, panel B is refreshingly simple and may be defined as "synchronized irregular bursting." Nevertheless, both activity patterns contain many subtle variations that frustrate quantification.

Figure 1.4 represents episodes of electronically integrated data showing "uncoordinated irregular bursting" in A and "synchronized irregular bursting" in B. Although panel A may well represent global "irregular" temporal bursting, it is quite apparent that almost every channel displays short spells of oscillatory (in some cases almost periodic) behavior. The more regular and highly synchronized pattern of B also

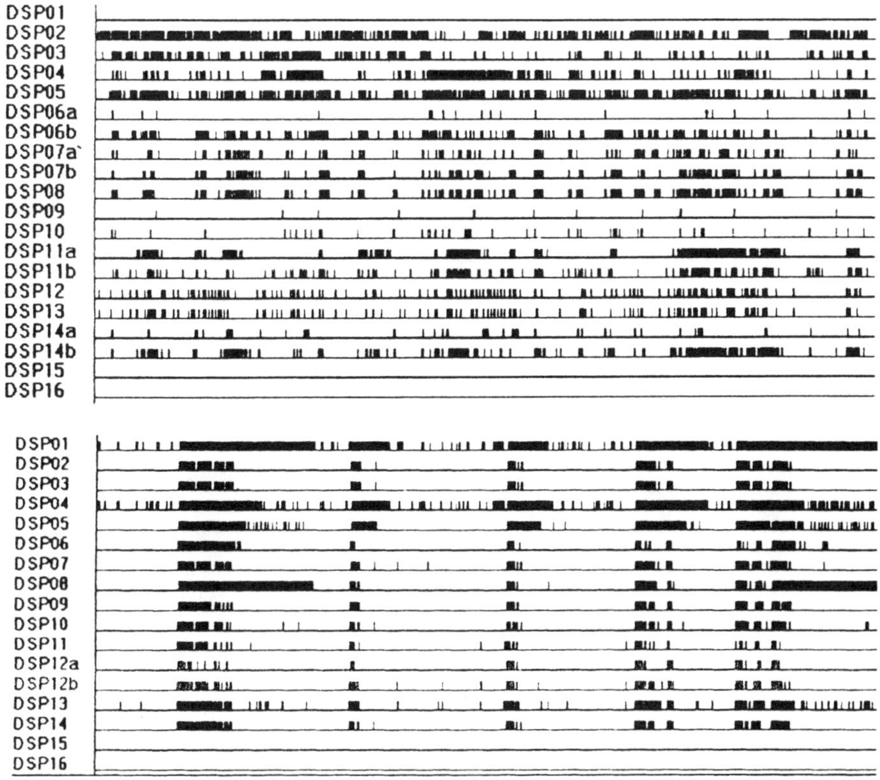

Fig. 1.3. Native oscillatory states. 30 sec periods of digitized spike data after action potential recognition and separation using the Spectrum Scientific (Dallas) MNAP software. Top: Irregular bursting activity with several subsets of partially synchronized activity patterns expressed simultaneously. Bottom: Synchronized irregular bursting.

shows episodes of specific activity that resist clear-cut classification. It is obvious that one must approach pattern identification initially as a search for common statistical features. Attention to every detail is not possible and should not be needed by effective classification schemes. Figure 1.4 also reveals that small amplitude bursts are rarely expressed on a majority of channels and can be considered "local" events. On the other hand, high-amplitude (intense) bursting leads to synchronization and often engages the entire network in a common, global pattern. The transition to such states has been termed "intensity recruitment." Figure 1.4(C) shows a sigmoidal recruiting relationship between channels 2 and 3 of another culture (Gross & Kowalski, 1991).

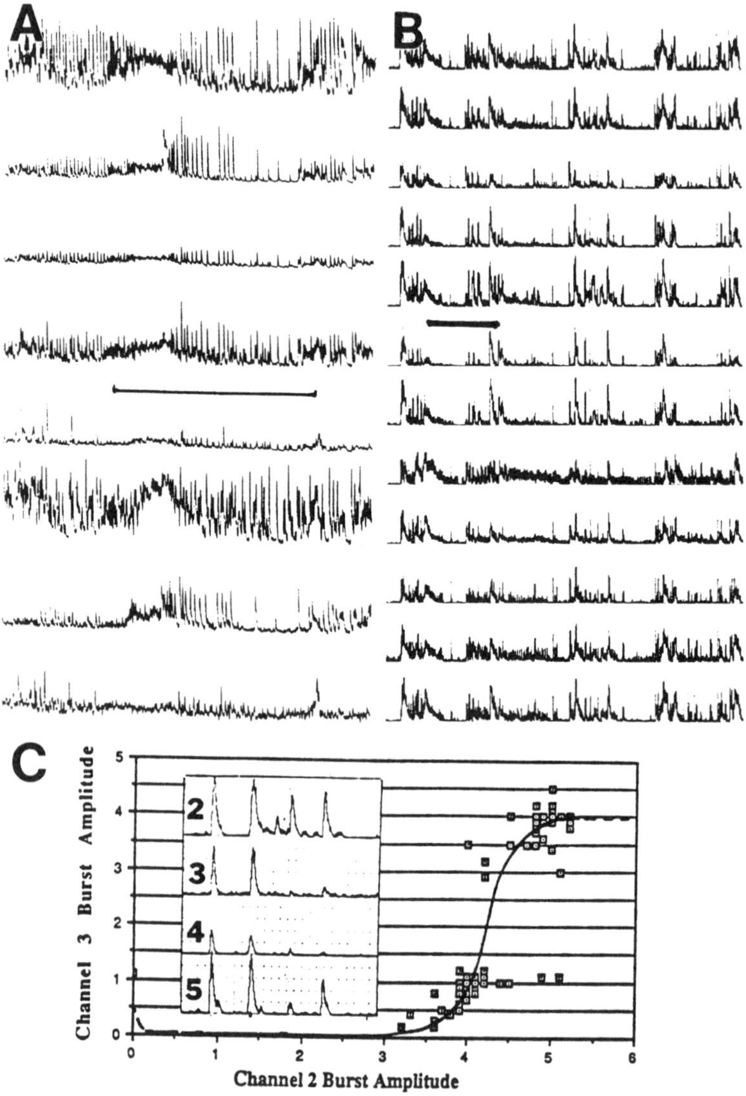

Fig. 1.4. Electronically (A) and digitally (B) integrated burst activity showing irregular temporal bursting but strong synchronization in B. Note short spells of oscillatory bursting in A and episodes of small amplitude activity that is not synchronized in B. (C) Sigmoidal recruitment of channel 3 by channel 2 (data set not shown). Integrated burst amplitudes (arbitrary units) reflect spike frequencies during the course of a burst. High spike frequencies in bursts are instrumental in generating global synchronization of most units in a network.

Complex intraburst oscillations are shown in Fig. 1.5. The temporal complexity in A is such as to make it difficult to define a "burst." Although one may be tempted to call the activity in A a sequence of four bursts, the fine structure of each burst is dominated by oscillatory activity in the form of short bursts, often riding on tonic spiking. Every rapid excursion of the integrated activity reflects a sudden acceleration of spiking presumably due to major synaptic events. For this reason, it is preferred to call the structures in A "burst complexes." Panel B, in contrast, consists of single short bursts with one large synchronized burst complex. The clonic segment is a damped oscillation of sequentially increasing periods but also with increasing amplitudes (arrows). The latter is a manifestation of spike frequency recovery upon slowing of the burst pattern.

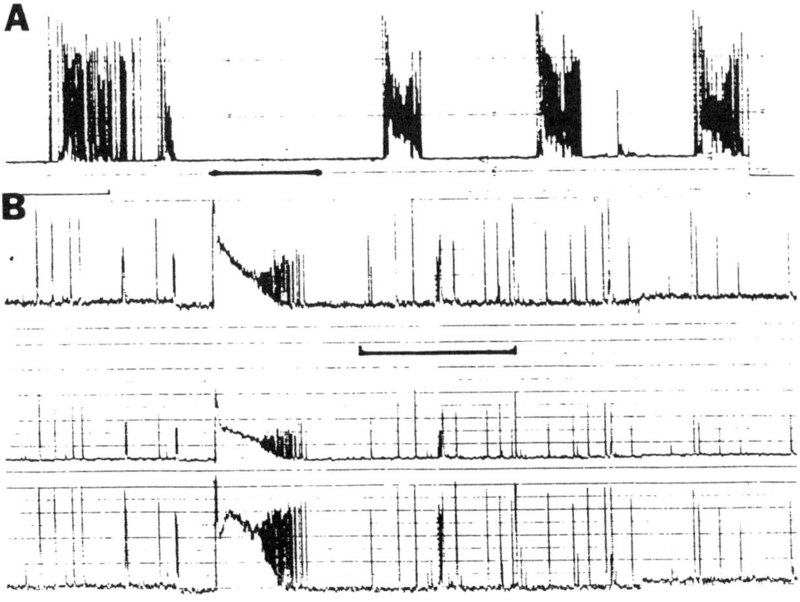

Fig. 1.5. Oscillatory activity in burst episodes. (A) Burst complexes and burst complex packets. Note that individual short bursts often ride on tonic activity. (B) Short synchronized bursting on three channels with one large burst episode. Tonic high frequency spiking in the burst breaks into high frequency bursting with damped periods. Burst amplitudes increase as quiet burst intervals develop, allowing neurons to recover from high frequency activity.

Oscillatory activity modes are therefore common "attractors" for the spontaneous, pharmacologically unmodified activity of most networks. However the network visits these attractors only transiently. As shown below, the blocking of inhibitory synapses can rapidly stabilize these attractors regardless of the mode of the initial activity, and can also enhance the regularity of existing oscillatory patterns.

3. INDUCED OSCILLATIONS

3.1. Network Oscillations after Disinhibition

In a spontaneously active network, the blocking of the inhibitory GABA and glycine receptors (with bicuculline and strychnine, respectively) generates nearly periodic oscillatory burst patterns of remarkable regularity in burst period and duration on most, and often all, electrodes. This is shown in Fig. 1.6 with a single channel stripchart record of integrated spike activity. It can be seen that the irregular oscillatory activity of the native state becomes regularized in burst period, amplitude, and duration after the addition of 5 μm strychnine. Figure 1.6(B) demonstrates that the oscillatory state, in the continued presence of strychnine, lasts for a long period of time, although the burst frequency and regularity can deteriorate substantially in 12 hours. Oscillatory activity under the influence of 40 μm bicuculline is shown in Fig. 1.7. Burst rates increase quickly after bicuculline and establish a relatively stable state at about 30 bpm. A cluster plot for burst period shows unorganized native activity with a transition to a tight oblong cluster with a mean period of 2 seconds. Channel synchronization and burst oscillations are shown in C. Despite the high degree of synchronization, the burst envelopes are not identical, reflecting variations in spike patterns within the bursts. The effects of strychnine and bicuculline are additive over a wide interval of concentrations (Hightower, 1988), and demonstrate the existence of separate inhibitory GABA and glycine circuits in these cultures.

Cultured networks are approximately 1,000-fold more sensitive to strychnine than to bicuculline. Whereas oscillatory behavior usually begins at 10 μm bicuculline and saturates at 30 μm, initial pattern changes are obtained with nanomolar concentrations of strychnine (Gross et al., 1992, Fig. 7). Both compounds tend to increase the burst rate when the native burst activity is low and decrease it when the native activity is high. In the latter case the increase in burst duration and concomitant rise in spike production per burst results in increased after-hyperpolarizations that lengthen the burst period. Burst fusion and intense spiking, produced by 5 to 10 μm NMDA (Gross, 1994), has never been observed with either compound. In addition, strychnine at concentrations above 20 μm reduces spike frequencies and amplitudes with irreversible damage to the culture if not removed. Disinhibition also has been observed to initiate activity in quiet cultures (network ignition) and almost always generates synchronized oscillatory states. Finally, periodic oscillatory responses are concentration-dependent and generally do not develop below 100 nm. Although both disinhibition and excitation (with glutamate and its analogs) increase total spike production, there is a clear asymmetry in the way networks respond: whereas excitation increases spike production within highly variable patterns, disinhibition almost always regularizes burst durations and periods and generates oscillatory states.

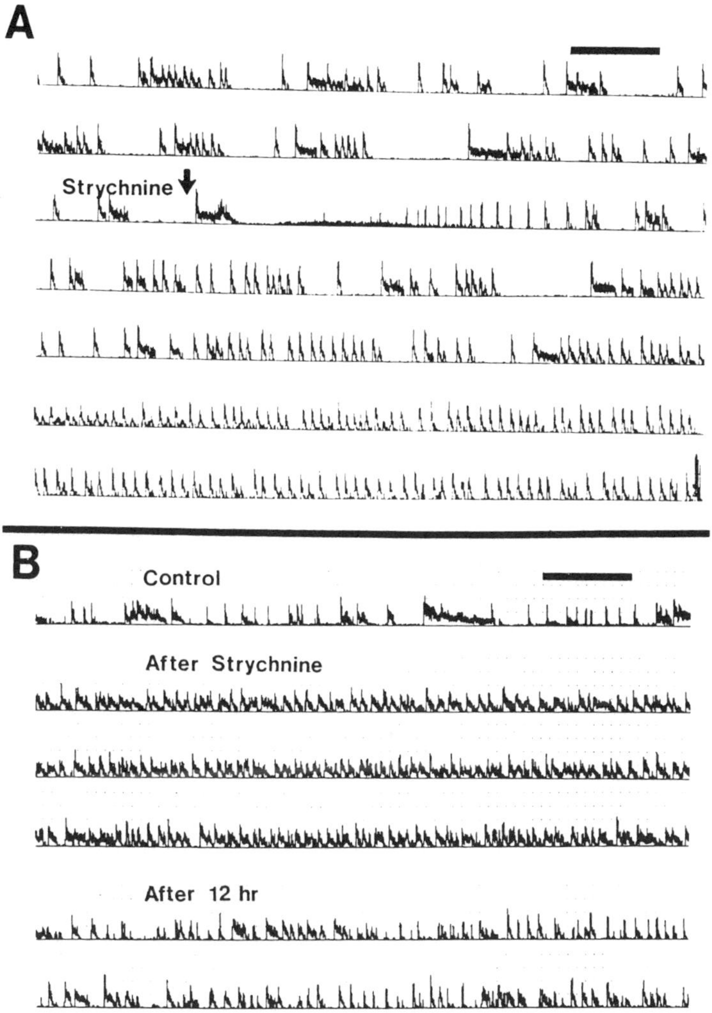

Fig. 1.6. Typical response of a single channel to the blocking of glycine receptors with 5 μm strychnine (A). Such network disinhibition generates nearly-periodic oscillatory burst patterns of remarkable regularity in burst period and duration on most, and often all, electrodes. (B) Oscillatory states, in the continued presence of strychnine, last for a long period of time, although the regularity deteriorates substantially in 12 hours.

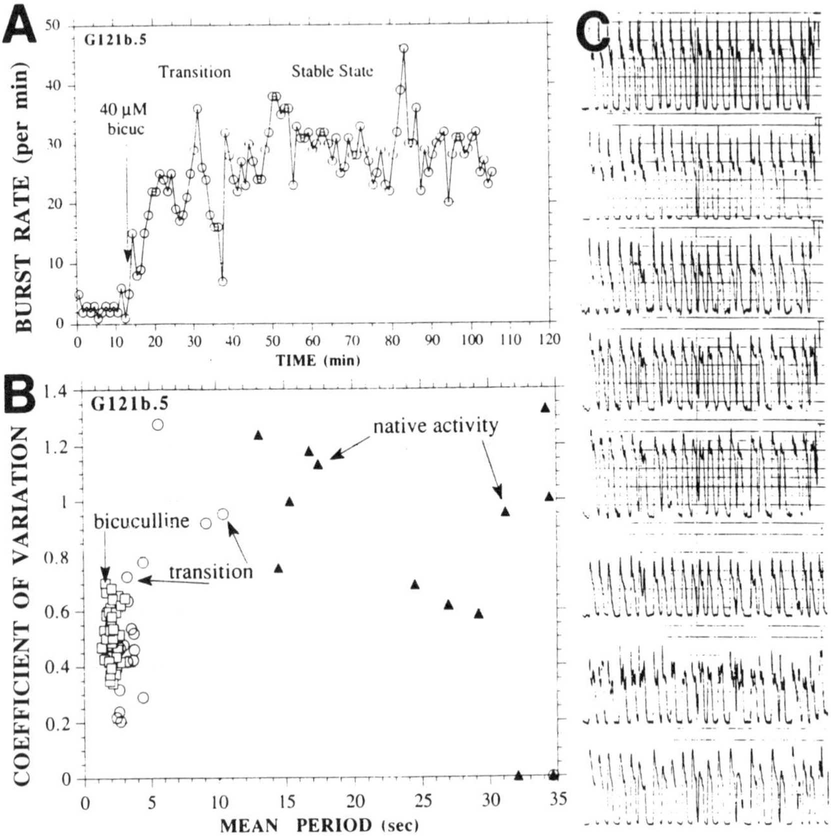

Fig. 1.7. Representative oscillatory activity under the influence of 40 µm bicuculline. (A) Burst rate increase after bicuculline and establishment of a relatively stable state near 30 bpm. (B) Cluster plot for burst period showing unorganized native activity with a transition to a more regular activity mode. (C) Chart record of integrated bursts showing channel synchronization and burst oscillations.

3.2. Pharmacological Modification of Oscillatory Activity Modes

Stable oscillatory states, once initiated by disinhibition, can be altered by general physical and chemical influences such as temperature and pH (Rhoades, Weil, & Gross,

1993) as well as by a large number of pharmacological compounds (Gross, 1994, Gross & Kowalski, 1991; Rhoades & Gross, 1994). In an attempt to investigate burst mechanisms, we have induced oscillatory states with bicuculline in order to regularize the burst patterns and establish a dynamic environment that can be readily quantified (Rhoades & Gross, 1994). The influences of neuroactive compounds were then investigated in terms of changes in the oscillatory pattern. These experiments are reviewed in Fig. 1.8 in which all initial activities (top traces) represent stationary oscillatory states induced by 60 µm bicuculline. This concentration is comfortably

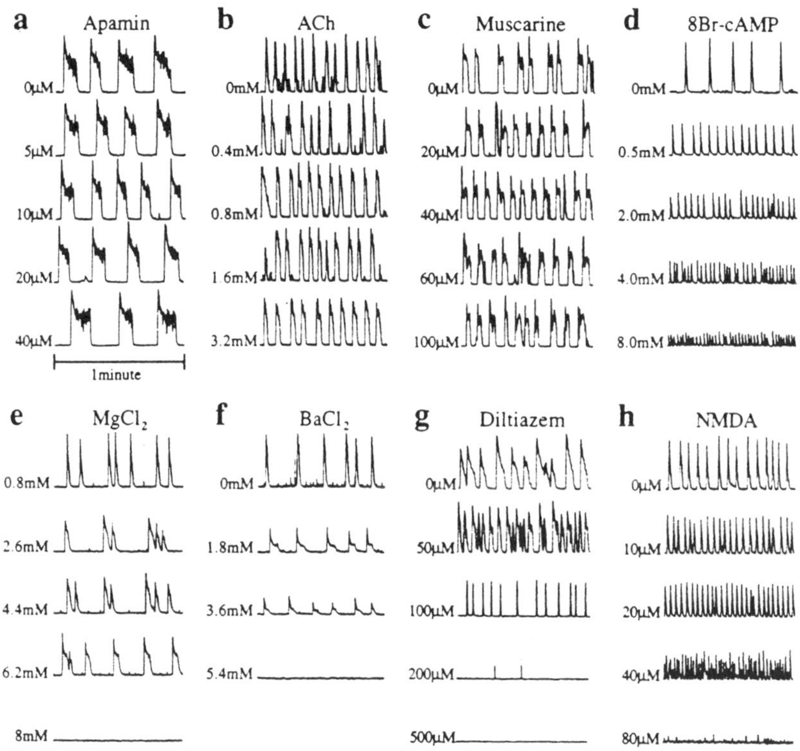

Fig. 1.8. Modification of bicuculline-induced oscillations (first trace in all panels) by neuroactive compounds. Effect on oscillatory states is both compound specific and concentration specific. (From Rhoades & Gross, 1994).

beyond saturation of the $GABA_A$ receptors that starts at 30 μm bicuculline and does not affect the culture adversely at higher concentrations (Jordan, 1992).

It can be seen from Fig. 1.8 that pharmacological influences differ greatly for different compounds with varying effects on burst parameters. Cessation of activity is also substance-specific. The substances investigated by Rhoades and Gross (1994) are summarized in Table 1.1 where additional information is listed on minimum effective concentrations, effects on three burst variables, and concentrations at which the activity

Substance	Function	Effect on Oscillating Culture				
		MEC	BR	BD	BA	Stops Act.
acetylcholine	neuromodulator/transmitter	?	-	+	0	no
4 aminopyridine	blocks voltage-gated K^+ conductance	10 μm	+++	---	--	no
apamin	blocks Ca^{++} dep. K^+ conducatnce	40 μm	-	0	0	no
barium chloride	blocks internal Ca^{++} dependent process	1 mm	0	++	---	5 mm
charybdotoxin	blocks Ca^{++} dep. K^+ conductance	100nm	++	-	-	no
cesium chloride	K^+ analog, K^+ channel conductance		+++	---	--	4 mm
choline chloride	Cl^- analog	5 mm	-	0	-	?
8-Br-cAMP	second messenger analog	100 μm	+++	-	---	10 mm
diltiazem	L-type calcium channel blocker	25 μm?	++	--	--	200 μm
magnesium chlor.	Ca^{++} channel blocker at synapses and NMDA channel blocker	2 mm	++	-	-	7 mm
muscarine	decreases Ca^{++} dep. K^+ conductance	0	0	0	0	?
NMDA	activates NMDA gluatamate receptors	1 μm	+++	-	--	60 μm
ouabain	blocks Na^+/K^+ pump	?	0	0	---	20 μm
potassium chlor.	depolarizes membrane potential	6 mm	+++	--	--	~15 mm
tetraethyl ammon.	inactivates K^+ channel (extracellular)	3 mm	0	--	---	50 mm
veratridine	activates Vg sodium channels	3 μm	---	0	--	6 μm

Table 1.1. Substances investigated by Rhoades and Gross, 1994. MEC: minimum effective concentration; BR: burst rate; BD: burst duration; BA: burst amplitude (from integrated burst envelopes)

terminated. It is important to note that these values are specific for oscillatory states elicited by bicuculline. Influences on native activity may show similar trends, but not identical effects on burst patterns. The effects on native activity are also more difficult to identify because the native pattern is not regularized.

3.3. Oscillations Induced by Electrical Stimulation

Single neurons, or a combination of neurons in the network can be selectively stimulated to determine their influence over the spontaneous network pattern or to generate an artificial *input* to the cultured network (Gross, Rhoades, & Kowalski, 1993). In this manner, a great variety of sensory input patterns (or feedback) can be simulated for the obvious purpose of ascertaining their influence on network development, generic spontaneous activity, and pharmacological responses, as well as for possible studies of network learning (Sparks & Gross, 1995).

Among a variety of responses to stimulation, oscillatory behavior is frequently seen and entrainment of a spontaneously active network to stimuli can be elicited routinely. Stimulation-induced oscillatory behavior is temporary and usually takes the form of damped repetitive bursting immediately after the stimulation episode (Gross et al., 1993). Network arousal with progressive increases in bursting and "clonic" after-stimulus oscillations that mimic the electrical induction of epileptiform activity *in vivo* is often observed. Entrainment to a stimulus is possible regardless of whether the network is spontaneously active in the native state or is under the influence of inhibitory circuit blockers such as bicuculline. Figure 1.9 shows the developing entrainment to regular stimulus pulses ranging in interval from 4.5 to 1 second. Immediate burst responses to the stimulus pulse (single biphasic pulse, 300 μs, 0.9 V at electrode) reaches a peak of 84% in the top three channels for the 2.3 second stimulation interval and falls off to approximately 30% at the 4.5- and 1-second intervals. The number of bursts per channel increases exponentially from 13 at the 4.5 second interval to 45 at the 1 second stimulus pulse interval.

It is pertinent to ask whether the observed synchronized oscillations in culture reflect epileptiform activity and whether such simple neural systems can make a contribution to the study of epilepsy. Many observations lead to a strong affirmative answer. Seizure-related (epileptiform) electrical activity in the CNS is characterized by hyperexcitability and hypersynchronization (Hochman, Baraban, Owens, & Schwartzkroin, 1995). "Excitability" and "hypersynchronization," however, are usually not clearly defined. Excitability could represent ease of triggering spiking, or more high frequency spiking in bursts, or both. In culture, it is the "burst intensity" (i.e., the magnitude of the spike frequency within a burst) that is of significance. High burst intensities force synchrony upon the network (see Fig. 1.7(C)). Conversely, excitability in terms of high burst frequencies at low intensities is not correlated with global synchronization. It is generally difficult to separate excitability and synchrony in epileptiform activity *in vivo* (Hochman et al., 1995), which mirrors the observations in culture. Also, as *in vivo,* the cultured system synchronizes and regularizes its pattern under the influence of rising extracellular K^+ (Rhoades & Gross, 1994).

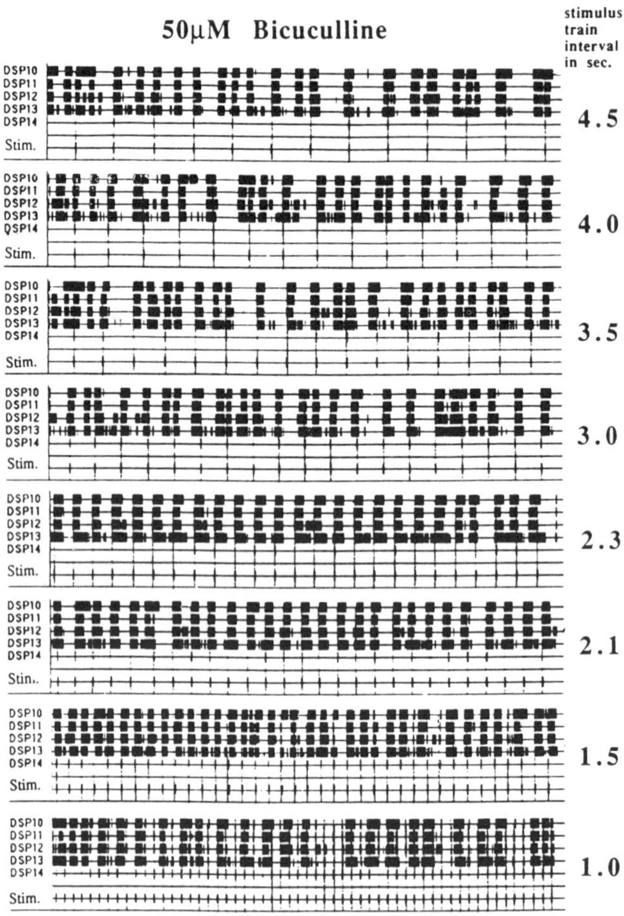

Fig. 1.9. Entrainment of network to electrical stimulation (single biphasic pulses, 300 μs, 0.9 V at electrode) reaches a peak of 76% for the 2.3 second interval and falls off to approximately 30% at the 4.5 second and 1 second intervals.

One difference between *in vivo* and *in vitro* responses is that epileptic seizures are generally short lived and self-terminating in animals, whereas similar bursting may last for long periods of time (hours) *in vitro*. This difference could be a result of the small extracellular volume in vivo which allows a rapid rise in K^+ concentration that, in turn, is instrumental in the termination of the oscillatory activity. *In vitro*, the large medium bath essentially holds the K^+ concentration constant. As was shown in Table 1.1, bursting stops at approximately 12-16 mM.

4. THEORETICAL CONSIDERATIONS

4.1. Modeling

Many independent investigations have confirmed that the neuronal culture environment together with array recording techniques are particularly suitable for the study of manifestations of nearly synchronized bursting activity. We want to stress that this methodology also provides an insight into mechanisms of *dynamical self-organization* of the underlying network into *variable and flexible subensembles with internally synchronized activity* a concept recently upgraded to one of the basic paradigms of biological neuronal networks (see, e.g., Simmers, Meyrand, & Moulins, 1995).

The challenge to theory is now concentrated around the following basic questions: (1) What is the minimal biologically realistic model of a neuronal network with such behaviors? (2) What are the basic mechanisms of local ensemble formation and local activity synchronization? (3) What are the basic mechanisms of global (network) ensemble formation and network activity synchronization? (4) What is the purpose and biological significance of synchronized periodic modes in contexts other than pacemaker functions? (5) Why is this mode often observed at the network developmental stage? (6) What role does it play in "information processing"? (7) When does a synchronized periodic mode represent pathological (epileptiform) activity?

Some of these questions were addressed by Kowalski, Albert, Rhoades, and Gross (1992) with a model of (1) "point-like" modified Hodgkin-Huxley type neurons which are not endogenous bursters but may display such behavior when externally driven by other units and/or injected currents, and (2) a simplified phenomenological model of chemical synapses where significant post-synaptic currents are generated only if there are rapid (spike-related) changes in the presynaptic membrane potential. It was demonstrated that such simplified models typically undergo transitions from quiescent to periodic synchronized bursting states if the interneuronal coupling parameters (synaptic strengths) exceed some critical value. In the simplest case, the dynamics of such a transition can be considered a Hopf bifurcation when the network equilibrium state becomes unstable above some critical coupling strengths and a new, stable network periodic state emerges. Much more complex activity modes are also possible in the framework of such models (including network "splitting" into synchronized subensembles with a significant phase shift between them, more than one stable activity state, period doubling, and synchronized chaotic modes. These behaviors are illustrated in Figs. 1.10-1.12.

The examples from our model show that synchronous, but not necessarily periodic, activity is one of the main modes for a network composed of essentially identical neurons with identical interconnnections. However, small changes in the neuronal parameters and/or synaptic efficacies often lead to nearly synchronous activity with small but fixed phase shifts between bursts. Our experimental data also show small phase differences during periodic bursting but the corresponding "phase differences" seem to be random variables with some generic distribution function for a given network (Gross & Kowalski, 1991). This may suggest that parts of real networks displaying nearly synchronous periodic bursting are, on average, structurally homogeneous but undergo small fluctuations of their parameters. The cluster plot method described is one of the simplest ways to demonstrate subtle changes in such weakly perturbed dynamical systems. In our model we did not include noise terms and/or any conduction delays, however we demonstrated that a random reduction of interconnections in a homogeneous network leads to desynchronization.

On a more complex level are states where the network is subdivided into two or more nearly synchronized subpopulations with essential phase differences between different groups. This is a "coarse-grain" phase lock sometimes observed for a finite length of time in our experiments. The presence of apparently chaotic, but synchronized modes was one of the most intriguing theoretical observations made by Kowalski, Albert, and Gross (1990) and Kowalski et al. (1992). The concept of "synchronous chaos" proved to be useful in many physical contexts such as coupled lasers and coding theory. However, the presence of truly chaotic states in biological neuronal networks is still an open question, due to the described problems with the system stationarity and usually strong noise components.

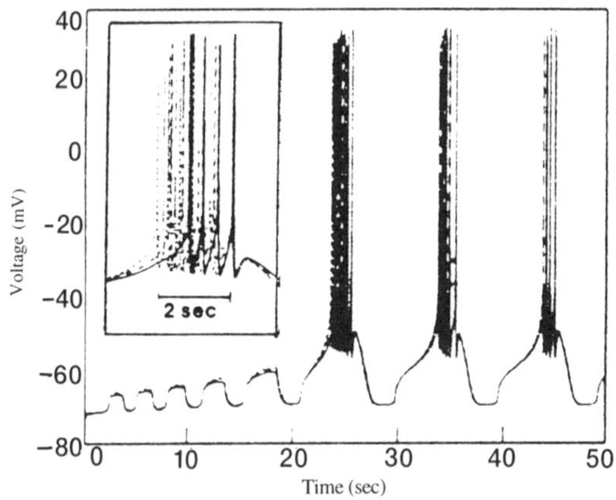

Fig. 1.10. Rapid synchronization to a stationary, periodic bursting state in a model network of 4 HH-type neurons with all-to-all, identical synaptic interactions. The inset shows the first network burst at a magnified time scale. The network enters the synchronized periodic bursting mode for a wide range of different initial membrane voltages (for the state presented, voltages were -50, -55, -60, -65 mV).

4.2. Mechanisms Underlying Oscillations in Cultured Networks: Experimental Considerations

Both experimental and modeling results support the existence of two or more coexisting temporal patterns with each roughly synchronized among a subset of channels. In the model, such "network splitting" arises spontaneously. In the experimental setting the question arises whether different patterns are generated by an interconnected network or reside in different, separate circuits. However, the number of different channel activity patterns is always reduced when such networks are disinhibited; in many, only one common pattern remains. Only if two patterns do not

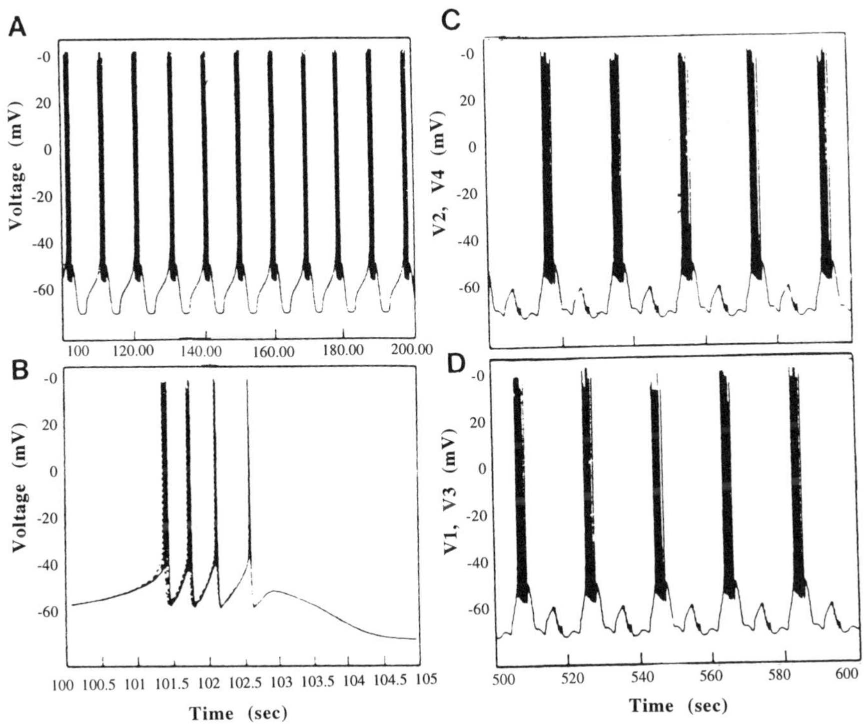

Fig. 1.11. (A & B) Approximate synchronization on a network of four neurons with identical synaptic efficacies but with different conductivities for each channel. The network enters the nearly synchronized state despite "individual differences" between neurons. (C & D) A network of four interacting neurons which entered a periodic bursting state with two pairs (C and D) of synchronized neurons. There is a significant phase shift between these synchronized subsets. Such behavior can be proven generic in large populations of coupled non-linear oscillators, and is also seen experimentally.

merge under disinhibition, then the underlying morphological substrate is not connected or is so weakly connected that it can be considered two separate networks.

It is interesting that strong bursting is often seen without any spiking in the interburst intervals in the native state, as well as after disinhibition (Droge et al., 1986; Gross, 1994; Gross & Kowalski, 1991; Gross & Lucas, 1982; Maeda et al., 1995). This implies that tonic inhibitory activity is not necessary to halt bursting and generate long quiet periods. In addition, it has been shown by Maeda et al. (1995) that the direction of propagation of activity within a cultured network varies from burst to burst and that a physical sectioning of a single network can generate independent spontaneous bursting in each part. These authors concluded that bursting is not controlled by the diffusion of an extracellular chemical factor and can be ignited in different regions of the network. These data are consistent with a picture where single cells or, most likely, cell clusters

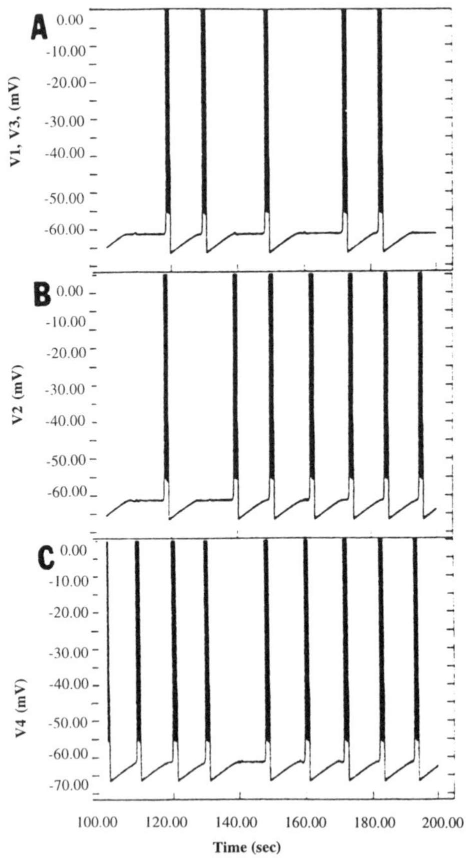

Fig. 1.12. Complex behavior in a network of four neurons with two of the neurons following the same pattern in A. The activity is chaotic (chaotic bursting).

generate suprathreshold spiking from subthreshold oscillations. This spiking, in turn, ignites local region into bursting that spreads through the network and transiently entrains other regions. Such a model suggests that networks are dominated by sensitive loci with high excitatory synaptic density, that there are several of such regions, that they compete for dominance, and that complex network patterns are as much a function of the superposition of circuit patterns and collision phenomena as they are shaped by inhibitory influences. The activity is mediated by chemical synapses because (1) network spontaneous activity in spinal cultures ceases in 6 to 10 mM magnesium (Droge et al., 1986; Rhoades & Gross, 1994); and (2) the search for gap junctions in mouse spinal cord cultures (Nelson, Neale, & Macdonald, 1981) and rat CNS cultures (Maeda et al., 1995) has met with negative results.

An initial investigation of burst mechanisms (Rhoades & Gross, 1994; see also Fig. 1.9) provided the following conclusions: (1) Oscillation is critically dependent on L-type (slow kinetic) calcium channels; (2) calcium-dependent intracellular processes help regulate burst timing (burst initiation); (3) oscillations are not influenced greatly by Ca^{++} regulated K^{+} conductances; (4) the specific empirical relationship between burst rate and $[K^{+}]_{O}$ is mediated principally through voltage-gated Ca^{++} channels, (5) the critical repolarizing Ca^{++} dependent process leading to burst termination is Ca^{++} inactivation of Ca^{++} conductances rather than Ca^{++} inactivation of K^{+} conductances. It is important to note that pharmacological effects are initially always interpreted on the cellular level, because of known influences on specific membrane mechanisms involved in burst pattern generation. However, superimposed on these cellular effects are network effects. The dynamic interaction between these two phenomena is complex and must be an important component of future research into the behavior and capabilities of networks.

5. SUMMARY AND CONCLUSIONS

Experimental results reported from cultured networks lead to a picture of networks containing many small, local neuronal ensembles composed of tens of neurons each with the main activity mode of nearly synchronized, nearly oscillatory spiking and bursting. Connected together, these groups (or nacelles) form a network displaying a rich repertoire of patterned bursting with the ability of transiently entraining to a common pattern or entering stable oscillatory states under disinhibition. Approximate synchronization is evident not only in stationary activity states of such networks, but is also typical for the observed transient states. The generic character of this phenomenon was stressed in our earlier papers (Droge et al., 1986; Gross, 1994; Gross & Kowalski, 1991; Kowalski et al., 1992) and has also been noticed in more recent independent investigations (Maeda et al., 1995; Robinson et al., 1993).

The creation of local, flexible, strongly interconnected neuronal sub-assemblies communicating with each other via long-range, sparse interconnections seems to be a solution for achieving system reliability and fault tolerance in mammalian networks operating with relatively unreliable nodes (or neurons) with variable connectivity. Local synchrony ensures a (necessary) multiplexing of the activity by spreading the pattern over many neurons and automatically duplicating the pattern in all axons leaving the network. This facilitates both local guiding (information) inputs as well as "read-out" by distant parts of the CNS.

A particular network may have a rich repertoire of stable oscillatory states (i.e. many attractors) that depend on the cellular constituents, the network circuitry, and its synaptic states. Each may be attained from a specific set of initial internal conditions and/or external stimuli applied to a specific location (basins of attraction). This leads to a picture where information processing depends on specific local disinhibition, emergence of local, strongly correlated excitation, and modulation of it by external or neighboring internal patterned activity.

Evolution generally uses all reproducible phenomena that emerge in various complex systems. If oscillations arise as noise driven phenomena in cell groups with strong excitatory interconnection (e.g., Douglas et al., 1995), then oscillatory states most likely have been employed effectively for a variety of tasks as long as they can be controlled by mechanisms such as inhibitory circuitry. The continual spontaneous activity in isolated, self-organized neuronal systems in culture, at ages ranging from 2 weeks to over 9 months, may well be maintained by an "engine" that is oscillatory in nature. This view is strengthened by the universal oscillatory responses that emerge as stable states when active inhibition is removed. It appears that *oscillation, and not quiescence, is the natural state of neural tissue.* Oscillations of neural systems are "ready states" that arise spontaneously and can be easily and rapidly modified by small external influences, providing that strong oscillatory bursting has not yet developed. To trigger a complex pattern from a quiescent state is more difficult, slower, and less precise because small perturbations usually lead only to a forced, entrained motion of the former equilibria. Well-developed bursting states also show this type of inertia. "Ready states" must, therefore, be limited to oscillatory spiking or weak oscillatory bursting.

ACKNOWLEDGMENTS

This work was supported by the Texas Advanced Research Program and by the Hillcrest Foundation of Dallas, Texas, founded by Mrs. W.W. Caruth, Sr.

REFERENCES

Abuzaid, M. A., Vithalani, P. V., Howard, L., Gosney, W. M., & Gross, G. W. (1991). A VLSI peripheral system for monitoring and stimulating action potentials of cultured neurons. *Proceedings of the First Great Lakes Symposium on VLSI, Kalamazoo, MI,* 170-173.

Alger, B. E. (1984). Hippocampus: Electrophysiological studies of epileptiform activity *in vitro.* In R. Dingledine (Ed.), *Brain Slices* (pp. 155-199). New York: Plenum Press.

Arbas, E. A., & Calabrese, R. L. (1987). Slow oscillations of membrane potential in interneurons that control heartbeat in the medicinal leech. *Journal of Neuroscience*, *7*, 3953-3960.

Babb, T. L., & Crandall, P. H. (1976). Epileptogenesis of human limbic neurons in psychomotor epileptics. *Electroencephalography and Clinical Neurophysiology*, *40*, 225-243.

Brown, T. A. (1914). On the nature of the fundamental activity of the nervous centres together with an analysis on the conditioning of the rhythmic activity in progression and a theory of the evolution of function in the nervous system. *Journal of Physiology*, *48*, 18-46.

Dichter, M. A. (1986). *Mechanisms of Epileptogenesis.* New York: Plenum Press.

Douglas, R. J., Koch, C., Mahowald, M., Martin, K. A. C., & Suarez, H. H. (1995). Recurrent excitation in neocortical circuits. *Science*, *268*, 981-985.

Droge, M. H., Gross, G. W., Hightower, M. H., & Czisny, L. E. (1986). Multielectrode analysis of coordinated, rhythmic bursting in cultured CNS monolayer networks. *Journal of Neuroscience*, *6*, 1583-1592.

Freeman, W. J. (1978). Spatial properties of an EEG event in the olfactory bulb and cortex. *Electroencephalography and Clinical Neurophysiology*, *44*, 586-605.

Freeman, W. J., & Schneider, W. (1982). Changes in spatial paterns of rabbit olfactory EEG with conditioning to odors. *Psychophysiology*, *19*, 44-56.

Gariano, R. F., & Groves, P. M. (1988). Burst firing induced in midbrain dopamine neurons by stimulation of the medial prefrontal and anterior cingulate cortices. *Brain Research*, *462*, 194-198.

Getting, P.A. (1989). Emerging principles governing the operation of neural networks. *Annual Review of Neuroscience*, *12*, 185-204.

Glass, L., & Mackey, M. C. (1989). *From Clocks to Chaos: The Rhythms of Life*. Princeton, NJ: Princeton University Press.

Gloor, P., Quesney, L. F., & Zumstein, H. (1977). Pathophysiology of generalized penicillin epilepsy in the cat: The role of cortical and subcortical structures. II. Topical applications of penicillin to the cerebral cortex and to subcortical structures. *Electroencephalography and Clinical Neurophysiology*, *43*, 79-94.

Gopal, K., & Gross, G. W. (1996a). Auditory cortical neurons *in vitro:* Cell culture and multichannel extracellular recording. *Acta Oto-Laryngologica*, *116*, 690-696.

Gopal, K., & Gross, G. W. (1996b). Auditory cortical neurons *in vitro*: Initial pharmacological studies. *Acta Oto-Laryngologica*, *116*, 697-704.

Gray, C. M., König, P., Engel, A. K., & Singer, W. (1989). Oscillatory responses in cat visual cortex exhibit inter-columnar synchronization which reflects global stimulus properties. *Nature*, *338*, 334-335.

Gray, C. M. (1994). Synchronous oscillations in neuronal systems: mechanisms and functions. *Journal of Computational Neuroscience*, *1*, 11-38.

Grillner, S., Buchanan, J. T. , Wallen, P., & Brodin, L. (1988). Neural control of locomotion in lower vertebrates. In A. H. Cohen, S. Rossignol, & S. Grillner (Eds.), *Neural Control of Rhythmic Movements in Vertebrates* (pp. 1-40). New York: Wiley.

Gross, G. W. (1994). Internal dynamics of randomized mammalian neuronal networks in culture. In D. A. Stenger & T. M. McKenna (Eds.), *Enabling Technologies for Cultured Neural Networks* (pp. 277-317). New York: Academic Press.

Gross, G. W., & Kowalski, J. M. (1991). Experimental and theoretical analysis of random nerve cell network dynamics. In P. Antognetti & V. Milutinovic (Eds.), *Neural Networks: Concepts, Applications, and Implementations, Vol. 4* (pp. 47-110). Englewood, NJ: Prentice-Hall.

Gross, G. W., & Lucas, J. H. (1982). Long-term monitoring of spontaneous single unit activity from neuronal monolayer networks cultured on photoetched multielectrode surfaces. *Journal of Electrophysiology Techniques*, *9*, 55-67.

Gross, G. W., Rhoades, B. K., & Jordan, R. J. (1992). Neuronal networks for biochemical sensing. *Sensors and Actuators*, *6*, 1-8.

Gross, G. W., Rhoades, B. K., Reust, D. L., & Schwalm, F. U. (1993). Stimulation of monolayer networks in culture through thin film indium-tin oxide recording electrodes. *Journal of Neuroscience Methods*, *50*, 131-143.

Gross, G. W., Rhoades, B. K., & Kowalski, J. M. (1993). Dynamics of burst patterns generated by monolayer networks in culture. In H. W. Bothe, M. Samii, & R. Eckmiller (Eds.), *Neurobionics* (pp. 89-121). Amsterdam: Elsevier.

Gross, G. W., & Schwalm, F. U. (1994). A closed chamber for long-term electrophysiological and microscopical monitoring of monolayer neuronal networks. *Journal of Neuroscience Methods*, *52*, 73-85.

Gross, G. W., Wen, W., & Lin, J. (1985). Transparent indium-tin oxide patterns for extra-cellular, multisite recording in neuronal culture. *Journal of Neuroscience Methods*, *15*, 243-252.

Gutnick, M. J., & Friedman, A. (1986). Synaptic and intrinsic mechanisms of synchronization and epileptogenesis in the neocortex. *Experimental Brain Research*, *14*, 327-335.

Hamburger, V., & Balaban, M. (1963). Observations and experiments on spontaneous rhythmical behavior in the chick embryo. *Developmental Biology*, *7*, 533-545.

Hatton, G. I. (1994). Hypothalamic neurobiology. In R. Dingledine (Ed.), *Brain Slices* (pp. 341-374). New York: Plenum Press.

Hightower, M. H. (1988). *Electrophysiological and morphological analyses of mouse spinal cord mini-cultures grown on multimicroelectrode plates*. Doctoral dissertation, Department of Biological Sciences, University of North Texas, Denton.

Hochman, D. W., Baraban, S. C., Owens, J. W. M., & Schwartzkroin, P. A. (1995). Dissociation of synchronization and excitability in furosemide blockade of epileptiform activity. *Science*, *270*, 99-102.

Jahnsen, H., & Llinas, R. (1994a). Electrophysiological properties of guinea-pig thalamic neurones: An *in vitro* study. *Journal of Neurophysiology*, *349*, 227-247.

Jahnsen, H., & Llinas, R. (1994b). Ionic basis for the electroresponsiveness and oscillatory properties of guinea-pig thalamic neurones *in vitro*. *Journal of Physiology*, *349*, 227-247.

Jobert, A., Bassant, M. H., & Lamour, Y. (1989). Hemicholinium-3 selectively alters the rhythmically bursting activity of septo-hippocampal neurons in the rat. *Brain Research*, *476*, 220-229.

Jordan, R. J. (1992). Investigation of inhibitory synaptic influences in neuronal monolayer networks cultured from mouse spinal cord. M.S. Thesis, Dept. of Biological Sciences, Univ. of North Texas, Denton.

Kowalski, J. M., Albert, G. L., & Gross, G. W. (1990). On the asymptotically synchronous chaotic orbits in systems of excitable elements. *Physical Review A*, *42*, 6260-6263.

Kowalski, J. M., Albert, G. L., Rhoades, B. K., & Gross, G. W. (1992). Correlated spontaneous activity in cultured neuronal networks as possible manifestations of synchronized chaos. In S. Vohara, M. Sapano, M. Schlesinger, L. Pecora, & W. Ditto (Eds.), *Proceedings of the 1st Conference on Experimental Chaos in Arlington, VA* (pp. 213-218). Singapore: World Scientific.

Kowalski, J. M., Albert, G. L., Rhoades, B. K., & Gross, G. W. (1992). Neuronal networks with spontaneous, correlated bursting activity: theory and simulations. *Neural Networks*, *5*, 805-822.

Lucas, J. H., Emery, D.G., Wang, G., Rosenberg-Schaffer, L. J., Jordan, R. S., & Gross, G. W. (1994). *In vitro* investigations of the effects of nonfreezing low temperatures on lesioned and uninjured mammalian spinal neurons. *Journal of Neurotrauma*, *11*, 35-61.

Maeda, E., Robinson, H. P. C., & Kawana, A. (1995). The mechanism of generation and propagation of synchronized bursting in developing networks of cortical neurons. *Journal of Neuroscience*, *15*, 6834-6845.

Malsburg, C. von der (1981). *The correlation theory of brain function*. Internal Report, Max-Planck-Institute of Biophysical Chemistry, Göttingen, Germany.

McCormick, D. A., & Feeser, H. R. (1990). Functional implications of burst firing and single spike activity in lateral geniculate relay neurons. *Neuroscience*, *1*, 103-113.

McCormick, D. A., & Pape, H. (1990). Properties of a hyperpolarization-activated cation current and its role in rhythmic oscillation in thalamic relay neurones. *Journal of Physiology*, *431*, 291-318.

Milner, P. (1974). A model for visual shape recognition. *Psychological Review*, *81*, 521-535.

Nelson, P. G., Neale, E. A., & Macdonald, R. L. (1981). Electrophysiological and structural studies of neurons in dissociated cell cultures of the central nervous system. In P. G. Nelson & M. Lieberman (Eds.), *Excitable Cells in Tissue Culture* (pp. 39-80). New York: Plenum Press.

Peterson, E. L. (1983a). Generation and coordination of heartbeat timing oscillation in the medicinal leech. I. Oscillation in isolated ganglia. *Journal of Neurophysiology*, *49*, 611-626.

Provine, R. R. (1971). Embryonic spinal cord: synchrony and spatial distribution of polyneuronal burst discharges. *Brain Research*, *29*, 155-158.

Raeva, S. W. N. (1990). Unit activity of the human thalamus during voluntary movements. *Stereotactical and Functional Neurosurgery*, *54-55*, 154-158.

Rhoades, B. K., Weil, J. C., & Gross, G. W. (1993). Spike train serial dependence, burst rate, burst regularity, and network synchrony all increase with increasing temperature in cultured spinal cord networks. *Society of Neuroscience Abstracts*, *19*, 656.12.

Rhoades, B. K., & Gross, G.W. (1994). Potassium and calcium channel dependence of bursting in cultured neuronal networks. *Brain Research*, *643*, 310-318.

Robinson, H. P. C., Kawahara, M., Jimbo, Y., Torimitsu, K., Kuroda, Y., & Kawana, A. (1993). Periodic synchronized bursting and intracelllular calcium transients elicited by low magnesium in cultured cortical neurons. *Journal of Neurophysiology*, *70*, 1606-1616.

Simmers, J., Meyrand, P., & Moulins, M. (1995). Dynamic network of neurons. *American Scientist*, *83*, 262-268.

Singer, W. (1990). Search for coherence: A basic principle of cortical self-organization. *Concepts in Neuroscience*, *1*, 1-26.

Sparks, C. A., & Gross, G. W. (1995). Reversible network responses to electrical stimulation: post-stimulation changes in spontaneous activity in cultured mammalian spinal networks. *Society of Neuroscience Abstracts*, *21*, 74.3.

Sporns, O., Tononi, G., & Edelman, G. M. (1991). Modeling perceptual grouping and figure-ground segregation of means of active reentrant connections. *Proceedings of the National Academy of Sciences*, *88*, 129-133.

Steriade, M., Curro Dossi, R., & Nuñez, A. (1991). Network modulation of a slow intrinsic oscillation of cat thalamocortical neurons implicated in sleep delta waves: cortically induced synchronization and brainstem cholinergic suppression. *Journal of Neuroscience*, *11*, 3200-3217.

Stewart, M., & Fox, S. E. (1989). Two populations of rhythmically bursting neurons in rat medial septum are revealed by atropine. *Journal of Neurophysiology*, *61*, 982-993.

Tell, F., & Jean, A. (1990). Rhythmic bursting patterns induced in neurons of the rat nucleus tractus solitarii, *in vitro*, in response to N-methyl-D-aspartate. *Brain Research*, *533*, 152-156.

2

Detection of Oscillations and Synchronous Firing in Neurons

David C. Tam
University of North Texas

ABSTRACT

We introduce a time-invariant neural spike train analysis method to detect oscillations in neurons, and a cross-interval—interspike-interval measure for detecting the synchronous spike firings between neurons. A renormalized measure of the ratio of interspike intervals, called firing trend index, is used to detect relative changes in firing rate so that true oscillations can be distinguished from other statistical local random fluctuations, while the cross-interval—interspike-interval analysis is used to detect the specific nature of the time-locked firing between neurons so that correlated spike firings can be distinguished from uncorrelated firings. Such a distinction of correlated firing is important to reveal whether the near-synchronous firings are tightly time-locked or uncorrelated due to chance coincidence. Simulation results showed that these analyses can uncover the spike generation process contributing to the phenomenon of oscillations and correlated synchronous firings in neurons.

1. INTRODUCTION

Recent interest in the phenomena of oscillations and synchronous firing in neurons has generated many interesting hypotheses concerning neural signal processing in the central nervous system. In order to address the nature of these phenomena, we need to quantitatively identify what oscillations and synchronous firing are. In this chapter, we introduce a method for distinguishing true oscillations from other random fluctuations in neuronal firing. We also introduce another method for detecting synchronous firings among neurons.

1.1. Oscillations

Oscillation of firing is a phenomenon that is often exhibited in the central nervous system (CNS). This oscillation can be observed in many different respects. In terms of the firing pattern of an individual neuron, oscillation can be observed in an increase of firing rate periodically, often seen as bursts of firing activity. In terms of the firing patterns of multiple neurons, oscillation can be observed in synchronous firing among these neurons. In other words, if the neurons in a network are not firing synchronously, oscillatory patterns will not be exhibited at the network level, even if each individual neuron is firing oscillatory patterns. Thus, it is important to first identify the oscillatory patterns of firing for a single neuron, and then identify the synchronous nature of spike firing for multiple neurons in a network.

We introduce a quantitative method for distinguishing true oscillations from random fluctuations in neuronal spike firing. Oscillations are generally considered as increases of firing patterns periodically, or semi-periodically, intermixed with periods of inactivity or decreased firing activities. These increased firing rates can also be considered as bursts of spike activities. These bursting activities exhibited in neurons can be occurring either randomly or deterministically at specific time intervals. Thus, it is our objective to distinguish the bursts of activity due to random fluctuations in firing from those bursts that represent oscillations in firing.

Given that we have identified the oscillations in firing for an individual neuron, we then address the issue of synchronous firing in a network of neurons. Synchronous firing is often observed in a network of neurons when a large number of individual neurons fire synchronously or when these neurons increase their bursting activities all at the same time. When these individual neurons are firing periodically, the synchronized firing will produce oscillations at the network level. But when the majority of the neurons fires desychronously, no oscillations will be observed at the network level even if these individual neurons are firing periodically. Thus, it is our second objective to detect the synchronicity of firing among neurons.

1.2. Synchronous Firings

Synchronized neural activity is often loosely defined with respect to the timing of the arrival of individual action potentials (or spikes) in the "synchronized" burst of activity transmitted along the neural pathways. Technically, the term *near-synchronous* or *near-coincident* more accurately describes the *synchrony* found in the biological nervous system since *absolute synchrony* (defined by the simultaneous arrival of action potentials without any time delay) rarely occurs in reality. It becomes important then to define what is meant by *synchrony*. Should bursts of activity synchronized within one millisecond, ten milliseconds, a hundred milliseconds or even a second be considered as synchrony? In other words, what is the time-scale that we consider as synchrony in spike firing?

Synchronized neural activity is often detected by electroencephalogram (EEG) or field potentials. These electrical records of neural activity are the summation of the action potentials generated by many neurons, often by the thousands. As a result, if these neurons are firing synchronously, the electrical signals will summate in-phase to produce large amplitude fluctuations. If these neurons are firing desynchronously, the electrical signals will summate out-of-phase, producing desynchronized patterns of electrical activities. Thus, it is important to examine the synchronicity of the firing of spikes in neurons to determine their in-phase and out-of-phase relationships.

Determining the time-scale of these in-phase and out-of-phase relationships is important. Since each action potential usually lasts less than a millisecond in vertebrates, the timing of the arrival of action potentials within a synchronized burst of activity can be resolved at the time-scale of milliseconds, whereas synchronized activity in EEG signals are resolved at a much longer time-scale, in the order of ten to hundred milliseconds. Thus, it is important to analyze the arrival of action potentials in a neuron where the precise timing of these signals can be measured exactly so that the in-phase and out-of-phase relationships can be determined. For instance, a neuron could be firing individual spikes out-of-phase with respect to another neuron in the time-scale of milliseconds, yet this out-of-phase relationship may not be detected at the EEG level when the time-resolution is in tens of milliseconds, thus interpreting this out-of-phase relationship as in-phase synchronous firing.

1.3. Correlated Spike Firings

Another important phenomenon resulting from the analysis of spike trains (or time-series of action potentials) is the difference between correlated firings and near-synchronous firings that are not correlated. *Correlated firings* mean that the timings of the arrival of action potentials from different neurons are correlated at specific time-latencies (i.e., time-locked or phase-locked), whereas *near-synchronous* firings imply that the timings of the arrival of action potentials are approximately the same, but not necessarily phase-locked, or correlated with the exact timing relationship between neurons. In fact, near-synchronous firings may be uncorrelated or a result of chance coincidence if the firings are not phase-locked or time-locked. Therefore, it is important to distinguish correlated firing activities from uncorrelated activities so that the specific interactions observed among the neurons can be quantified. Thus, we will concentrate on identifying the correlated activity in neurons when we address the synchronization issue of the spike firing in the CNS.

1.4. Spike Train Analyses

Since the firings of neurons can be quantified by a spike train, the analysis of such spike trains is commonly called spike train analysis. Spike train analysis provides a powerful tool in examining the dynamical interactions among neurons. There are many existing traditional spike train analyses such as the conventional auto-correlation technique (Perkel et al., 1967a; Rodieck et al., 1962) and cross-correlation techniques (Perkel et al., 1967b). Other spike train analytical techniques were also developed for the detection of specific conditional interactions among neurons such as temporal integration (Tam, 1998), cross-interval analyses (Tam et al., 1988; Tam & Gross, 1994), logical conditional correlation among neurons (Tam, 1993a), spatio-temporal correlation among neurons (Tam, 1993b), time-delayed neural network equivalence of cross-correlation computation (Tam, 1993d), artificial neural network implementation of enhanced cross-correlation computation (Tam, 1993e), gravitation clustering algorithm (Gerstein & Aertsen, 1985; Gerstein et al., 1985; Lindsey et al., 1989), snowflake analysis (Perkel et al., 1975), vectorial analysis (Tam, 1992a, 1992b, 1993c), joint interspike interval difference analysis (Fitzurka & Tam, 1995), first-order interspike interval difference phase plane analysis (Fitzurka & Tam, 1996a), second-order interspike interval difference phase plane analysis (Fitzurka & Tam, 1996b), and time-scale invariant method of detecting changes and oscillations (Tam, 1996).

We present two separate analyses. First, the "firing trend indices," h_1, h_2, and k, are used to detect changes in the firing patterns of neurons independent of the absolute time scale being considered such that patterns such as oscillations can easily be detected. Second, an integrated correlation method, called ISI—CI analysis, is presented to extract the firing probability of a neuron before and after a *reference* neuron has fired. The timing relationships between the firing of two neurons can be established where the correlation between these two neurons can be extracted. Thus, this analysis can be used to determine the synchronized relationship between neurons and how the firing of one neuron is correlated to the firing of another neuron.

2. METHODS

2.1. Interspike Intervals

Figure 2.1 depicts a schematic diagram of two idealized spike trains showing the times of occurrence of the spikes. Let a spike train A (with a total of N_A spikes) be represented by:

$$f_A(t) = \sum_{n=1}^{N_A} \delta(t - t_n) \tag{1}$$

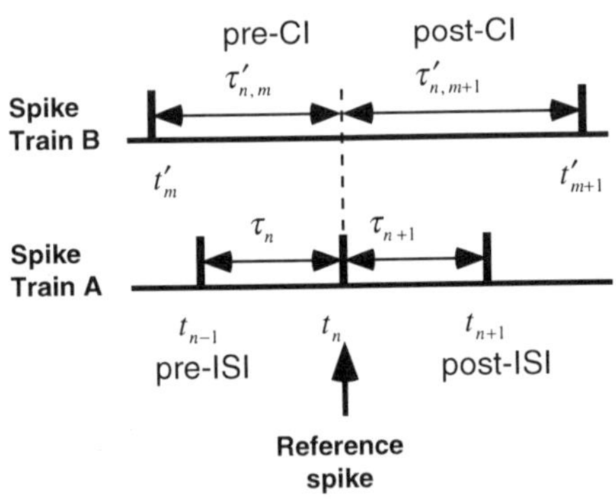

Fig. 2.1. Schematic diagram showing two idealized spike trains and the relationships between spike firing times: pre-ISI, post-ISI, pre-CI and post-CI for the two spike trains A and B.

where t_n is the time of occurrence of nth spikes in spike train A, and δ is a Dirac delta function denoting the occurrence of spikes. The first-order interspike interval (ISI) with respect to the nth reference spike (τ_n) is defined as

$$\tau_n = |t_{n-1} - t_n| \tag{2}$$

for $t_n > t_{n-1}$, and the second-order ISI with respect to the nth reference spike (τ_n'') is defined as

$$\tau_n'' = \tau_{n+1} + \tau_n. \tag{3}$$

2.2. Firing Trend Indices

The local variations in firing rate can be quantified by the following firing trend indices. These indices are used to establish the trend of changes in firing rate, such as an increasing trend and a decreasing trend. The local firing trend is defined as the changes in instantaneous firing rates between adjacent ISIs. By tracing the local firing trend, long-term oscillations can be distinguished from local random fluctuations of spike firings.

The firing trend index (h_1) is defined as the ratio between the first-order ISI and the second-order ISI relative to the nth reference spike (Tam, 1996),

$$h_1 = \frac{\tau_n}{\tau_n^{//}} = \frac{\tau_n}{\tau_n + \tau_{n-1}} \tag{4}$$

Note that the value of h_1 can be shown to be bounded by 0 and 1 (i.e., $0 < h_1 < 1$). Therefore, comparison between how firing intervals change can be made independent of the absolute time-scale of the interspike intervals. When h_1 approaches to the asymptotic value of 0 ($h_1 \rightarrow 0$), extreme change from a long ISI to a short ISI consecutively is revealed (i.e., $\tau_{n-1} >> \tau_n$). Similarly, when h_1 approaches to the asymptotic value of 1 ($h_1 \rightarrow 1$), extreme change from a short ISI to a long ISI consecutively is revealed (i.e., $\tau_{n-1} << \tau_n$). Finally, when h_1 is at the mid-point ($h_1 = 0.5$), no change in the consecutive ISIs is revealed (i.e., $\tau_{n-1} = \tau_n$)).

Another index, h_2, is defined as the ratio between the first-order ISI relative to the $n-1^{st}$ reference spike and the second-order ISI relative to the nth reference spike,

$$h_1 = \frac{\tau_{n-1}}{\tau_n^{//}} = \frac{\tau_{n-1}}{\tau_n + \tau_{n-1}} \tag{5}$$

where h_1 and h_2 are related by the following equation:

$$h_2 = 1 - h_1 \tag{6}$$

with the value of h_2 bounded by 0 and 1 (i.e., $0 < h_2 < 1$).

Alternatively, another firing trend index (k) can be defined as the ratio of the difference between the two adjacent ISIs (called the interspike interval difference or ISID) (Fitzurka & Tam, 1995, 1999) to the second-order ISI,

$$k = \frac{\Delta\tau_n}{\tau_n^{//}} = \frac{\tau_n - \tau_{n-1}}{\tau_n + \tau_{n+1}} \tag{7}$$

where $\Delta\tau_n$, the ISID, is defined as:

$$\Delta\tau_n = \tau_n - \tau_{n-1}. \tag{8}$$

Note that the value of k is bounded by -1 and 1 (i.e., $-1 < k < 1$). The above three indices are related with the following equation:

$$k = h_1 - h_2. \tag{9}$$

Using this k index, no change in firing in consecutive intervals is indicated by $k = 0$ (i.e., $\Delta\tau_n = 0$). Extreme lengthening in consecutive ISIs (i.e., $\tau_{n-1} \leq \tau_n$) is indicated by $k \to 1$, and extreme shortening in consecutive ISIs, (i.e., $\tau_{n-1} \geq \tau_n$) is indicated by $k \to -1$. Thus, by plotting these indices with respect to time would provide a clear indication of the evolution of serial trends in firing (see Figs. 2.2-2.4). Note that oscillations, which may or may not be periodic, can be revealed by these indices clearly. Because the indices h_1, h_2, and k are related by Equations (6) and (9), the analyses below will illustrate examples using the index h_1 only.

In summary, these firing trend indices are used to quantify local variations in firing rate independent of the time-scale of the firing patterns by examining the relative changes using a renormalized measure. These analyses can be applied to the spike trains of individual neurons to quantify the variations of firing patterns, such as oscillations. In order to detect the synchrony of firing among neurons, a different analysis is needed.

2.3. Cross-Intervals

In order to characterize the synchronicity of spike firings among neurons, the relationship between the firing times of spikes in different neurons needs to be established. The cross-interval analysis provides a quantitative measure to reveal the specific timing relationship of spike firings between two neurons. When the timing relationships are established, the in-phase firing relationship can be quantified.

Let us consider two spike trains (as depicted in Fig. 2.1), and choose spike train A as the reference, and spike train B as the compared, then the ISIs and the cross-intervals (CIs) can be defined as follows. The pre-ISI (τ_n), relative to the nth reference spike in the reference spike train, A, is defined as

$$\tau_n = |t_{n-1} - t_n|, \tag{10}$$

and post-ISI (τ_{n+1}), relative to the nth reference spike in the reference spike train A is defined as

$$\tau_{n+1} = |t_{n+1} - t_n| \tag{11}$$

(see Fig. 2.1). The pre-CI ($\tau'_{n,m}$) of spike train B, relative to the nth reference spike in spike train A, is defined as

$$\tau'_{n,m} = |t_m' - t_n| \tag{12}$$

such that $t_n \geq t_m'$ and $t_n < t_{m+1}'$, and the post-CI ($t_n \geq t_{m+1}'$) of spike train B, relative to the nth reference spike in spike train A, is defined as

$$\tau'_{n,m+1} = |t_{m+1}' - t_n| \tag{13}$$

such that $t_n \geq t_m'$ and $t_n < t_{m+1}$ (see Fig. 2.1). The timing relationship between the ISIs and CIs between the two spike trains is illustrated in Fig. 2.1.

2.4. Interspike Interval — Cross-Interval Analysis

The timing relationships between the firing of a spike in one neuron with respect to that of another neuron can be quantified by the ISI—CI analysis. The ISI represents the recurring firing times of spikes in an individual neuron, whereas the CI represents the latency of the spike occurrence between two neurons. Thus, by quantifying the relationship between the times of spike occurrence within a neuron and between two neurons, the in-phase and out-of-phase coupling between neurons can be established.

There are six possible combinations between the ISI and CI pairs when the intervals (both ISIs and CIs) preceding and succeeding a reference spike is considered in the reference spike train, A. The relationship between these six pairs of intervals can form graphs that are illustrated in Fig. 2.5: pre-ISI vs. post-ISI, pre-CI vs. post-CI, pre-ISI vs. post-CI, post-ISI vs. post-CI, pre-ISI vs. pre-CI, and post-ISI vs. pre-CI.

When these ISI and CI pairs are used as the *xy*-coordinates, they can be plotted on an *xy*-plot to show the relationship between the firing intervals graphically. The timing relationship between these intervals is represented by the coordinate of the point in the *xy*-plot. The construction of these *xy*-scatter plots can be done by representing the corresponding ISI and CI pairs as the (x,y)-coordinates in the *xy*-plots by considering all spikes sequentially in the reference spike train, A. That is, each point in the *xy*-scatter plot represents the corresponding ISI and CI pair.

When the pre-ISI and post-ISI pair is plotted as the *xy*-coordinates, the *xy*-plot (Fig. 2.5A) corresponds to the conventional joint interspike interval (JISI) analysis (Rodieck et al., 1962). The graph illustrates the relationship between the consecutive firing of two spikes within spike train A. That is, the graph shows the serial relationship of the recurrence spike firings in an individual neuron. The sequence of spike firing can be traced by this graph, which represents the serial relationship between adjacent ISIs. This graph can be used to quantify repetitive firing patterns in a neuron, such as oscillations.

The *xy*-plot of the pre-CI and post-CI pair (Fig. 2.5B) corresponds to the cross-interspike interval analysis described by Tam et al. (1988). The coordinate of the point in the graph represents the serial relationship between the firing of a reference spike in the reference spike train, *A*, and the pre- and post-CIs in the compared spike train, *B*. This graph can be used to infer the mutually reciprocal firing relationship between these two neurons, that is, the timing relationship of firing between the two neurons before and after the reference spike.

The *xy*-plot of the pre-ISI and post-CI pair (Fig. 2.5C) corresponds to the temporal integration of doublets analysis described by Tam (1998). The graph displays the relationship between the subsequent firing of a spike in the compared spike train *B* relative to the preceding firing of a spike prior to the reference spike in the reference spike train, *A*. This graph can be used to detect the temporal integration period of a doublet (two consecutive spikes) in the reference neuron that may contribute to the firing of the next spike in the compared neuron. Thus, the specific in-phase firing relationship between two neurons with respect to the integration period can be established by this graph.

The *xy*-plot of the post-ISI and post-CI pair (Fig. 2.5D) corresponds to the post-conditional cross-interval analysis (Tam, 1993f; Tam & Gross, 1994). This graph can be used to show the relationship between the subsequent firing of a spike in the compared spike train *B* relative to the next firing of a spike after the reference spike in the reference spike train *A*.

The *xy*-plot of the pre-ISI and pre-CI pair (Fig. 2.5E) corresponds to the pre-cross-interspike interval analysis (Tam & Fitzurka, 1995). This graph can be used to quantify the relationship between the prior firing of a spike in the compared spike train *B* relative to the previous firing of a spike prior to the reference spike in the reference spike train *A*. This analysis can be used to detect spatial summation of spikes that may contribute to the generation of the next spike firing.

The *xy*-plot of the post-ISI and pre-CI pair (Fig. 2.5F) corresponds to the cross-interval analysis described by Tam et al. (1988) and Gross and Tam (1994). This graph can be used to show the relationship between the prior firing of a spike in the compared spike train *B* relative to the subsequent firing of a spike after the reference spike in the reference spike train *A*. This analysis can be used to detect the in-phase firing relationship of a compared neuron in relation to the subsequent spike firing of the reference neuron.

Finally, four of the above six ISI-CI analyses can be combined into a single graph to capture the essential coupled firing times between two neurons. The *xy*-plots of ISI and CI pairs represented in Figs. 2.5C-2.5F can be re-integrated in a single *xy*-plot illustrated in Fig. 2.6. In this case, the negative *x*-axis represents the pre-ISI, the positive *x*-axis represents the post-ISI, the negative *y*-axis represents the pre-CI and the positive *y*-axis represents the post-CI in a single plot. This composite *xy*-plot is called the ISI-CI plot since the *x*-axis represents the ISI and the *y*-axis represents the CI.

2.5. Interpretations of the ISI-CI Plots

Each point in the ISI-CI plot represents the coordinate of the ISI-CI pair revealing the relationship between the ISI and CI. Thus, clusters of points in ISI-CI scatter plot suggest that there is a similar relationship between the ISI and CI pair. In other words, clusters of points indicate that the same firing pattern is repeated. This shows that the consecutive firing between the compared neuron and the reference neuron is constant, that is, phase-locked. In this way, repetitive firing patterns between the compared and reference spike trains can be graphically revealed by this analysis. Clustering of bands of points found in this graph can be used to indicate that the spike firings between the compared and reference neurons are correlated.

A horizontal band of points found in the ISI-CI plot suggests that there is a specific constant firing relationship between the compared and reference neurons (as indicated by the constant CI). This relationship is, however, independent of the consecutive firing of spikes within the reference neuron (as indicated by the ISIs).

A vertical band of points found in the ISI-CI plot suggests that the firing of consecutive spikes in the reference neuron is a constant (as indicated by the ISIs), while this relationship is independent of the firing of adjacent spikes in the compared neuron (as indicated by the CIs). In this case, the timing of the spike firing between these two neurons is not correlated, even though the neurons by themselves fire characteristically as revealed by the ISI distribution.

3. RESULTS

3.1. Detection of Oscillations or Changes in Firing Rate Using Firing Trend Indices

We provide results from spike trains simulated with known stochastic spike generating processes to illustrate true oscillations can be distinguished from random fluctuations using the firing trend index analysis. Without quantitative analysis, such as the one introduced here, local random fluctuations in firing rate can be interpreted as oscillations. We will use three example cases to illustrate the differences between (a) pseudo-oscillations, (b) random fluctuations, and (c) quasi-random fluctuations.

3.1.1. Detection of Fluctuations from Pseudo-Oscillations in Periodic Firing. Our first example is neuron A firing with a periodic spike train whose period fluctuates with a Gaussian variance. This is a typical example of pacemaker neuron that can be found in the central nervous system. This periodic spike train is simulated with a mean firing rate of 5 ms, modulated with a Gaussian variance around the mean.

The simulated spike train is shown in Fig. 2.2A showing the Gaussian modulated spike firing for the neuron. The plot of time versus ISI (τ) is shown in Fig. 2.2B showing the variability of the ISIs with respect to time. Local fluctuation of spike firings can be seen in this graph. The large fluctuations of firing rate can be seen in this analysis of serial ISIs (τ). This observation can be mistaken for oscillations in the neuron's firing sequence, yet this simulated neuron simply fired periodically with a constant mean ISI varied with a Gaussian variance.

With further analysis using the introduced renormalized firing trend index, h_1 (see Fig. 2.2C), the variations in firing rate are revealed to be relatively constant rather than fluctuating widely as in Fig. 2.2B. This is consistent with the fact that the neuron was simulated with a constant mean and a constant Gaussian variance. Thus, this "further analysis" shows that this apparent oscillation is merely an artifact. Therefore, it is fundamentally important to use quantitative analyses to determine whether the spike firing rate is truly oscillating or fluctuating due to random variability.

As discussed earlier, when the same data is re-plotted using the firing trend index h_1 instead of τ in Fig. 2.2C, a strikingly "stable" trend can be observed. The fluctuations or oscillations in firing intervals seen in Fig. 2.2B appear to be more stable when this time-invariant measure, h_1, is used (cf. Fig. 2.2C). The *constancy* of the firing trend is revealed using this renormalized measure, h_1, of ISI, as expected for a Gaussian process.

Using this analysis, the h_1 index truly reflects the characteristics of a relatively constant variation of ISIs centered around the "mean" (displayed horizontally in the plot)

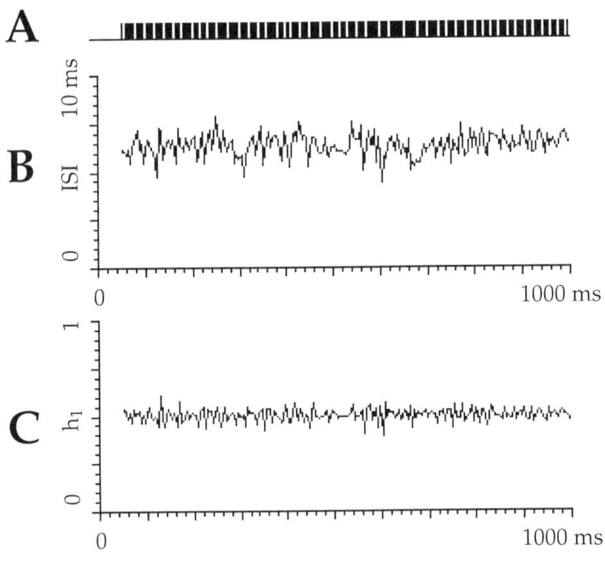

Fig. 2.2. (A) A graphical display of the simulated Gaussian varied periodic spike train. (B) A plot of time versus ISI, τ, for the same spike train. (C) A plot of time versus the firing trend index, h_1, for the same spike train.

when the ISIs are renormalized. This renormalization restores the appearance of the periodic nature (i.e., constant ISI, τ) of the original spike train when the h_1 measure is used (Fig. 2.2C) as compared with using the original ISI (τ) measure (Fig. 2.2B). The long-range fluctuations in ISIs (or pseudo-oscillations) are eliminated from the h_1 plot (see Fig. 2.2C).

Furthermore, the firing trend index can detect transient changes in firing rate. The abrupt changes in firing rate (appearing as large consecutive deviations from the mean) can be detected more clearly using the h_1 measure (Fig. 2.2C) than the ISI (τ) measure (Fig. 2.2B). This shows that the abrupt changes are much better detected as transients using the firing trend index (h_1) measure than the ISI (τ) measure. This clearly illustrates how the firing trend index analysis can be used to distinguish not only pseudo-oscillations from true oscillations but also detect transient changes more quantitatively.

3.1.2. Detection of True Random Renewal Firings from Non-Random Fluctuations. Next, we want to distinguish the firing patterns that are generated by a truly random process (i.e., a renewal process such as the Poisson process), from a process that may appear random. Such random spike firing patterns are often exhibited by neurons in the central nervous system, especially the auditory neurons. Therefore, we simulate neuron *B* with a spike train generated by a Poisson process with a mean ISI of 5 ms. This is used to illustrate the characteristics of a truly random spike train. Figure 2.3A shows the random firing patterns of the Poisson neuron, and Fig. 2.3B shows the random fluctuations of ISIs by plotting the time versus ISIs (τ). Notice that there are more short ISIs than long ISIs, as expected for a Poisson process. This is because a Poisson distribution resembles a negative exponential function with more frequent occurrences of short intervals than long intervals (giving a *burst-like* sequence of spike firing). Thus, it is congruent with the expected theoretical prediction that the ISIs tends to *hover* around shorter ISIs (i.e., closer to the x-axis in the serial τ plot (Fig. 2.3B) with a few occasional long ISIs intersperse between these "quasi-bursts"). These "quasi-bursts" of spike firing can be seen clearly in the spike train shown in Fig. 2.3A.

The random nature of firing for a Poisson process is also shown to be time-independent using our time-invariant firing trend index which eliminates the underlying time-scale of the firing process. When the ISI (τ) is renormalized using the h_1 index (Fig. 2.3C), this renormalized measure of ISI is shown to fill the entire range of values between 0 and 1. No *preferred* firing trends are observed using the h_1 index (as revealed by the rather uniform distribution of the h_1 index spanning the whole range between 0 and 1). This is congruent with the truly random, renewal process which spans the entire range of all possible firing trends.

On the other hand, when the ISI, τ, is used as the measure (Fig. 2.3B), *preferred* firing intervals of short ISIs are found, giving rise to the *burst-like firing patterns* which are not true bursts since these short ISIs are coincidental for a Poisson process. Again, the neuron can be mistaken as exhibiting non-periodic fluctuations or oscillations in firing when burst-like firing patterns are occasionally observed. These non-periodic pseudo-oscillations are misleading because a neuron firing with a truly-random Poisson process always appears to fire in a series of short ISIs (giving the *burst-like* appearance) followed by long pauses (long ISIs). Therefore, it is important to use quantitative

A

B

C

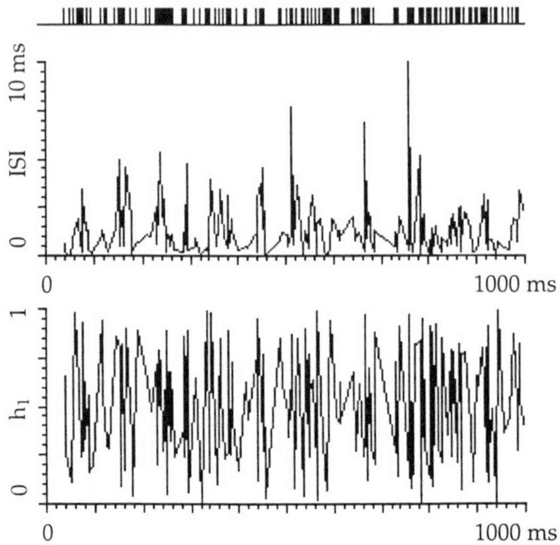

Fig. 2.3. (A) A graphical display of the simulated Poisson spike train. (B) A plot of time versus ISI, τ, for the same spike train. (C) A plot of time versus the firing trend index, h_1, for the same spike train.

analysis, such as the h_1 index, to distinguish non-periodic oscillations from random fluctuations that span the entire range of possible firing trends (ranging between 0 and 1 for the h_1 index).

3.1.3. Detection of Quasi-Random Firings from Local Fluctuations. Finally, neuron *C* is simulated with a quasi-random firing pattern (uniformly distributed random pattern) with a mean ISI of 5 ms (Fig. 2.4A). Although a spike train generated using such uniformly distributed ISIs is non-physiological and highly artificial, it serves the purpose of illustrating some very interesting phenomena for the detection of fluctuations in firing trends.

Figure 2.4 clearly shows the uniformity in the distribution of ISIs as seen from the spike train representation (Fig. 2.4A). The uniformly distributed nature of the original spike train is clearly revealed in the plot of serial ISIs, which is expected to span the entire range of ISIs between 0 and 5 ms (Fig. 2.4B). Yet when the ISI is renormalized by the h_1 index and plotted for this spike train (Fig. 2.4C), a constant trend of firing fluctuating around a "mean" (h_1 = 0.5). Comparing this analysis with that of the Gaussian spike train (Fig. 2.2C), the range of fluctuation is greater for this example, as expected.

A

B

C

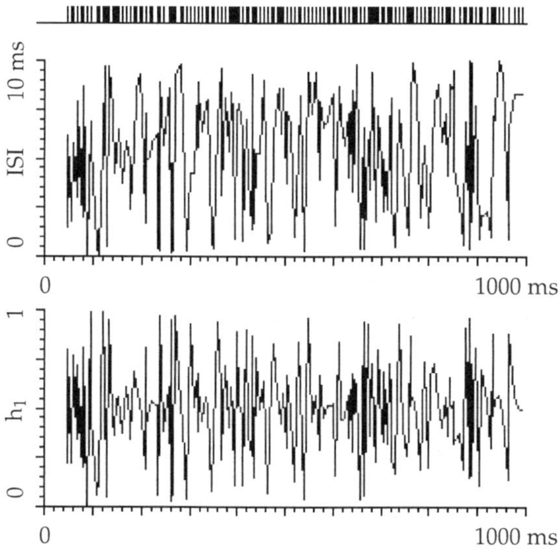

Fig. 2.4. (A) A graphical display of an artificial spike train generated with uniformly distributed ISIs. (B) A plot of time versus ISI, τ, for the same spike train. (C) A plot of time versus the firing trend index, h_1, for the same spike train.

Additionally, this firing trend analysis also detects the times where abrupt changes (large deviations) occur (comparing Figs. 2.4A and 2.4C), whereas such abrupt changes are difficult to distinguish using the conventional ISI measure (comparing Figs. 2.4A and 2.4B).

The wide excursions of h_1 value in Fig. 2.4C, which correspond to the abrupt changes in firing intervals, are correlated with the sudden changes in firing trend (cf. Fig. 2.4A) much more readily than the ISI measure (cf. Fig. 2.4B). This illustrates the advantage of using h_1 to detect oscillations and abrupt changes in firing intervals for a pseudo-random firing pattern.

3.2. ISI-CI Analyses

While the preceding firing trend index analyses can uncover the difference between pseudo-oscillations and true oscillations, the correlation analyses described below will illustrate the difference between correlated, time-locked responses and those that are uncorrelated. We will use the ISI-CI analyses to extract the relationship between the firing times of neurons. We will use a set of connected neurons to illustrate the intriguing coupling between the firing times of the neurons. The neurons are simulated using a stochastic spike train generation process.

The analyses of timing relationships between the ISIs and CIs in various combinations are shown in Figs. 2.5 and 2.6 for two connected neurons, *D* and *E*. Neuron *D* is a randomly firing neuron whose spike train is generated with Poisson process. Neuron *E* is coupled with the firing of neuron *D* at a latency of 2.5 ms and a 50% probability of synaptic coupling strength. Neuron *E*'s firing is generated by temporally integrating two incoming spikes within a 10 ms time-window.

3.2.1. The Pre-ISI vs. Post-ISI Analysis. First, the JISI plot (pre-ISI vs. post-ISI) is shown in Fig. 2.5A to reveal the relationship between consecutive firing in neuron *D*, which is used as the reference neuron in the cross-correlation analyses below. A negative exponential distribution of points can be seen in this JISI plot, which is congruent with the random firing characteristic of this Poisson neuron.

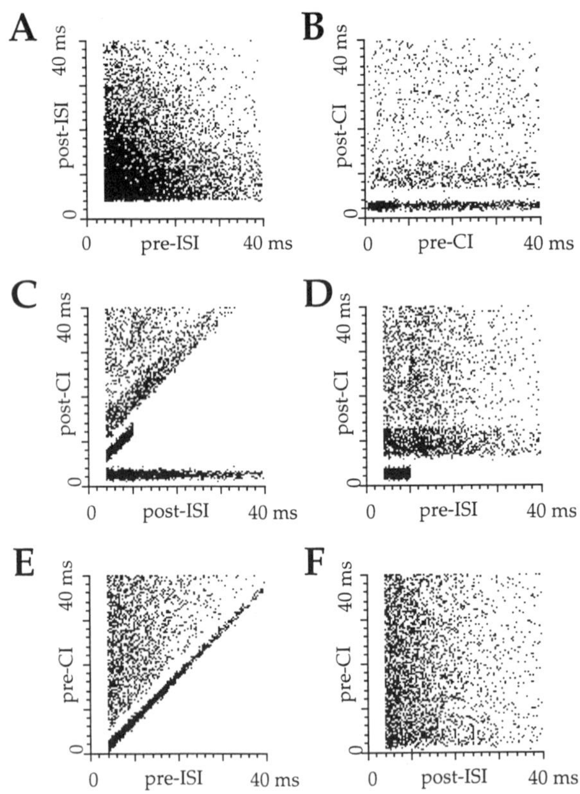

Fig. 2.5. The *xy*-plots of the six different ISI-CI analyses for neurons.

3.2.2. The Pre-CI vs. Post-CI Analysis. The scatter plot of pre-CI vs. post-CI for this neuron-pair is displayed in Fig. 2.5B, which shows the timing relationships between the firing of these two neurons. The relative times of spike arrival before and after the firing of a reference spike in the reference neuron are shown in this plot. A horizontal band of points along the 2.5 ms post-CI in this plot shows that there is a preference for neuron *E* to fire 2.5 ms after a spike has fired in neuron *D* (i.e., they are time-locked together with a 2.5 ms cross-interval). This is congruent with the simulation parameters in which the neurons are coupled together with a latency of 2.5 ms. This analysis clearly reveals the correlated spike firing between these two neurons. Their firings are coupled, and are in near-synchrony. Although the firing pattern of neuron *D* is random as simulated, this analysis reveals the synchronicity of firing between these two neurons that may not be detected otherwise.

This analysis also shows that there is a time-locked relationship between the spike firing in the reference neuron and the subsequent firing in the compared neuron. There is no such time-locked synchrony with respect to the preceding firing in the compared neuron. Thus, this pre-CI vs. post-CI analysis shows that even for this neuron pair, the near-synchronous firing is not reciprocal. The correlated time-locked firing pattern is preceded by the firing in the reference neuron, followed by the firing in the compared neuron, but not vice versa. This clearly reveals that the intriguing coupled firing relationship between these two neurons may have significant implications in the interpretation of the signal processing among neurons in the network that are not reciprocal. This uni-directional time-locked coupling in spike firing between neurons is not generally revealed by examining the near-coincidence of firing in neurons without specifically addressing the particular correlational relationship between the timing of spike firing in these neurons.

3.2.3. The Post-ISI vs. Post-CI Analysis. Next, the scatter plot of post-ISI vs. post-CI of the same two neurons is shown in Fig. 2.5C. Again, a cluster of points along the horizontal band of 2.5 ms post-CI can be seen. This indicates that there is a preference for the compared neuron to fire 2.5 ms after a spike has fired in the reference neuron, similar to what was shown in the cross-interval (pre-CI vs. post-CI) analysis (Fig. 2.5B). The preferred time-locked firing interval between these two neurons is independent of the previous firing of a spike prior to the occurrence of the reference spike (pre-ISI) in the reference neuron. The diagonal band of points reflects that the two neurons are coupled not only with respect to the first spike but also with respect to the second spike. This is congruent with the fact that neuron *E*'s firing involves temporal integration of two preceding spikes from neuron *D*.

3.2.4. The Pre-ISI vs. Post-CI Analysis. Figure 2.5D shows the pre-ISI vs. post-CI scatter plot for the two neurons. Again, the preferential firing of neuron *E* 2.5 ms after a spike has fired in the reference neuron is revealed. This coupling relationship lasts only for the duration of 10 ms of pre-ISI, which is congruent with the 10- ms temporal integration period for neuron *E* to generate a spike. Thus, the time-locked firing pattern between these two neurons (as indicated by the horizontal band of points along constant post-CI) is limited to the firing interval (pre-ISI) of 10 ms for this neuron-pair. This analysis reveals the coupled firing relationship between these two neurons is confined to a specific integration period. Therefore, the exact condition in which the two neurons are coupled is extracted by this analysis which may not be revealed if specific quantitative analyses are not applied.

3.2.5. The Pre-ISI vs. Pre-CI Analysis. Figure 2.5E displays the pre-ISI vs. pre-CI scatter plot. A diagonal band of points is observed in this graph. This is due to the near-coincident, correlated firing between two neurons. This result reveals similar interpretations of the time-locked coupling relationship between these two neurons.

3.2.6. The Post-ISI vs. Pre-CI Analysis. Last, but not least, Fig. 2.5F shows the post-ISI vs. pre-CI scatter plot for these two neurons. No particular clustering or band of points are found in this analysis, which shows that these particular intervals are not correlated. In other words, the pre-CI is not correlated with the post-ISI of the neuron, which is congruent with the fact that the firing of neuron *E* would have no effects on the next firing of neuron *D*, since neuron *E* is driven by neuron *D*, but not vice versa. Thus, the above analyses clearly reveal that the firing of the neuron pair was coupled not just near-synchronously, but also in very specific non-reciprocal manner.

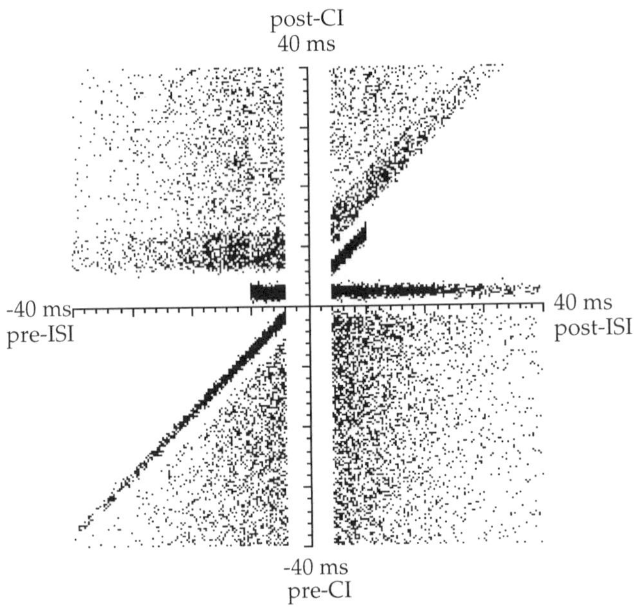

Fig. 2.6. The composite ISI/CI plot of the same neuron pair shown in Figs. 2.5C-F, with the pre-ISI and pre-CI plotted as negative.

3.2.7. The Composite ISI-CI Analysis. To summarize the foregoing results, a composite plot is shown in Fig. 2.6 representing four of the earlier analyses (by combining Figs. 2.5C-F). This new representation provides a better visualization of the relationship between the CIs and ISIs. The horizontal and diagonal bands of points can be seen spanning the positive and negative axes. Note that the lack of points between the pre-ISI of 4 ms and the post-ISI of 4 ms is an indication of the refractory period of neuron D.

In summary, the time-locked firing between these two neurons can be revealed by the horizontal band of points with respect to the preceding or succeeding spike firing in neuron E relative to a reference spike in neuron *D*. The "truncated" band of points indicates the duration of the above time-locked firing. Thus, not only is the near-synchronous firing between these two neurons revealed, but also the conditions in which they are coupled are also uncovered specifically.

4. CONCLUSION

Two separate spike train analyses were introduced to detect oscillations and synchronous firing in neurons. The firing trend indices is used as a time-invariant method for detecting changes of firing patterns or oscillation patterns in neurons. Since they renormalize the time scale producing a relative measure of time with respect to the local trend, these analyses allow us to differentiate between pseudo-oscillations and true oscillations in spike firing.

The ISI-CI analyses can be applied to provide a clear indication of the specific relationship between the preferred firing intervals (ISIs) within a neuron and between the time-correlated cross-intervals (CIs) in relation to these two neurons. Thus, the correlation relationship between any neuron pair can be revealed based on the relative timing of the spike firing between two neurons. Reciprocal and non-reciprocal relationships can also be revealed by these analyses.

Based on these correlation patterns, the synchronized firing or near-coincident firing of spikes between neurons can be assessed. When a cluster of points is found in the ISI-CI plots, the specific dependence relationship between the firing intervals can be established. Thus, correlated firing patterns as well as synchronized firing characteristics between neurons can be assessed based on the consecutive firing of spikes between any pair of neurons in a network.

This chapter shows that it is important to examine the oscillations and synchronous firing in neurons more closely with quantitative analyses so that subtle phenomena that are not obvious at first glance may be revealed. The functional significance of these oscillations and synchronous firing can then be assessed with these quantitative analyses.

ACKNOWLEDGMENTS

This research was supported in part by ONR Grant numbers N00014-93-1-0135 and N00014-94-0686 and by the University of North Texas Faculty Research Grant.

REFERENCES

Fitzurka, M. A., & Tam, D. C. (1995). A new spike train analysis technique for detecting trends in the firing patterns of neurons. In J. M. Bower (Ed.), *The Neurobiology of Computation* (pp. 73-78). Boston: Kluwer.

Fitzurka, M. A., & Tam, D. C. (1996a). First order interspike interval difference phase plane analysis of neuronal spike train data. In J. M. Bower (Ed.), *Computational Neuroscience* (pp. 429-434). San Diego: Academic Press.

Fitzurka, M. A., & Tam, D. C. (1996b). Second order interspike interval difference phase plane analysis of neuronal spike train data. In J. M. Bower (Ed.), *Computational Neuroscience* (pp. 435-440). San Diego: Academic Press.

Fitzurka, M. A., & Tam, D. C. (1999). A joint interspike interval difference stochastic spike train analysis: Detecting sequential changes in the firing trends of single neurons. *Biological Cybernetics*, in press.

Gerstein, G. L., & Aertsen, A. (1985). Representation of cooperative firing activity among simultaneously recorded neurons. *Journal of Neurophysiology*, *54*, 1513-1528.

Gerstein, G. L., Perkel, D. H., & Dayhoff, J. E. (1985). Cooperative firing activity in simultaneously recorded populations of neurons: Detection and measurement. *Journal of Neuroscience*, *5*, 881-889.

Gross, G. W., & Tam, D. C. (1994, June). Pre-conditional correlation between neurons in cultured networks. *Proceedings of the World Congress on Neural Networks, San Diego, CA* (Vol. 2, pp. 786-791). Hillsdale, NJ: Lawrence Erlbaum Associates.

Lindsey, B. G., Shannon, R., & Gerstein, G. L. (1989). Gravitational representation of simultaneously recorded brainstem respiratory neuron spike trains. *Brain Research*, *483*, 373-378.

Perkel, D. H., Gerstein, G. L., & Moore, G. P. (1967a). Neuronal spike trains and stochastic point process. I. The single spike train. *Biophysical Journal*, *7*, 391-418.

Perkel, D. H., Gerstein, G. L., & Moore, G. P. (1967b). Neuronal spike trains and stochastic point process. II. Simultaneous spike trains. *Biophysics Journal*, *7*, 419-440.

Perkel, D. H., Gerstein, G. L., Smith, M. S., & Tatton, W. G. (1975). Nerve-impulse patterns: A quantitative display technique for three neurons. *Brain Research*, *100*, 271-296.

Rodieck, R. W., Kiang, N. Y.-S., & Gerstein, G. L. (1962). Some quantitative methods for the study of spontaneous activity of single neurons. *Biophysical Journal*, *2*, 351-368.

Tam, D. C. (1992a, June). Vectorial phase-space analysis for detecting dynamical interactions in firing patterns of biological neural networks. *Proceedings of the International Joint Conference on Neural Networks* (Vol. 3, pp. 97-102). Piscataway, NJ: IEEE.

Tam, D. C. (1992b, November). A novel vectorial phase-space analysis of spatio-temporal firing patterns in biological neural networks. *Proceedings of the Simulation Technology Conference*, pp. 556-564.

Tam, D. C. (1993a, July). A new conditional correlation statistics for detecting spatio-temporally correlated firing patterns in a biological neuronal network. *Proceedings of the World Congress on Neural Networks* (Vol. 2, pp. 606-609). Hillsdale, NJ: Lawrence Erlbaum Associates.

Tam, D. C. (1993b). Novel cross-interval maps for identifying attractors from multi-unit neural firing patterns. In B. H. Jansen & M. E. Brandt (Eds.), *Nonlinear Dynamical Analysis of the EEG* (pp. 65-77). River Edge, NJ: World Scientific Publishing Co.

Tam, D. C. (1993c). A multi-neuronal vectorial phase-space analysis for detecting dynamical interactions in firing patterns of biological neural networks. In F. H. Eeckman & J. M. Bower (Eds.), *Computational Neural Systems* (pp. 49-53). Norwell, MA: Kluwer.

Tam, D. C. (1993d). Computation of cross-correlation function by a time-delayed neural network. In C. H. Dagli, L. I. Burke, B. R. Fernandez & J. Ghosh (Eds.), *Intelligent Engineering Systems through Artificial Neural Networks: Vol. 3* (pp. 51-55). New York: American Society of Mechanical Engineers Press.

Tam, D. C. (1993e). A hybrid time-shifted neural network for analyzing biological neuronal spike trains. In O. Omidvar (Ed.), *Progress in Neural Networks: Vol. 2* (pp. 129-146). Norwood, NJ: Ablex.

Tam, D. C. (1993f). A new post-conditional correlation method for extracting excitation-inhibition coupling between neurons. *Society for Neuroscience Abstracts*, 19, 1598.

Tam, D. C. (1996). A Time-scale invariant method for detection of changes and oscillations in neuronal firing intervals. In J. M. Bower (Eds.), *Computational Neuroscience* (pp. 465-470). San Diego: Academic Press.

Tam, D. C. (1998). A cross-interval spike train analysis: The correlation between spike generation and temporal integration of doublets. *Biological Cybernetics*, *78*, 95-106.

Tam, D. C., Ebner, T. J., & Knox, C. K. (1988). Cross-interval histogram and cross-interspike interval histogram correlation analysis of simultaneously recorded multiple spike train data. *Journal of Neuroscience Methods*, *23*, 23-33.

Tam, D. C., & Fitzurka, M. A. (1995) A stochastic time-series analysis for detecting excitation-inhibition couplings among neurons in a network. In M. Witten & D. J. Vincent (Eds.), *Computational Medicine, Public Health and Biotechnology: Building a Man in the Machine Mathematical Biology and Medicine, Vol. 5* (pp. 921-931).

Tam, D. C., & Gross, G. W. (1994, June). Post-conditional correlation between neurons in cultured neuronal networks. *Proceedings of the World Congress on Neural Networks* (Vol. 2, pp. 792-797). Hillsdale, NJ: Lawrence Erlbaum Associates.

Tam, D. C., & Gross, G. W. (1994). Dynamical changes in neuronal network circuitries using multi-unit spike train analysis. In T. McKenna & D. A. Stenger (Eds.), *Enabling Technologies for Cultured Neural Networks* (pp. 319-345). San Diego: Academic Press.

3

Coexisting Stable Oscillatory States in Single Cell and Multicellular Neuronal Oscillators

Douglas A. Baxter and Hilde A. Lechner
The University of Texas Medical School at Houston

Carmen C. Canavier
University of New Orleans

Robert J. Butera, Jr.
National Institutes of Health

Anthony A. DeFranceschi, and John W. Clark, Jr.
Rice University

John H. Byrne
The University of Texas Medical School at Houston

ABSTRACT

The dynamical behavior of individual neurons and of neural circuits emerges from the interactions among multiple nonlinear processes at the molecular, cellular, synaptic and network levels. Thus, characterizing the dynamical performance of a complex system of nonlinear elements is fundamental to an understanding of neural function. This chapter illustrates how some of the concepts and analytical techniques of nonlinear dynamical systems were applied to computational and experimental analyses of single cell and multicellular neuronal oscillators. The results of these studies provided additional insights into how neurons and neural circuits might exploit nonlinear dynamics at the cellular level to generate and control oscillatory patterns of electrical activity and to process and store information.

1. INTRODUCTION

Oscillatory patterns of electrical activity play many important roles in the neural functions. They underlie the generation of rhythmic movements (for recent reviews see

Calabrese, 1995; Dean & Cruse, 1994; Grillner, Wallen, & Vianna di Preisco, 1990; Harris-Warrick, 1993; Harris-Warrick, Marder, Selverston, & Moulins, 1992; Jacklet, 1989; Pearson, 1993; Rossignol & Dubuc, 1994), contribute to processing of sensory information (e.g., Eckhorn, Reitboeck, Arndt, & Dicke, 1990; Freeman, 1994; Ghose & Freeman, 1992; Gray, 1994; McKenna, McMullen, & Shlesinger, 1994; Singer, 1993a, 1993b; Malsburg, 1995), influence arousal and attention (e.g., Crick, 1984; Lopes da Silva, 1991; Steriade, Jones, & Llinas, 1990) and may play a role in learning and memory (e.g., Crick & Mitchison, 1983; Eckhorn, Schanze, Brosch, Salem, & Bauer, 1992; Freeman, 1992; Hobson, 1988; Huerta & Lisman, 1993, 1995; Klimesch, Schimke, & Pfurtscheller, 1993; Liljenstrom & Hasselmo, 1995; Singer, 1993b). Indeed, some have speculated that synchronized neural oscillations play a much broader role in nervous systems and form the basis for higher cognitive functions and consciousness (e.g., Crick, 1994; Crick & Koch, 1990; Haken & Stadler, 1990; Llinas & Pare, 1991; Llinas & Ribary, 1993). Thus, investigating the mechanisms underlying the generation, control and synchronization of neuronal oscillations is critical to understanding many aspects of neural function.

Two approaches, one computational and the other experimental, are being used to investigate neural oscillations. A widespread approach to modeling oscillatory activity has involved the construction and analysis of systems of coupled nonlinear oscillators (for recent reviews see Ermentrout, 1994; Kopell, 1988, 1995; Kuramoto, 1995; Rand, Cohen, & Holmes, 1988). Generally, such assemblies incorporate oscillatory elements that exhibit a single and asymptotically stable limit cycle (i.e., the elements are monostable), and it is assumed that the limit cycle that characterizes the dynamics of the individual oscillators continues to exist after the oscillators are coupled together (Rand et al., 1988) and that this coupling simply advances or delays the phase of activity in each oscillator. The dynamical behavior of systems of such nonlinear oscillators is relatively well understood provided that the individual oscillators are monostable, that the number of oscillators is small and/or there is a high degree of symmetry and that the coupling among oscillators is more-or-less symmetrical and stationary. Despite their relatively simple features, assemblies of coupled nonlinear oscillators manifest a number of biologically relevant phenomena, such as generating oscillatory patterns that correspond to various features of rhythmic movements (e.g., Buchanan, 1992; Cohen et al., 1992; Collins & Stewart, 1993; Gottschalk, Ogilvie, Richter, & Pack, 1994; Lansner & Edeberg, 1994; Rowat & Selverston, 1993; Williams, 1992; Yuasa & Ito, 1990), processing sensory information (e.g., Chawanya, Aoyagi, Nishikawa, Okuda, & Kuramoto, 1993; Eckhorn et al., 1990; Grossberg & Somers, 1991; Li & Hopfield, 1989; Niebur, Koch, & Rosin, 1993; Sompolinsky, Golomb, & Kleinfeld, 1990; Malsburg & Buhmann, 1992; Yamaguchi & Shimizu, 1994), and encoding memories (e.g., Hayashi, 1994; Horn & Usher, 1991; Mori, Davis, & Nara, 1989; Wang, Buhmann, & Malsburg, 1990).

Experimental analyses have demonstrated that biological oscillators make use of cellular and synaptic elements that are more complex and diverse than those commonly simulated in computational studies. In general terms, biological oscillatory activity results from reciprocal interactions between excitatory and inhibitory processes. Such reciprocal interactions may occur at the level of a single cell by coupling between excitatory and inhibitory membrane conductances or at the level of a neural circuit by synaptic connections among cells. In the former case, the cells can exhibit autonomous oscillatory firing patterns (e.g., Adams & Benson, 1989; Baxter & Byrne, 1991; Benson & Adams, 1987; Canavier, Clark, & Byrne, 1991; Connors & Butnick, 1990; Destexhe, Babloyantz, & Sejnowski, 1993; Jacklet, 1989; Llinas, 1990; McCormick, Huguenard, & Strowbridge, 1992). In the latter case, the oscillatory behavior is an emergent property of the network architecture (e.g., Bower, 1992; Getting, 1989; Harris-Warrick et al., 1992; Jacklet, 1989; Nadim, Olsen, DeSchutter, & Calabrese, 1995; Pearson, 1993; Raymond, Baxter, Buonomano, & Byrne, 1992; Selverston, 1992; Sharp, Skinner, & Marder, 1996; Traub & Miles, 1992). In many cases, however, oscillatory activity emerges from a combination of both cellular and network mechanisms (e.g., Destexhe et al., 1993; Elson & Selverston, 1992; Pearson, 1993; Sejnowski, McCormick, & Steriade, 1995; Steriade, McCormick, & Sejnowski, 1993; von Krosigk, Bal, & McCormick, 1993).

An intriguing possibility, which we are pursuing, is that additional and possibly novel insights to neural oscillations will emerge from computational studies of neurons and neural circuits that more realistically reflect the nonlinear dynamical properties of individual neurons and synaptic connections. In this chapter, we will describe some of our current research on how diverse dynamical behaviors emerge from the nonlinear properties of single cell and multicellular neuronal oscillators. Both computational and experimental analyses were used to demonstrate that an autonomously bursting neuron can support multistability; that is, a proliferation of coexisting periodic attractors within the phase space of the cell (Butera, Clark, & Byrne, 1996; Byrne, Canavier, Lechner, Clark, & Baxter, 1994; Canavier, Baxter, Clark, & Byrne, 1993, 1994; Lechner, Baxter, Clark, & Byrne, 1996; see also Bertram, 1993).[1] Each of these attractors corresponded to a different pattern of oscillatory activity, and brief perturbations (e.g., synaptic inputs) could switch the electrical activity of the cell from one stable pattern of oscillation to another. These mode transitions did *not* require any changes in the parameters of the model and such parameter-*in*dependent transitions provided an enduring response to a transient input. Similarly, multistability was demonstrated in small multicellular

---

[1] It may be useful to define some of the terms that we have used to characterize the dynamics of this neuronal model. The "phase space" of a dynamical system is a mathematical space with independent coordinates representing the dynamic variables needed to specify the instantaneous state of the system. Often dynamical systems have many variables, which makes the phase space of the complete system multidimensional and highly complex. Thus, a common practice is to choose only two of the state variables and make a two dimensional projection of the phase space, i.e., a phase-*plane* projection. Because the state variables change in a continuous manner, "trajectories" emerge that provide a two-dimensional representation of the solutions of the multi-dimensional model (e.g., Fig 3.3). An "attractor" is a trajectory (or point) in phase-space to which the system will converge from a set of initial coordinates. Several different types of attractors can emerge from a nonlinear system. For example, if an oscillatory trajectory periodically repeats itself such that the orbits around the attractor overlay each other, then the attractor is referred to as a "limit cycle." In contrast, some attractors have complex structures such that successive orbits diverge exponentially in time. Such aperiodic attractors are referred as "strange" or "chaotic" (for reviews see Baker & Gollub, 1990; Ermentrout, 1994, 1995; Guckenheimer, Gueron, & Harris-Warrick, 1993; Moon, 1992; Rinzel & Ermentrout, 1989; Wang & Rinzel, 1995).

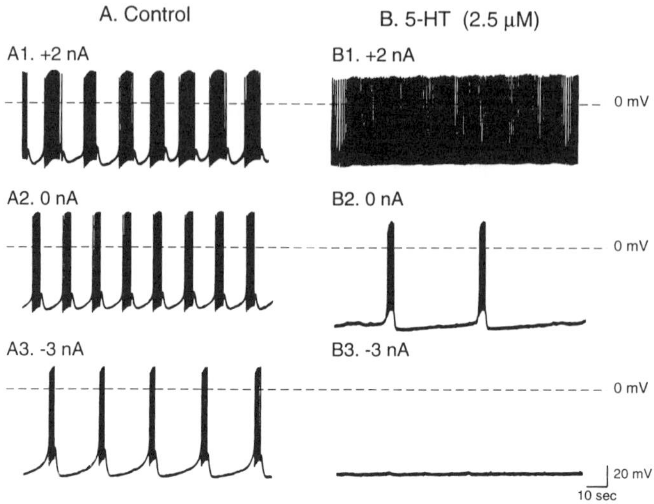

Fig. 3.1. Parameter-dependent changes in electrical activity of neuron R15. Intracellular recordings from an R15 neuron in the absence (A, Control) and in the presence of serotonin (B, 5-HT). R15 is an endogenously bursting neuron that can exhibit different modes of electrical activity, ranging from a silent state, to various bursting modes, to continuous spiking (i.e., beating). In the absence of any external inputs (A2), the cell exhibits regular bursting activity. The electrical activity changes in a parameter-dependent manner for different levels of bias current. Applying a depolarizing bias current (A1) shifted the activity of R15 to a different bursting mode in which the bursts were more intense and the interburst hyperpolarization was reduced. Applying a hyperpolarizing bias current (A3) shifted R15 into different bursting mode in which the duration of the bursts was reduced and the interburst hyperpolarization was increased. The mode of activity in R15 also can be modified by applying modulatory transmitter, such as 5-HT, which modulates the anomalous-rectifier potassium current and the slow-inward calcium current. In the presence of 5-HT (B2), the activity of the cell is shifted to a bursting mode that is characterized by an increase the interburst hyperpolarization, an increase in the frequency of action potentials during the burst and a decrease in the duration of the each burst. The response of the cell to bias currents was also altered by 5-HT. In the presence of 5-HT, the depolarizing bias current shifted the electrical activity of the cell to a beating mode (constant spiking; B1), whereas the hyperpolarizing bias current shifted the cell into a silent mode (B3).

neuronal oscillators (Baxter, Canavier, Butera, Clark, & Byrne 1996; Canavier, Baxter, Clark, & Byrne, 1995; Canavier, Butera, Dror, Baxter, Clark, & Byrne, 1997), and thus, brief perturbations could induce parameter-*in*dependent transitions between distinct oscillatory modes of activity. These studies have provided novel insights into how nonlinear dynamical processes can contribute to generation and control of oscillations in neural systems as well as potential functional roles for multistability in neural systems.

2. R15: A SINGLE-CELL NEURONAL OSCILLATOR

The primary subject of our analysis has been the R15 neuron, which is located in the abdominal ganglion of the marine mollusc *Aplysia* (for review see Adams & Benson, 1989). R15 has intrigued neurobiologists for decades, principally because of its intrinsic ability to produce bursting activity (e.g., Figs. 3.1 and 3.6). During the burst, the frequency of action potentials increases, and reaches a peak about midway through the burst. Thereafter, the frequency decreases; hence, R15 is often referred to as a parabolic burster. After the last spike, there is a characteristic depolarizing afterpotential, which is followed by a post-burst (or interburst) hyperpolarization. The hyperpolarization relaxes and the cycle repeats itself. In the absence of external stimulation or synaptic input, R15 produces rather regular bursting activity for many hours in the isolated abdominal ganglia preparation. Indeed, the R15 neuron can be removed from the ganglia, maintained in culture and the cell still expresses bursting behavior (Lechner, Baxter, & Byrne, personal observation; Parsons, Salzberg, Obaid, Raccuia-Behling, & Kleinfeld, 1991).

Another intriguing feature of R15 is its capability to exhibit many different modes of oscillatory activity. Previous experimental studies have demonstrated two conventional methods of shifting the activity of R15 between these different modes. The first method is illustrated in Fig. 3.1A. One can alter the activity of R15 by intracellularly injecting a constant bias current. In the absence of any bias current (Fig. 3.1A2), R15 produced a regular bursting pattern. Applying a depolarizing bias current (Fig. 3.1A1) shifted the activity of R15 to a different bursting mode in which the bursts were more intense and the length and depth of the interburst hyperpolarization was reduced. In contrast, hyperpolarizing bias currents (Fig. 3.1A3) shifted R15 into yet another bursting mode in which the duration of the bursts was shortened and the length and depth of the interburst hyperpolarization was increased.

The second method is illustrated in Fig. 3.1B. The mode of activity in R15 can also be modified by applying modulatory transmitters such as serotonin (5-HT) (for recent reviews see Bertram, 1993; Butera, Clark, Canavier, Baxter, & Byrne, 1995). Figure 3.1B2 illustrates that a low concentration of 5-HT (2.5 μM) shifted the activity of R15 into a mode of bursting in which the length and depth of the interburst hyperpolarization was increased, the frequency of action potentials during the bursts was increased and the duration of the bursts was decreased. In addition, the presence of 5-HT altered the manner in which R15 responded to bias currents. In the presence of 5-HT, the depolarizing bias current (Fig. 3.1B1) shifted the activity of R15 into a beating mode (i.e., continues spiking), whereas the hyperpolarizing bias current (Fig. 3.1B3) shifted the cell into a silent mode. Thus, the mode of activity in R15 can be changed by modifying one or more of the biophysical parameters (e.g., membrane conductances or externally applied bias current) that govern the oscillatory activity in R15.

3. MULTISTABILITY: COEXISTING DYNAMICAL STATES IN A MODEL OF R15

Enduring changes in the electrical activity of neurons, such as the parameter-dependent changes illustrated in Fig. 3.1, generally have been attributed to persistent modulation of the biophysical parameters that govern neuronal membrane conductances (for reviews see Kaczmarek & Levitan, 1987; Marder, 1993). An implicit assumption has been that once all parameters are fixed, the ultimate mode of electrical activity exhibited is determined, and that the only way to alter the activity is to change one or more of the biophysical parameters. An alternative possibility is that several stable modes of activity coexist at a single set of parameters, and that transient perturbations could switch the neuron from one stable mode of activity to another. Although coexisting stable oscillatory states (i.e., multistability) are a well-known mathematical phenomenon (e.g., Guckenheimer & Holmes, 1983), their potential existence and functional significance have not been extensively investigated in plausible models of neurons.

We have been using a Hodgkin-Huxley type model of the R15 neuron and computer simulations to investigate whether multiple modes of activity can indeed coexist in neuronal oscillators. The specific details of the model are beyond the scope of this chapter, but they can be found in Canavier et al. (1991, 1993; see also Butera et al., 1995). Briefly, the structure and parameters for the model were derived from the extensive experimental data that is available from biophysical analyses of membrane currents in R15. In the model (Fig. 3.2A), the action potentials are mediated by three currents, a fast sodium current (I_{Na}), a fast calcium current (I_{Ca}) and a delayed-rectifier potassium current (I_K). The slow membrane oscillations that underlie the bursting rhythm is mediated primarily by a slow-inward calcium current (I_{SI}). In parallel with the ionic conductances is a membrane capacitance and currents generated by ion exchanges and pumps. In addition, the ability to apply an extrinsic bias current was incorporated into the model as well as a description of a synaptic conductance. Some of these ionic conductances are also regulated by intracellular levels of calcium and/or second messengers (Fig. 3.2B). For example, I_{SI} undergoes calcium-dependent inactivation. Thus, the model also includes a lumped parameter description of the regulation of intracellular calcium such that calcium accumulates in an intracellular pool and is removed via ion exchanges, pumps, and a buffer system. Finally, some of the conductances are modulated by transmitters. For example, the actions of 5-HT can be simulated by increasing in the maximum conductances of I_{SI} and an anomalous rectifier potassium current (I_R). Prior studies (Butera et al., 1995; Byrne et al., 1994; Canavier et al., 1991) have demonstrated that this model accurately simulated many of the salient features of the electrical activity of R15, including its basic bursting behavior as well as parameter-dependent changes in activity (e.g., responses to external bias currents and modulatory transmitters).

Figure 3.3 illustrates a novel method for shifting the activity of the R15 model among different modes of oscillatory activity. Panel A illustrates a simulation that exhibited a beating mode of activity, Panel B illustrates a simulation that exhibited a

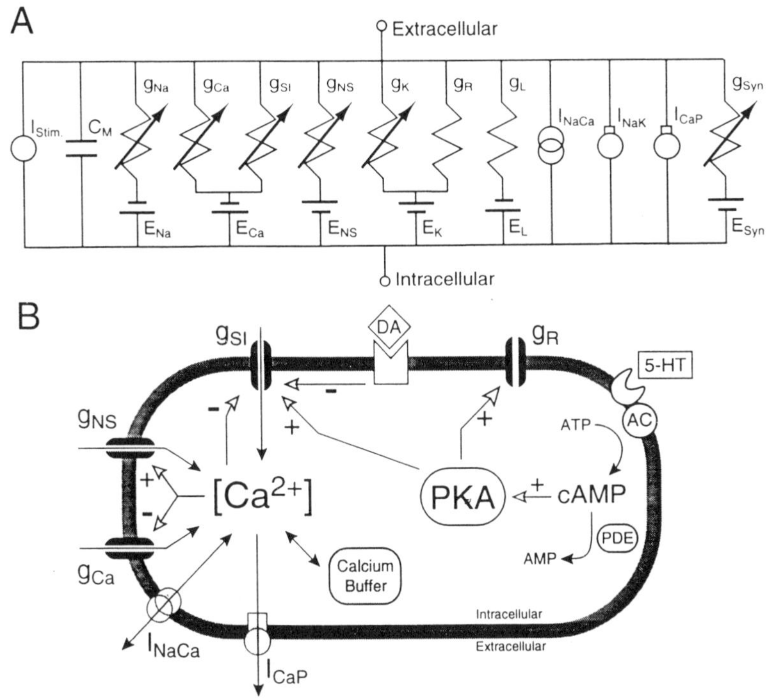

Fig. 3.2. Model of R15. A: Hodgkin-Huxley type equivalent electrical circuit of the cell membrane. Nonlinear conductances are indicated by variable resistors, each associated with a specific equilibrium potential (E). In parallel with membrane capacitance (C_M) are seven ionic conductances: fast sodium conductance (g_{Na}); fast calcium conductance (g_{Ca}); slow-inward calcium conductance (g_{SI}); nonspecific inward current (g_{NS}); delayed-rectifier potassium conductance (g_K); anomalous-rectifier potassium conductance (g_R); and leakage conductance (g_L). The model also includes three background currents generated by a sodium-calcium exchanger (I_{NaCa}); a sodium-potassium pump (I_{NaK}); and a calcium extrusion pump (I_{CaP}). Application of extrinsic bias current is represented by $I_{Stim.}$ and synaptic inputs by g_{Syn}. Time-dependent change in membrane potential (V) is described by the differential equation $dV/dt = -(I_{Na} + I_{Ca} + I_{SI} + I_{NS} + I_K + I_R + I_L + I_{NaCa} + I_{NaK} + I_{CaP} + I_{Syn} - I_{Stim.})/C_M$. Hodgkin-Huxley type gating variables are described by solutions of first-order equations of the general form $dz/dt = (z_\infty - z)/\tau_z$, where z_∞ is steady-state value and τ_z time constant associated with each gating variable. B: calcium fluid compartment model and intracellular regulatory pathways. Ca^{2+} concentration in the extracellular fluid compartment is considered constant. Net change in concentration of intracellular Ca^{2+} is determined by Ca^{2+} fluxes generated by Ca^{2+} components of ionic currents and pumps/exchangers, and uptake and release of Ca^{2+} by a calmodulin-type Ca^{2+} buffer. Several ionic conductances (g_{SI}, g_{NS}, g_{Ca}) are regulated by intracellular Ca^{2+} concentration. Adenylyl cyclase (AC) is activated by serotonin (5-HT) and catalyzes production of cAMP. Degradation of cAMP occurs by cleavage of cAMP by phosphodiesterase (PDE). Conductances g_{SI} and g_R are increased by cAMP, through phosphorylation of channel proteins via cAMP-dependent protein kinase A (PKA). Mechanisms by which dopamine (DA) decreases g_{SI} have not been elucidated fully. In the model, modulation of g_{SI} by DA is depicted as acting directly on the channel. Filled arrows represent fluxes and open arrows regulatory/modulatory interactions. Regulatory/modulatory interactions that increase an ionic conductance (or increase PKA activity) are indicated by + and those that decrease an ionic conductance by −. The full set of model equations and parameters is in Butera et al. (1995) or Canavier et al. (1991, 1993).

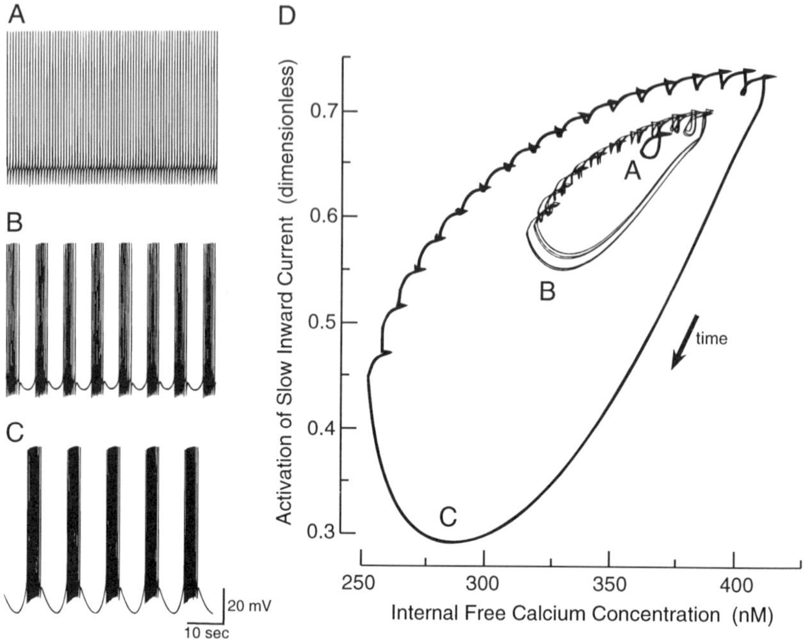

Fig. 3.3. Coexisting modes of dynamical activity in a model of R15. Three different simulations, each using the *same* set of values for the parameters in the model but with slightly different initial values for some of the state variables, produced three distinct modes of dynamical activity: beating (A), bursting (B), and a different type of bursting (C). The bursting modes clearly differed in appearance, most notably in the intensity and frequency of bursting and length and depth of the interburst hyperpolarization. D: phase-plane projection of the periodic attractors that define the coexisting oscillatory modes. The evolution of two of the most slowly changing state variables in the model (activation of a slow inward current and internal calcium concentration) was plotted. Time is implicit, but its direction is indicated by the arrow labeled "time." The attractor labeled "*C*" corresponds to the bursting activity in Panel C. The smooth part of the curve corresponds to the interburst interval, whereas the convoluted loops correspond to the spikes. Although it appears as if only a single line is plotted (i.e., a single orbit around the attractor), in fact, 200 sec of simulated time are plotted, which corresponds to ~20 orbits. The orbits exactly overlay each other, thus this attractor represents a limit cycle. The attractor labeled "*B*" corresponds to the bursting in Panel B. The orbits of this attractor do not overlay each other, which suggests this may be a chaotic . The limit cycle labeled "*A*" corresponds to the beating mode in Panel A.

bursting mode, and Panel C illustrates a simulation that exhibited a different mode of bursting. What is surprising is that all three of these simulations used the same set of values for the parameters in the model; that is, these three modes of activity were coexistent. These three different modes of activity resulted from only slight alterations in the initial values for some of the state variables. The stability of each mode of activity was determined by simulating large epochs (~6 hr) of simulated time (not shown). Thus, depending on how the state variables of model were initialized, the model exhibited either a beating mode or one of several distinct bursting modes.

To gain some insights into the dynamical behavior of this model and the emergence of these multiple, coexisting modes of activity, we found it useful to examine attractors within the system using a phase-plane analysis. Phase-plane projections containing two of the most slowly changing variables, the activation gating variable for the slow inward calcium current (s) and the internal concentration of calcium ($[Ca]_i$), were the most informative (see Canavier et al., 1993). Panel D of Fig. 3.3 illustrates the phase-plane projections for the three coexisting modes of activity. The outermost loop, which is labeled "*C*," is the attractor that is associated with the bursting mode illustrated in Panel C. Each phase of this attractor represents a different phase of the burst. For example, the upper left phase of the attractor is associated with the spike discharge; a period in time when the activation of the calcium current is increasing as is the calcium concentration. The burst terminates at the upper right. The lower portion of the loop begins the interburst hyperpolarization; a phase of the burst when the calcium activation is decreasing as is the calcium concentration. Nested within this outer attractor is the attractor labeled "B," which is associated with bursting activity illustrated in Panel B, and nested within this second bursting attractor is the attractor for beating activity, which is labeled "A." Although not illustrated in this figure, eight distinct modes of stable oscillatory activity have been observed using same the set of values for the parameters in the model that generated the data illustrated in Fig. 3.3 (Byrne et al., 1994; Canavier et al., 1993, 1994; see also Butera et al., 1996). Thus, this empirically derived model of R15 exhibited multistability in that several distinct modes of oscillatory activity coexisted for a single set of parameter values.

3.1. Parameter-Independent Transitions Between Distinct Modes of Oscillatory Activity

Admittedly, generating different modes of oscillatory activity by altering initial conditions of each simulation is somewhat arbitrary, and perhaps unphysiological. But implicit in the concept of attractors is the notion that a perturbation of one or more of the variables would propel the trajectory off the attractor. If the displacement was sufficiently small, the system would return to the stable attractor. In presence of multiple attractors, however, a sufficiently large perturbation could propel the system into the basin of attraction for a nearby attractor. Thus, the perturbation would shift the ongoing activity of the cell from one mode to another. This suggests that it may be possible to produce these types of transitions, not by altering initial conditions, but rather, by introducing brief perturbations, such as synaptic inputs.

To test this possibility we introduced a synaptic conductance into the model and presented the cell with simulated postsynaptic potentials (PSPs; see Fig. 3.2 and Canavier et al., 1993). Figure 3.4 illustrates a transition from bursting activity to beating activity that was induced by a brief synaptic input. Prior to the perturbation, the model exhibited stable bursting activity. The attractor that was associated with this bursting activity is illustrated in Panel A. The perturbation propelled the trajectory of the system off this stable bursting attractor (Panel B) and after a brief transient, the system settled onto the stable beating attractor (Panel C), which coexisted with the bursting attractor in the phase space. Once established, the new mode persisted indefinitely or until subsequent synaptic input perturbed the neuron into another mode of activity (not shown). Moreover, we found that such parameter-*in*dependent transients could be induced between adjacent attractors or between far removed attractors.

The data described above indicate that there are two fundamentally different ways of producing enduring change the mode of oscillatory activity in R15. One way was parameter dependent (e.g., Fig. 3.1), whereas the second method was parameter *in*dependent (e.g., Figs. 3.3 and 3.4). Parameter-*in*dependent changes in the mode of activity emerged from the proliferation of attractors in the phase space of this nonlinear system and brief perturbations could elicit transitions from one stable mode of oscillatory activity to another stable mode.

3.2. Phase Sensitivity of Parameter-Independent Transitions Between Dynamical States

Although not illustrated in this chapter (see Canavier et al., 1993), the effects of a perturbation were highly sensitive to its phase as well being dependent on its sign (depolarizing vs. hyperpolarizing), magnitude, frequency, and duration. Generally, perturbations that tended to dampen the burst or the interburst hyperpolarization propelled the trajectories toward the innermost attractors, whereas perturbations that augmented the burst or the interburst hyperpolarization propelled the trajectories in the opposite direction, toward the outermost attractors.

Insights into the ways that the phase of a perturbation might effect this system can be gained by examining the attractors of the system that are illustrated in Fig. 3.3D. Assume, for example, that the oscillatory activity of the system resides on the attractor labeled "*B*." If a perturbation was delivered during interburst hyperpolarization phase of attractor and if the perturbation tended to increase the hyperpolarization (e.g., a hyperpolarizing current pulse or an inhibitory PSP), then the system would be propelled toward the outer attractor (e.g., *C*). Conversely, if the perturbation tended to decrease the interburst hyperpolarization (e.g., a depolarizing current pulse or an excitatory PSP), then the system would propelled toward the inner attractor (e.g., *A*). Similarly, if the perturbation was delivered during the burst phase of the attractor and the perturbation tended to increase, or enhance, the burst (e.g., a depolarization), then the system would be propelled toward the outer attractor (e.g., *C*). And conversely, a perturbation that tended to decrease the burst (i.e., a hyperpolarization) would propel the system toward the inner attractor (e.g., *A*). The perturbation, however, must be sufficiently large to "knock" the system out of one basin of attraction into another, otherwise the system will simply return to the original attractor after a transient.

3.3. Regulation of Multistability by Modulatory Transmitters

We also investigated how the coexistence of multiple attractors was affected by changes in two parameters in the model: the anomalous rectifier conductance (g_R) and the slow inward calcium conductance (g_{SI}). The details of these analyses are not presented in this chapter, but are available in Byrne et al. (1994), Butera et al. (1996) and Canavier et al. (1994). These two conductances are the target for modulatory transmitters, such as 5-HT and dopamine (see Fig. 3.2B). Previous simulations illustrated how altering the parameters affected the intrinsic activity of R15 (Butera et al., 1995; Canavier, 1991). In addition, modulating these parameters also regulated the ability of the neuron to exhibit parameter-*in*dependent mode transitions. We found that small changes in these parameters can annihilate some of the coexisting modes of oscillatory activity. Indeed, for some values of the parameters only a single mode was exhibited. Thus, modulatory transmitters have the ability to regulate the number of modes that the neuron can exhibit and, hence, how the neuron will respond to synaptic inputs.

For example, during the simulation illustrated in Fig. 3.4, the model cell was positioned in a region of its parameter space that supported multiple coexisting attractors. Hence, a synaptic input was able to shift the activity of the cell to a different stable mode. If on the other hand, the actions of a modulatory transmitter had moved the cell into a region of its parameter space that supported only a single attractor, then the same synaptic input would have failed to induce an enduring change in the mode of activity. Rather, the perturbation would have induced a transient change in the dynamical activity of the cell, but the activity of the cell must eventually return to the one stable attractor present in the phase space. Similarly, a modulatory agent by setting the steady-state value of a key conductance can affect the ways in which the cell will respond to a subsequent perturbations that are induced by brief application of a modulatory agent (for examples see Byrne et al., 1994; Canavier et al., 1994).

4. BISTABILITY IN CELL R15

We also have conducted electrophysiological experiments to test two key predictions of the computational studies (Lechner et al., 1996). First, we examined whether the oscillatory electrical activity of R15 exhibited multistability. Second, we examined whether modulatory transmitters regulated multistability in R15. Conventional two-electrode current-clamp techniques were used to record electrical activity from the R15 neuron in isolated abdominal ganglia. Brief current pulses (5 to 10 nA; 1 to 1.5 sec) were used to perturb the membrane potential at approximately the maximum of the interburst hyperpolarization. As in the computational studies, it was also possible to use a phase-plane analysis to visualize the dynamic responses of R15 to the perturbations. The circuit illustrated in Fig. 3.5 was used to transform the recorded membrane voltages for the phase-plane projection (see also Butera et al., 1995; Pinsker & Bell, 1981). First, high frequencies were attenuated with a low-pass filter, which dramatically reduced amplitude of the action potentials but not the waveform of the slow oscillations underlying the bursting activity. The filtered voltage (V_{out}) was used to drive the horizontal input of an *xy*-plotter. The filtered voltage was also differentiated and the first derivative of the filtered voltage (dV_{out}/dt) was used to drive the vertical input of the *xy*-plotter (see Fig. 3.6).

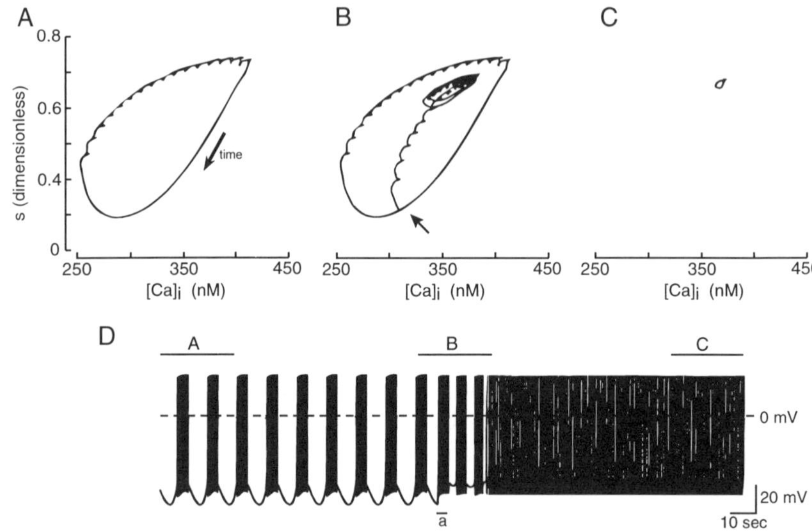

Fig. 3.4. Parameter-*in*dependent transition between distinct modes of dynamical activity in the R15 model. An example of a phase-plane analysis illustrating a transition from bursting to beating. A: trajectory plotting the limit cycle of the burst labeled "*A*" in Panel D. B: a brief perturbation during the hyperpolarizing phase (arrow) caused the trajectory to leave the bursting attractor and fall onto a coexistent beating attractor, which is illustrated in Panel C. D: simulated electrical activity in the model of R15. Initially, the model expressed stable bursting activity. A brief current pulse (bar labeled "a") caused a transition from bursting to beating. Following the transition, the stability of the beating mode was confirmed by continuing the simulation for six hours of simulated time. Data from the three portions of this record that are denoted with the bars labeled "*A*," "*B*," and "*C*" were used to create the phase-plane plots illustrated in Panels A, B, and C.

Figure 3.5 illustrates an apparent parameter-*in*dependent transition in the oscillatory activity of R15 from bursting to beating. Prior to the perturbation, the cell exhibited stable bursting activity, and the attractor associated with this mode of oscillatory activity is illustrated in Panel A. The perturbation propelled the trajectory of the cell off the bursting attractor (Panel B) and after a brief transient, the cell settled onto the a beating attractor (Panel C), which appeared to have been coexistent in the phase

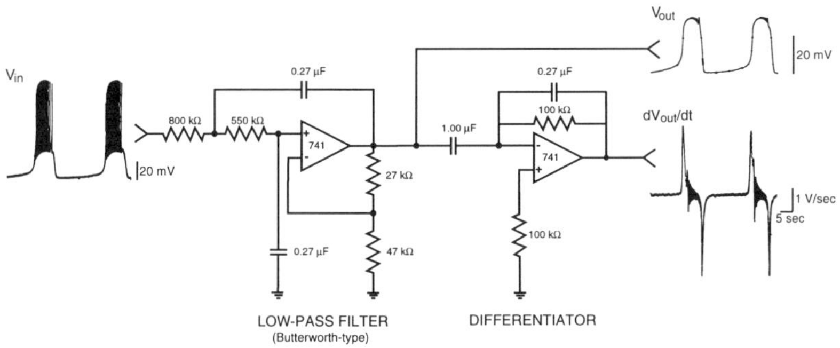

Fig. 3.5. Filter and differentiator. This circuit was used to transform experimental data for a phase-plane analysis. Intracellular recordings from cell R15 (V_{in}) were first conditioned with a low-pass filter that eliminated frequencies higher than ~0.65 Hz. The spikes were attenuated, whereas the slow wave oscillation that underlies the bursting activity was not (V_{out}). The second operational amplifier produced the first derivative of the filtered voltage (dV_{out}/dt). To create a phase-plane plot, dV_{out}/dt was then plotted against V_{out} (see Fig. 3.6).

space. Once established, the beating mode was relatively stable and this new mode of oscillatory activity persisted for ~5 min. In some preparations, the induced beating activity persisted (up to 40 min) until a second perturbation was applied, which re-established the original bursting mode (not shown). Although in physiological experiments it is not possible to control all of the parameters governing the dynamics of the system, analyses of 13 preparations indicated that perturbations induced a significant increase in the duration of continuous spiking activity. These results were consistent with the notion of parameter-*in*dependent shifts of oscillatory activity between coexisting bursting to beating modes.

Given that R15 exhibited bistability (i.e., coexisting bursting and beating modes), we also examined whether 5-HT regulated the eligibility of R15 for multistability. Analyses of 10 preparations indicated that a low concentration of 5-HT (1 μM) significantly increased the likelihood that a perturbation would induce a mode shift and that 5-HT significantly increased duration of the induced beating activity (i.e., he stability of the beating attractor). Taken together, the above results demonstrated that neuron R15 can exhibit bistability in that transitions between bursting and beating oscillatory modes could be triggered by brief perturbations. Moreover, this effect was enhanced in the presence of 5-HT. These findings support the predictions obtained from our computational studies that the level of a modulator can influence the number and/or stablility of coexisting attractors within the dynamical activity of a neuron.

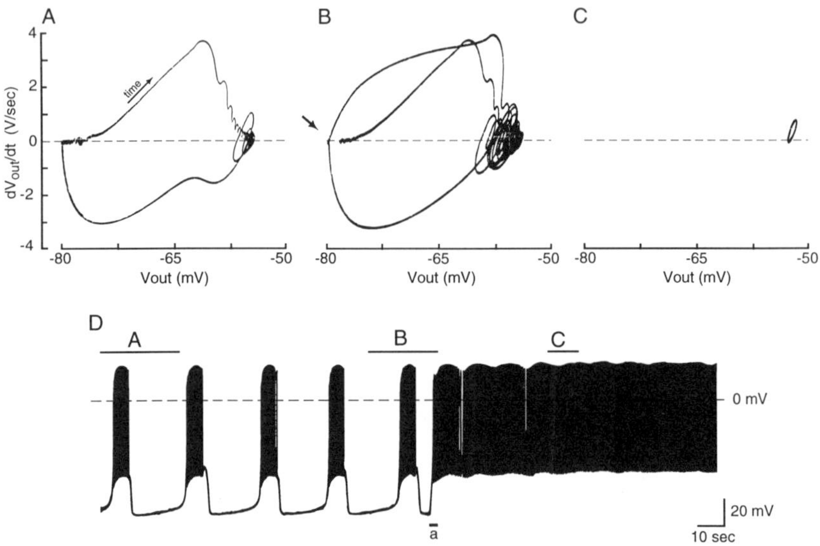

Fig. 3.6. Parameter-*in*dependent transition between distinct modes of electrical activity in cell R15. An example of a phase-plane analysis illustrating a transition from bursting to beating. A: trajectory plotting the limit cycle of the burst, labeled "*A*" in Panel D. Three phases can be distinguished: a depolarizing phase ($dV/dt>0$), the attenuated spiking activity at membrane potentials between −60 and −50 mV and the interburst hyperpolarization at membrane potentials below −65 mV. Time is implicit, but its direction is indicated by the arrow labeled "time." B: brief perturbation during the hyperpolarizing phase (arrow) caused the trajectory to leave the bursting attractor and fall onto a coexistent beating attractor, which is illustrated in Panel C. D: intracellular recordings from a R15 neuron. Initially, the cell expressed stable bursting activity. A brief current pulse (bar labeled "a") caused a transition from bursting to beating. The induced beating activity was relatively stable and persisted for ~5 min, after which the electrical activity returned to the original bursting pattern (not shown). The three portions of this record that are denoted with the bars labeled "A," "B," and "C" were first conditioned with the circuit illustrated in Fig. 3.5 and were then used to create the phase-plane plots illustrated in Panels A, B, C.

5. MULTISTABILITY IN MULTICELLULAR NEURONAL OSCILLATORS

Recently, we have begun to extend our analyses of the dynamics of neuronal oscillators to include examinations of multicellular oscillators. These preliminary analyses have focused on two general circuit architectures: a homogenous circuit composed of diverse cellular and synaptic elements. In addition, we have begun to use physiological experiments to examine some of the predictions of these recent computer studies.

5.1. Bistability in a Homogenous Neural Ring Network

Using computer simulations, the first circuit that we examined was a three cell ring network (Fig. 3.7A). Each of the three cells had identical properties as did each of the three synaptic connections. The cells were our current model of the R15 neuron (Butera et al., 1995) and the parameter values that were used in these simulations positioned the cells in a region of their parameter space that supported only a single attractor, which was a bursting limit cycle. Thus, the individual circuit elements by themselves did not support multistability. The ring network, however, did exhibit multistability (Fig. 3.7). Panel B illustrates a simulation in which the cells fired in the

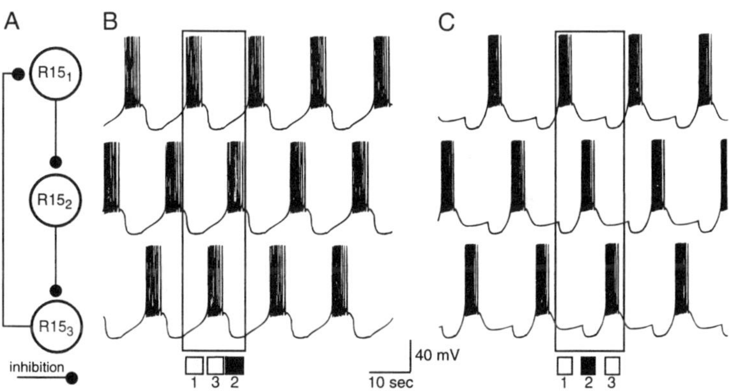

Fig. 3.7. Coexisting modes of dynamical activity in a model of a neural ring network. A: network configuration. In this homogenous network, the properties of all three cells were identical as were the properties of all three synaptic connections. Two different simulations (B, C), each using the *same* set of values for the parameters in the model but slightly different initial values for some of the state variables, produced two distinct modes of dynamical activity. The two modes can be most easily distinguished by comparing the sequence of firing of the cells. B: the large, open box outlines a single cycle of patterned activity in the ring network and the smaller, shaded boxes indicate the relative phases and durations of activity in the three cells. In this mode of activity, the cells fire in the sequence $R15_1 \rightarrow R15_3 \rightarrow R15_2$. C: in this mode of activity, the cells fire in the sequence $R15_1 \rightarrow R15_2 \rightarrow R15_3$.

sequence $R15_1 \rightarrow R15_3 \rightarrow R15_2$. Panel C illustrates a second simulation that used the identical set of parameter values but slightly different initial values for some of the state variables. This second simulation exhibited a different pattern of oscillatory activity in which the cells fire in the sequence $R15_1 \rightarrow R15_2 \rightarrow R15_3$. Thus, at least two stable patterns of oscillatory activity coexisted within the phase space of this ring network.

Figure 3.8 illustrates that the ring network could be switched between these different oscillatory patterns by brief perturbations. Prior to the first perturbation, the network exhibited a stable pattern of activity in which the cells fired in the sequence $R15_1 \rightarrow R15_2 \rightarrow R15_3$ (Panel A). A brief perturbation applied to cell $R15_2$ switched the pattern of network activity to the firing sequence $R15_1 \rightarrow R15_3 \rightarrow R15_2$ (Panel B). Finally, a second perturbation applied to cell $R15_2$ returned the activity of the ring network to its original sequence (Panel C). The two patterns of activity exhibited by this network differed not only in the sequence of firing but also in the period of each cycle of activity, and the duration and intensity of bursting in each of the cells. Our more recent work has illustrated that as the number of cells in the ring network was increased, and the number of coexisting patterns also increased (Baxter et al., 1996; Canavier et al., 1995, 1997).

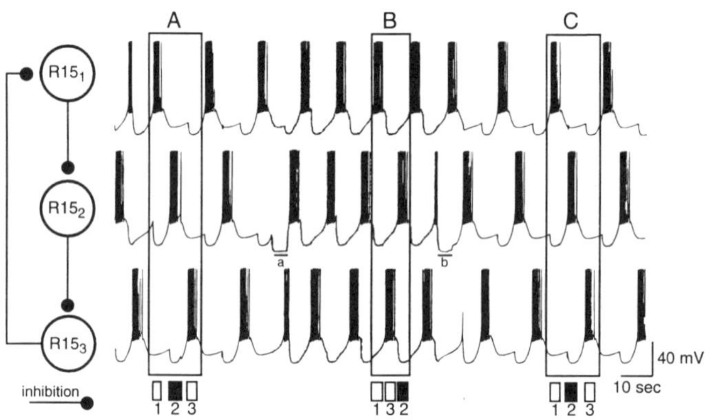

Fig. 3.8. Parameter-*in*dependent transitions between distinct modes of dynamical activity in a model of a neural ring network. The oscillatory activity of a the three cell network could be switched between two distinct modes by applying a brief perturbation to any of the neurons. In this example, the perturbations (bars labeled "a" and "b") were applied to cell $R15_2$. A: prior to the first perturbation, the network expressed a mode of activity with a firing sequence of $R15_1 \rightarrow R15_2 \rightarrow R15_3$. B: the first perturbation (bar labeled "a") switched the mode of activity to a firing sequence of $R15_1 \rightarrow R15_3 \rightarrow R15_2$. In addition to expressing a different sequence of firing, this mode also had a shorter period. The mode outlined in Panels A and C had a period of ~15 sec, whereas the mode outlined in Panel B had a period of ~11 sec. C: a second perturbation (bar labeled "b") switched the pattern of activity back to the original mode (i.e., $R15_1 \rightarrow R15_2 \rightarrow R15_3$).

Similarly, if the parameters values for the individual cells were modified such that the cells themselves became multistable, then the number and diversity of coexisting oscillatory patterns dramatically increased (Baxter et al., 1996; Canavier et al., 1995, 1997; see also Pasemann, 1995).

In a preliminary series of physiological experiments, we have begun to examine the predictions of these computational studies by artificially creating a three cell ring network with R15 neurons (Fig. 3.9). The abdominal ganglion of *Aplysia* contains a single R15 neuron. Thus, to create a three cell network with R15 cells, three abdominal ganglia were isolated and placed in a recording chamber. The inhibitory synaptic connections between cells were artificially created by using the action potentials recorded in one cell (i.e., the "presynaptic cell") to trigger the injection of a brief hyperpolarizing current pulse into its "postsynaptic target." Thus, the R15 neurons could be coupled together to form a three cell ring network.

This artificial ring network of coupled R15 cells exhibited a stable pattern of oscillatory activity in which the cells fired in the sequence $R15_1 \rightarrow R15_2 \rightarrow R15_3$ (Fig. 3.10, Panel A). A brief perturbation applied to cell $R15_2$ switched the pattern of activity to a firing sequence of $R15_1 \rightarrow R15_3 \rightarrow R15_2$ (Panel B). This pattern persisted for several minutes, at which time a second perturbation returned the network to its original pattern of activity (not shown).

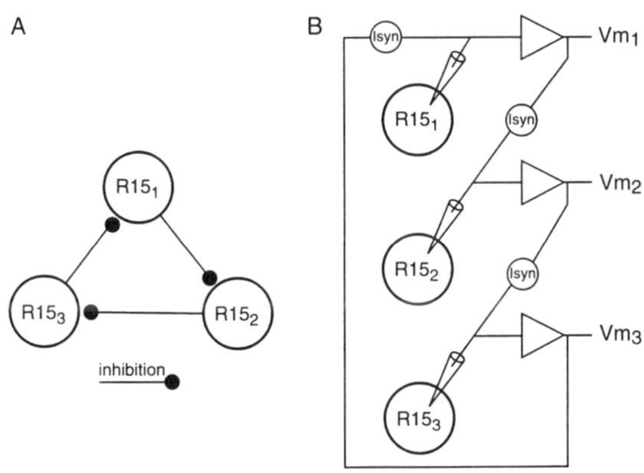

Fig. 3.9. Experimental methods for creating a ring network with three R15 neurons. A: network configuration. The abdominal ganglion of *Aplysia* contains a single R15 neuron. Thus, to create a three cell network, three abdominal ganglia were placed in a single recording chamber, and each R15 neuron was penetrated with an intracellular microelectrode that was used both to record membrane voltage and to injection current pulses (see Panel B). B: to create an artificial inhibitory synaptic connection, the action potentials that were recorded in one cell (e.g., Vm_1) triggered the injection of a brief hyperpolarizing current pulse (I_{syn}) into a second cell (e.g., $R15_2$). The strength of the inhibitory connections were adjusted to elicit ~5 mV hyperpolarization of the membrane potential of the postsynaptic cell.

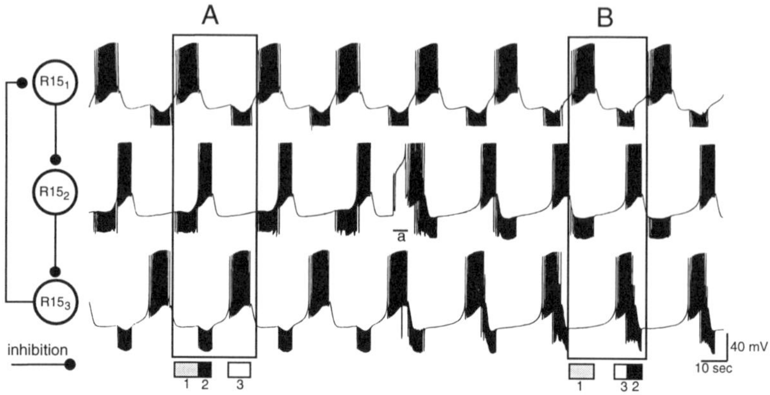

Fig. 3.10. Parameter-*in*dependent transitions between distinct modes of dynamical activity in a network R15 cells. The oscillatory activity of a network comprised of three R15 cells (see Fig. 9) could be switched between two distinct modes by brief perturbations. A: prior to the first perturbation, the network expressed a stable mode of activity with a firing sequence of $R15_1 \rightarrow R15_2 \rightarrow R15_3$. B: a perturbation applied to cell $R15_2$ (bar labeled "a") switched the mode of activity to a firing sequence of $R15_1 \rightarrow R15_3 \rightarrow R15_2$. This new mode of activity appeared to be relatively stable and persisted for several minutes, at which time a second perturbation was applied and the activity in the network returned to the original pattern (not shown).

The general features of the oscillatory neuronal activity generated by these ring networks are similar to the cyclical patterns of bursting activity that mediate many rhythmic movements (e.g., the alternating pattern of burst that characterize motor programs mediating locomotion; see also Collins & Stewart, 1993). Thus, multistability and parameter-*in*dependent shifts between distinct patterns of neural activity may be mechanisms contributing to switching between different behavioral states. To examine this possibility further, we have begun to examine multistability in a more realistic model of neuronal circuit that functions as a central pattern generator (CPG).

5.2. Bistability in a Heterogeneous Neural Network

As a result of work in our laboratory and by others, many of the neuronal elements of the CPG that controls aspects of feeding behavior in *Aplysia* have been identified and characterized (Fig. 3.11). Unlike the more theoretical ring networks that were examined earlier, the cells in this CPG have complex and distinctive electrophysiological properties. For example, cell B31 does not support conventional overshooting action potentials and brief depolarizations elicit a prolonged plateau-like potential; cell B35 is not spontaneously active and exhibits regenerative firing, cell B52 exhibits post-hyperpolarization rebound, and cell B64 is not spontaneously active and exhibits plateau-like potential and regenerative firing. Moreover, the synaptic connections also have complex and distinctive properties, including the expression of multicomponent synaptic

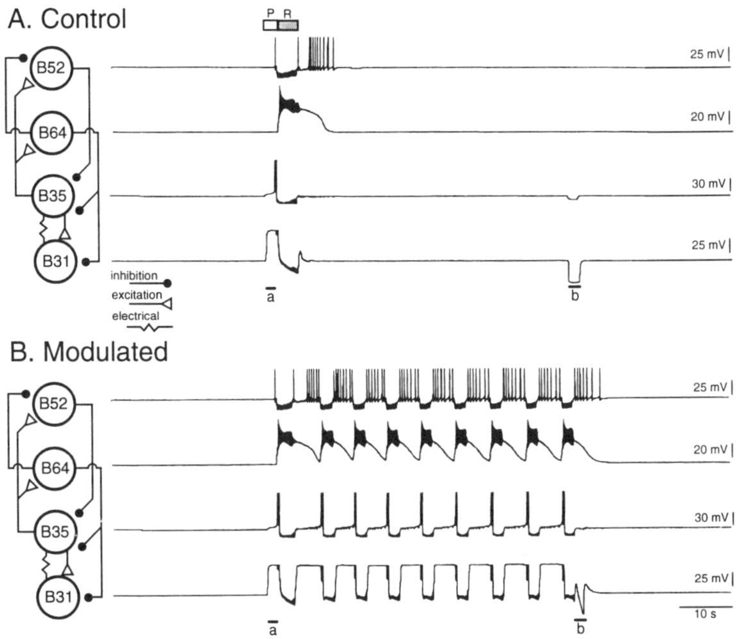

Fig. 3.11. Parameter-*in*dependent transitions between distinct modes of activity in a model of a heterogeneous network. The schematic diagram summarizes some of the cells and synaptic connections used in these simulations of the CPG. A complete description of the model was provided in Ziv et al. (1994; see also Kabotyanski et al., 1994). The electrical activities of four cells (B52, B64, B35 and B31) are plotted. A: in absence of any external input, the network was silent. After ~30 s, a depolarizing current pulse (bar labeled 'a') was injected into cell B31. This brief perturbation elicited only a single cycle of electrical activity in the network. The basic features of the feeding behavior that is mediated by this CPG involves rhythmic protractions and retractions of the feeding organs. The protraction phase of the neuronal activity is characterized by a sustained depolarization of cell B31 and is indicated by the open box labeled "P." The retraction phase is characterized by a sustained depolarization of cell B64 and is indicated by the shaded box labeled "R." After ~60 s, a hyperpolarizing current pulse (bar labeled "b") was injected into B31. This second perturbation did not elicit any patterned electrical activity. B: the actions of a modulatory transmitter were simulated by decreasing the maximum value of a slow depolarizing conductance in cell B64 from 0.5 μS to 0.4 μS. Under these conditions (i.e., in the simulated presence of the modulator) the brief depolarizing current pulse (bar labeled "a") elicited sustained oscillatory activity in the network, and the brief hyperpolarizing current pulse (bar labeled "b") switched the circuit back into the silent mode. Such transitions were equivalent to shifting the model of electrical activity between a stable limit cycle (oscillatory state) a stable fixed point (non-oscillatory state). Thus, some regions of the parameter space for this CPG supported bistability.

potentials (e.g., combined excitatory and inhibitory PSPs or PSPs with both fast and slow components) and different forms of plasticity (e.g., facilitation and depression). Thus, this network incorporates many heterogeneous neuronal and synaptic elements, and hence, provides an opportunity to examine whether the nonlinear properties of such a heterogeneous circuit can support multistability, and if so, what factors might control the multistability. The specific details of our model of this CPG are provided in Ziv, Baxter, and Byrne (1994; see also Kabotyanski, Ziv, Baxter, & Byrne, 1994).

In the first simulation, the values of the model parameters were set to recreate control conditions (Fig. 3.11A). In the absence of any external inputs, the circuit was silent. Two perturbations (i.e., brief current pulses injected into cell B31) were applied to the circuit. The first current pulse, which was a depolarizing current, elicited only a single cycle of patterned electrical activity in the circuit, and the second pulse, which was a hyperpolarizing current, failed to elicit any patterned electrical activity. The second simulation incorporated one of the actions of the modulatory transmitter dopamine, which decreases the excitability of cell B64 (Kabotyanski et al., 1994). To simulate this action of dopamine, the maximum value for a slow depolarizing conductance in cell B64 was decreased slightly. Following this modification (i.e., in the simulated presence of dopamine), the circuit remained in a silent mode in the absence of any external inputs (Fig. 3.11B). Two brief perturbations, which were identical to those used in the previous simulation, were again applied to cell B31. Now the first perturbation propelled the circuit into a stable oscillatory mode. [Long-duration simulations confirmed that both the silent and oscillatory modes were stable (data not shown).] After about 60 seconds of this oscillatory mode, the second perturbation was applied. Now the circuit switched back into the silent mode. Such transitions between coexistent oscillatory and silent modes are often referred to as hard excitation and annihilation, and are equivalent to a mode shift between activity associated with a stable limit cycle and that associated with a stable fixed point (non-oscillatory) in the phase space of the system. Thus, some regions of the parameter space for this CPG can support a simple form of multistability. Moreover, a modulatory transmitter could, in theory, regulate the eligibility of the CPG for multistability and thereby profoundly alter the responsiveness of the circuit to brief perturbations, such as synaptic inputs from higher-order neurons (e.g., command neurons) or from sensory neurons.

6. SUMMARY AND CONCLUSIONS

The computational and physiological studies that were reviewed in this chapter found that single cell and multicellular neuronal oscillators possessed multiple, coexistent modes of electrical activity. These modes of activity corresponded to multiple stable attractors, whose existence in phase space was an emergent property of the nonlinear dynamics of these neuronal oscillators. Brief perturbations could switch the activity of the neuronal oscillators between different modes. These mode transitions did not require any changes in the biochemical or biophysical parameters of the neurons, provided an enduring response to a transient input, as well as a mechanism for phasic sensitivity (i.e., temporal specificity). Finally, the multistability of these neuronal oscillators was found to be regulated by modulatory transmitters. By modulating membrane conductances, transmitters could position the neuronal oscillators in different regions of their parameter space; some regions supported multistability, whereas others did not.

Although the function of multistability in neuronal oscillators is speculative, these results raise the intriguing possibility that the nonlinear dynamical processes endow individual neurons and small neural circuits with the potential for more sophisticated information processing and storage than has generally been appreciated. At the very least, the proliferation of attractors that is associated with nonlinear systems could greatly amplify the effect of a presynaptic neuron on the activity of the postsynaptic neuron.

For example, it is generally believed that the generation of sustained oscillatory activity in a CPG and the generation of different patterns of electrical activity by a CPG requires a persistent presynaptic input (for reviews see Getting, 1989; Harris-Warrick et al., 1992; Marder, 1993; Marder et al., 1993; Nusbaum, 1994; Selverston, 1992; Weimann & Marder, 1994). The simulations describedearlier offer an alternative method for inducing permanent changes in the electrical activity of a CPG. This method exploits the multistability that can emerge from the nonlinear dynamical properties of the cellular and synaptic elements of the circuit. Thus, a transient synaptic input can switch a CPG between coexisting silent and oscillatory modes of electrical activity. Of particular interest was the emergence of oscillatory patterns with different phase relationships in the electrical activity of the elements. These different patterns of activity, in turn, could underlie distinct behaviors (e.g., different gaits in locomotion). Thus, by inducing parameter-*in*dependent transitions between different patterns, control signals (e.g., synaptic inputs from higher-order neurons such as command neurons) could switch the output of the CPG between distinct behaviors without the need to rewire the neural network.

Similarly, multistability could also be important in understanding the mechanics of inducing and maintaining changes in electrical activity in neurons that may be associated with some examples of learning and memory, as well as provide insights into some aspects of temporal specificity. Large numbers of coexisting stable periodic attractors could represent a method for storing temporally encoded information, and phase-sensitive, parameter-*in*dependent transitions between attractors could serve as a method for retrieving the information based on stable periodic attractors (see also Baird, 1986; Freeman, 1994; Li & Hopfield, 1989; Mpitsos, 1988).

Finally, it should be pointed out that electrical activity comprises only a portion of the nonlinear dynamical activity in neurons. Many biochemical reactions and second messenger systems include highly nonlinear and feedback processes. Moreover, both computational and experimental studies have demonstrated both simple and complex oscillations as well as multistability in several biochemical reactions and second messenger systems (e.g., Aon, Cortassa, Hervagault, & Thomas, 1989; Goldbeter, 1996; Raymond & Pocker, 1991; Schiffmann, 1989; Shen & Larter, 1994; Smolen, Baxter & Byrne, 1996; Thron, 1996). Thus, it seems possible that parameter-*in*dependent transitions at the molecular level could also serve as a substrate for information processing and storage.

ACKNOWLEDGMENTS

This work was supported in part by National Institutes of Health Grant R01-RR11626 to DAB, Air Force Office of Scientic Research Grant F49620-93-1-0272 to JHB, Office of Naval Research Grant N00014-95-0579 to JHB and JWC, and National Institute of Mental Health award K05-MH-000649 to JHB.

REFERENCES

Aon, M. A., Cortassa, S., Hervagault, J. F., & Thomas, D. (1989). pH-induced bistable dynamic behavior in the reaction catalysed by glucose-6-phosphate dehydrogenase and conformation hysteresis of the enzyme. *Biochemical Journal*, *262*, 795-800.

Baker, G. L., & Gollub, J. P. (1990). *Chaotic Dynamics: An Introduction*. Cambridge, UK: Cambridge University Press.

Baird, B. (1986). Nonlinear dynamics of pattern formation and pattern recognition in rabbit olfactory bulb. *Physica D*, *22*, 150-175.

Baxter, D. A., & Byrne, J. H. (1991). Ionic conductance mechanisms contributing to the electrophysiological properties of neurons. *Current Opinion in Neurobiology*, *1*,105-112.

Baxter, D. A., Canavier, C. C., Butera, R. J., Clark, J. W., & Byrne, J. H. (1996). Complexity in individual neurons determines which patterns are expressed in a ring circuit model of gait generation. *Sociey for Neuroscience Abstracts*, *22*, 1437.

Bertram, R. (1993). A computational study of the effects of serotonin on a molluscan burster neuron. *Biological Cybernetics*, *69*, 257-267.

Bower, J. M. (1992). Relations between the dynamical properties of single cells and their networks in piriform (olfactory) cortex. In T. McKenna, J. Davis, & S. F. Zornetzer (Eds.), *Single Neuron Computation* (pp. 437-462). New York: Academic Press.

Buchanan, J. T. (1992). Neural network simulations of coupled locomotor oscillators in the lamprey spinal cord. *Biological Cybernetics*, *66*, 367-374.

Butera, R. J., Jr., Clark, J. W., Jr., & Byrne, J. H. (1996). Dissection and reduction of a modeled bursting neuron. *Journal of Computational Neuroscience*, *3*, 199-223.

Butera, R. J., Jr., Clark, J. W., Jr., Canavier, C. C., Baxter, D. A., & Byrne, J. H. (1995). Analysis of the effects of modulatory agents on a modeled bursting neuron: Dynamic interactions between voltage and calcium dependent systems. *Journal of Computational Neuroscience*, *2*, 19-44.

Byrne, J. H., Canavier, C. C., Lechner, H., Clark, J. W., Jr., & Baxter, D. A. (1994). Role of nonlinear dynamical properties of a modeled bursting neuron in information processing and storage. *Netherlands Journal of Zoology*, *44*, 339-356.

Calabrese, R. L. (1995). Oscillation in motor pattern-generating networks. *Current Opinion in Neurobiology*, *5*, 816-823.

Canavier, C. C., Baxter, D. A., Clark, J. W., Jr., & Byrne, J. H. (1993). Nonlinear dynamics in a model neuron provide a novel mechanism for transient synaptic inputs to produce long-term alterations of postsynaptic activity. *Journal of Neurophysiology*, *69*, 2252-2257.

Canavier, C. C., Baxter, D. A., Clark, J. W., Jr., & Byrne, J. H. (1994). Multiple modes of activity in a model neuron suggest a novel mechanism for the effects of neuromodulators. *Journal of Neurophysiology*, *72*, 872-882.

Canavier, C. C., Baxter, D. A., Clark, J. W., Jr., & Byrne, J. H. (1995). Networks of physiologically-based neuronal oscillators may provide improved models of pattern generation. *Society for Neuroscience Abstract, 21*, 147.

Canavier, C. C., Butera, R. J., Dror, R. O., Baxter, D. A., Clark, J. W., & Byrne, J. H. (1997). Phase response characteristics of model neurons determine which patterns are expressed in a ring circuit model of gait generation. *Biological Cybernetics*, *77*, 367-380.

Canavier, C. C., Clark, J. W., Jr., & Byrne, J. H. (1991). Simulation of the bursting activity of neurons R15 in *Aplysia*: Role of ionic currents, calcium balance, and modulatory transmitters. *Journal of Neurophysiology*, *66*, 2107-2124.

Chawanya, T., Aoyagi, T., Nishikawa, I., Okuda, K., & Kuramoto, Y. (1993). A model for feature linking via collective oscillations in the primary visual cortex. *Biological Cybernetics*, *68*, 483-490.

Cohen, A. H., Ermentrout, G. B., Kiemel, T., Kopell, N., Sigvardt, K. A., & Williams, T. L. (1992). Modeling of intersegmental coordination in the lamprey central pattern generator for locomotion. *Trends in Neuroscience, 15*, 434-438.

Collins, J. J., & Stewart, I. N. (1993). Coupled nonlinear oscillators and the symmetries of animal gaits. *Nonlinear Science*, *3*, 349-392.

Connors, B. W., & Butnick, M. J. (1990). Intrinsic firing patterns of diverse neocortical neurons. *Trends in Neuroscience*, *13*, 99-104.

Crick, F. (1984). Function of the thalamic reticular complex: The searchlight hypothesis. *Proceeding of the National Academy of Sciences, USA*, *81*, 4586-4590.

Crick, F. (1994). *The Astonishing Hypothesis: The Scientific Search for the Soul.* New York: Maxwell Macmillan International.

Crick, F., & Koch, C. (1990). Towards a neurobiological theory of consciousness. *Seminars in Neuroscience*, *2*, 263-275.

Crick, F., & Mitchison, F. (1983). The function of dream sleep. *Nature*, *304*, 111-114.

Dean, J., & Cruse, H. (1995). Motor pattern generation. In M. A. Arbib (Ed.), *Handbook of Brain Theory and Neural Networks* (pp. 600-605). Cambridge, MA: MIT Press.

Destexhe, A., Babloyantz, A., & Sejnowski, T. J. (1993). Ionic mechanism for intrinsic slow oscillations in thalamic relay neurons. *Biophysical Journal*, *65*, 1538-1552.

Eckhorn, R., Reitboeck, H. J., Arndt, M., & Dicke, P. (1990). Feature linking via synchronization among distributed assemblies: Simulations of results from cat visual cortex. *Neural Computation*, *2*, 293-307.

Eckhorn, R., Schanze, T., Brosch, M., Salem, W., & Bauer, R. (1992). Stimulus-specific synchronizations in cat visual cortex: Multiple microelectrode and correlation studies from several cortical areas. In E. Basar & T. H. Bullock (Eds.), *Induced Rhythms in the Brain* (pp. 47-80). Boston: Birkäuser.

Elson, R. C., & Selverston, A. (1992). Mechanisms of gastric rhythmic generation in the isolated stomatogastric ganglion of spiny lobsters: Bursting pacemaker potentials, synaptic interactions, and muscarinic modulation. *Journal of Neurophysiology*, *68*, 890-907.

Ermentrout, B. (1994). An introduction to neural oscillators. In F. Ventriglia (Ed.), *Neural Modeling and Neural Networks* (pp. 79-110). New York: Pergamon.

Ermentrout, B. (1995). Phase-plane analysis of neural activity. In M. A. Arbib (Ed.), *The Handbook of Brain Theory and Neural Networks* (pp. 732-738). Cambridge, MA: MIT Press.

Freeman, W. J. (1992). Prediction on neocortical dynamic derived from studies in paleocortex. In E. Basar, & T. H. Bullock (Eds.), *Induced Rhythms in the Brain* (pp. 183-199). Boston: Birkäuser.

Freeman, W. J. (1994). Qualitative overview of population neurodynamics. In F. Ventriglia (Ed.), *Neural Modeling and Neural Networks* (pp. 185-215). New York: Pergamon.

Getting, P. A. (1989). Emerging principles governing the operation of neural networks. *Annual Review of Neuroscience*, *12*, 185-204.

Ghose, G. M., & Freeman, R. D. (1992). Oscillatory discharge in the visual system: Does it have a function? *Journal of Neurophysiology*, *68*, 1558-1574.

Goldbeter, A. (1996). *Biochemical Oscillations and Cellular Rhythms: The Molecular Bases of Periodic and Chaotic Behavior*. Cambridge, UK: Cambridge University Press.

Gottschalk, A., Ogilvie, M. D., Richter, D. W., & Pack, A. I. (1994). Computational aspects of the respiratory pattern generator. *Neural Computation*, *6*, 56-68.

Gray, C. M. (1994). Synchronous oscillations in neuronal systems: Mechanisms and function. *Journal of Computational Neuroscience*, *1*, 11-38.

Grillner, S., Wallen, P., & Vianna di Preisco, G. (1990). Cellular network underlying locomotion as revealed in a lower vertebrate model: Transmitters, membrane properties, circuitry, and simulation. *Cold Spring Harbor Symposium on Quantitative Biology*, *55*, 779-789.

Grossberg, S., & Somers, D. (1991). Synchronized oscillations during cooperative feature linking in a cortical model of visual perception. *Neural Networks*, *4*, 453-466.

Guckenheimer, J., Gueron, S., & Harris-Warrick, R. M. (1993). Mapping the dynamics of a bursting neuron. *Philosophical Transaction of the Royal Society of London B*, *341*, 345-359.

Guckenheimer, J., & Holmes, P. (1983). *Nonlinear Oscillations, Dynamical Systems, and Bifurcation of Vector Fields*. New York: Springer-Verlag.

Haken, H., & Stadler, M. (Eds.). (1990, June). *Synergistics of Cognition: Proceedings of the International Symposium at Schloss Elmau, Bavaria*. New York: Springer-Verlag.

Harris-Warrick, R. M. (1993). Pattern generation. *Current Opinion in Neurobiology*, *4*, 894-902.

Harris-Warrick, R. M., Marder, E., Selverston, A.I., & Moulins, M. (Eds.). (1992). *Dynamic Biological Networks: The Stomatogastric Nervous System*. Cambridge, MA: MIT Press.

Hayashi, Y. (1994). Oscillatory neural networks and learning of continuously transformed pattern. *Neural Networks*, *7*, 219-231.

Hobson, J. A. (1988). *The Dreaming Brain*. New York: Basic Books.

Horn, D., & Usher, M. (1991). Parallel activation of memories in an oscillatory neural network. *Neural Computation*, *3*, 31-43.

Huerta, P. T., & Lisman, J. E. (1995). Bidirectional synaptic plasticity induced by a single burst during cholinergic theta oscillation in CA1 in vitro. *Neuron*, *15*, 1053-1063.

Huerta, P. T., & Lisman, J. E. (1993). Heightened synaptic plasticity of hippocampal CA1 neurons during a cholinergically induced rhythmic state. *Nature*, *364*, 723-725.

Jacklet, J. W. (Ed.). (1989). *Neuronal and Cellular Oscillations*, New York: Marcel Dekker.

Kabotyanski, E. A., Ziv, I., Baxter, D. A., & Byrne, J. H. (1994). Experimental and computational analyses of a central pattern generator underlying aspects of feeding behavior in *Aplysia*. *Netherlands Journal of Zoology, 44*, 357-373.

Kaczmarek, L. K., & Levitan, I. B. (Eds.). (1987). *Neuromodulation*. Oxford, UK: Oxford University Press.

Klimesch, W., Schimke, H., & Pfurtscheller, G. (1993). Alpha frequency, cognitive load and memory performance. *Brain Topography*, *5*, 241-251.

Kopell, N. (1988). Toward a theory of modeling central pattern generators. In A. H. Cohen, S. Rossignol, & S. Grillner (Eds.), *Neural Control of Rhythmic Movements in Vertebrates* (pp. 369-413). New York: Wiley.

Kopell, N. (1995). Chains of coupled oscillators. In M. A. Arbib (Ed.), *The Handbook of Brain Theory and Neural Networks* (pp. 178-183). Cambridge, MA: MIT Press.

Kuramoto, Y. (1995). Collective behavior of coupled oscillators. In M. A. Arbib (Ed.), *The Handbook of Brain Theory and Neural Networks* (pp. 203-206). Cambridge, MA: MIT Press.

Lansner, A., & Edeberg, Ö. (1994). Neuronal network models of motor generation and control. *Current Opinion in Neurobiology*, *4*, 903-908.

Lechner, H. A., Baxter, D. A., Clark, J. W., Jr., & Byrne, J. H. (1996). Bistability and its regulation by serotonin in the endogenously bursting neuron R15 in *Aplysia Journal of Neurophysiology*, *75*, 957-962.

Li, Z., & Hopfield, J. J. (1989). Modeling the olfactory bulb and its neural oscillatory processing. *Biological Cybernetics*, *61*, 379-392.

Liljenstrom, H., & Hasselmo, M. E. (1995). Cholinergic modulation of cortical oscillatory dynamics. *Journal of Neurophysiology*, *74*, 288-297.

Llinas, R. R. (1990). Intrinsic electrical properties of nerve cells and their role in network oscillation. *Cold Spring Harbor Symposium on Quantitative Biology*, *55*, 933-938.

Llinas, R. R., & Pare, D. (1991). Of dreaming and wakefulness. *Neuroscience*, *44*, 521-535.

Llinas, R. R., & Ribary, U. (1993). Coherent 40-Hz oscillations characterizes dream state in humans. *Proceedings of the National Academy of Sciences, USA*, *90*, 2078-2081.

Lopes da Silva, F. (1991). Neural mechanisms underlying brain waves: From neural membranes to networks. *Electroencephalography and Clinical Neurophysiology*, *79*, 81-93.

Malsburg, C. von der, & Buhmann, J. (1992). Sensory segmentation with coupled neural oscillators. *Biological Cybernetics*, *67*, 233-242.

Malsburg, C. von der (1995). Binding in models of perception and brain function. *Current Opinion in Neurobiology*, *5*, 520-526.

Marder, E. (1993). Modulating membrane properties of neurons: Role in information processing. In T. A. Poggio & D. A. Glaser (Eds.). *Exploring Brain Functions: Models in Neuroscience* (pp. 27-42). New York: Wiley.

Marder, E., Abbott, L. F., Buchholtz, F., Epstein, I. R., Golowasch, J., Hooper, S. L., & Kepler, T. B. (1993). Physiological insights from cellular and network models of the stomatogastric nervous system of lobsters and crabs. *American Zoologist*, *33*, 29-39.

McCormick, D. A., Huguenard, J., & Strowbridge, B. W. (1992). Determination of state-dependent processing in thalamus by single neuron properties and neuromodulators. In T. McKenna, J. Davis, & S. F. Zornetzer (Eds.), *Single Neuron Computations* (pp. 259-290). New York: Academic Press.

McKenna, T. M., McMullen, T. A., & Shlesinger, M. F. (1994). The brain as a dynamic physical system. *Neuroscience*, *60*, 587-605.

Moon, F. C. (1992). *Chaos and Fractal Dynamics: An Introduction for Applied Scientists and Engineers*. New York: Wiley.

Mori, Y., Davis, P., & Nara, S. (1989). Pattern retrieval in an asymmetric neural network with embedded limit cycles. *Journal of Physics*, *A22*, L525-L532.

Mpitsos, G. J. (1988). Connectionist networks learn to transmit chaos. *Brain Research Bulletin*, *21*, 539-546.

Nadim, F., Olsen, Ø. H., DeSchutter, E., & Calabrese, R. L. (1995). Modeling the leech heartbeat elemental oscillator: I. Interactions of intrinsic and synaptic currents. *Journal of Computational Neuroscience*, *2*, 215-235.

Niebur, E., Koch, C., & Rosin, C. (1993). An oscillation-based model for the neuronal basis of attention. *Vision Research*, *33*, 2789-2802.

Nusbaum, M. P. (1994). Presynaptic control of neurones in pattern-generating networks. *Current Opinion in Neurobiology*, *4*, 909-914.

Parsons, T. D., Salzberg, B. M., Obaid, A. L., Raccuia-Behling, F., & Kleinfeld, D. (1991). Long-term optical recordings of patterns of electrical activity in ensembles of cultured *Aplysia* neurons. *Journal of Neurophysiology, 66*, 316-33.

Pasemann, F. (1995). Characterization of periodic attractors in neural ring networks. *Neural Networks*, *8*, 412-429.

Pearson, K. G. (1993). Common principles of motor control in vertebrates and invertebrates. *Annual Review of Neuroscience*, *16*, 265-297.

Pinsker, H. M., & Bell, J. (1981). Phase plane description of endogenous neuronal oscillators in *Aplysia*. *Biological Cybernetics*, *39*, 211-221.

Rand, R. H., Cohen, A. H., & Holmes, P. J. (1988). Systems of coupled oscillators as models of central pattern generators. In A. H. Cohen, S. Rossignol, & S. Grillner (Eds.), *Neural Control of Rhythmic Movements in Vertebrates* (pp. 333-365). New York: Wiley.

Raymond, J. L., Baxter, D. A., Buonomano, D. V., & Byrne, J. H. (1992). A learning rule based on empirically-derived activity-dependent neuromodulation supports operant conditioning in a small network. *Neural Networks*, *5*, 789-803.

Raymond, K. W., & Pocker, Y. (1991). Bistability and the ordered bimolecular mechanism. *Biochemistry and Cell Biology*, *69*, 661-664.

Rinzel, J., & Ermentrout, G. B. (1989). Analysis of neuronal excitability and oscillations. In C. Koch & I. Segev (Eds.), *Methods in Neuronal Modeling: From Synapse to Networks* (pp. 135-169). Cambridge, MA: MIT Press.

Rowat, P. F., & Selverston, A.I. (1993). Modeling the gastric mill central pattern generator of the lobster with a relaxation-oscillation network. *Journal of Neurophysiology*, *70*, 1030-1053.

Schiffmann, Y. (1989). Bistability and control for ATP synthase and adenylate cyclase is obtained by the removal of substrate inhibition. *Molecular and Cellular Biochemistry*, *86*, 19-40.

Sejnowski, T., McCormick, D. A., & Steriade, M. (1995). Thalamocortical oscillations in sleep and wakefulness. In M. A. Arbib (Ed.), *The Handbook of Brain Theory and Neural Networks* (pp. 976-980). Cambridge, MA: MIT Press.

Selverston, A. I. (1992). Pattern generation. *Current Opinion in Neurobiology*, *2*, 776-780.

Sharp, A. A., Skinner, F. K., & Marder, E. (1996). Mechanism of oscillation in dynamic clamp constructed two cell half-center circuits. *Journal of Neurophysiology*, *76*, 867-883.

Shen, P., & Larter, R. (1994). Role of substrate inhibition kinetics in enzymatic chemical oscillations. *Biophysical Journal*, *67*, 1414-1428.

Singer, W. (1993a). Neuronal representations, assembles and temporal coherence. *Progress in Brain Research*, *95*, 461-474.

Singer, W. (1993b). Synchronization of cortical activity and its putative role in information processing and learning. *Annual Review of Physiology*, *55*, 349-374.

Smolen, P., Baxter, D. A., & Byrne, J. H. (1996). Computational models of cAMP-dependent activation and repression of gene transcription involved in long-term memory formation. *Society for Neuroscience Abstracts*, *22*, 1880.

Sompolinsky, H., Golomb, D., & Kleinfeld, D. (1990). Global processing of visual stimuli in neural networks of coupled oscillators. *Proceedings of the National Academy of Sciences, 87*, 7200-7204.

Steriade, M., Jones, E. G., & Llinas, R. (1990). *Thalamic Oscillations and Signaling*. New York: Wiley.

Steriade, M., McCormick, D., & Sejnowski, T. (1993). Thalamocortical oscillations in the sleeping and aroused brain. *Science*, *262*, 679-685.

Thron, C. D. (1996). A model for a bistable biochemical trigger of mitosis. *Biophysical Chemistry*, *57*, 239-251.

Traub, R. D., & Miles, R. (1992). Synchronized multiple bursts in the hippocampus: A neuronal population oscillation uninterpretable without accurate cellular membrane kinetics. In T. McKenna, J. Davis, & S. F. Zornetzer (Eds.), *Single Neuron Computation* (pp. 463-476). New York: Academic Press.

von Krosigk, M., Bal, T., & McCormick, D. A. (1993). Cellular mechanism of a synchronized oscillation in the thalamus. *Science*, *261*, 361-364.

Wang, D., Buhmann, J.., & Malsburg, C. von der (1990). Pattern segmentation in associative memory. *Neural Computation*, *2*, 94-106.

Wang, X.-J., & Rinzel, J. (1995). Oscillatory and bursting properties of neurons. In M. A. Arbib (Ed.), *The Handbook of Brain Theory and Neural Networks* (pp. 686-691). Cambridge, MA: MIT Press.

Weimann, J. M., & Marder, E. (1994). Switching neurons are integral members of multiple oscillatory networks. *Current Biology*, *4*, 896-902.

Williams, T. L. (1992). Phase coupling by synaptic spread in chains of coupled neuronal oscillators. *Science*, *258*, 662-665.

Yuasa, H., & Ito, M. (1990). Coordination of many oscillators and generation of locomotory patterns. *Biological Cybernetics*, *63*, 177-184.

Ziv, I., Baxter, D. A., & Byrne, J. H. (1994). Simulator for neural networks and action potentials: Description and application. *Journal of Neurophysiology*, *71*, 294-308.

4
Oscillatory Local Field Potentials

Martin Stemmler
Humboldt Universität zu Berlin

Marius Usher
University of Kent

Christof Koch
California Institute of Technology

ABSTRACT

Although cortical oscillations in the 30-to-70-Hz range are robust and commonly found in local field potential measurements in both cat and monkey visual cortex (Eckhorn, Frien, Bauer, Woelbern, & Kehr, 1993; Gray, König, Engel, & Singer, 1989), they are much less evident in spike trains recorded from behaving monkeys (Bair, Koch, Newsome, & Britten, 1994; Young, Tanaka, & Yamane, 1992). We show that a simple neural network with spiking "units" and a plausible excitatory-inhibitory interconnection scheme can explain this discrepancy. The discharge patterns of single units is highly irregular and the associated single-unit power spectrum flat with a dip at low frequencies, as observed in cortical recordings in the behaving monkey (Bair et al., 1994). However, if the local field potential, defined as the summed spiking activity of all "units" within a particular distance, is computed over an area large enough to include direct inhibitory interactions among cell pairs, a prominent peak around 30-50 Hz becomes visible.

1. INTRODUCTION

The existence and putative significance of neuronal oscillations in the 30-to-70-Hz range in mammalian cortex are among the most hotly debated topics of systems neuroscience in recent years (for an overview see Singer, 1993). Although both single-cell and local field potential oscillations are routinely observed in cat visual cortex (Eckhorn et al., 1988; Freiwald, Kreiter, & Singer, 1995; Gray et al., 1989; Jagadeesh, Gray, & Ferster, 1992), oscillations are more elusive in primates. A number of groups report high frequency oscillations in visual and sensorimotor cortex in the awake monkey (Eeckman & Freeman, 1990; Kreiter & Singer, 1992; Livingstone, 1996; Murthy & Fetz, 1992; Sanes & Donoghue, 1993), while other researchers are unable to find strong evidence for high frequency oscillations (Bair et al., 1994; Tovee & Rolls,

1992; Young et al., 1992). In general, these oscillations are much more readily visible in the local field potential than in the spiking activity of single cells (Eckhorn et al., 1993). Detailed analysis reveals that the firing patterns of single neurons in cortical areas V1 (primary visual cortex) and motion area MT of the behaving monkey are highly irregular even at high discharge frequencies, with a coefficient of variability close to unity (Softky & Koch, 1993).

Taken together, these results pose a challenge for neural modeling: What kind of dynamic process can generate oscillations in local field variables *without* strongly oscillatory single-cell discharge patterns, as indicated by an absence of any oscillatory peak in the power spectrum of spike trains? Because all models of spiking neurons are, by definition, nonlinear oscillators, generating non-oscillatory model spike train spectra is a nontrivial matter, even when the synaptic input is noisy (Usher, Stemmler, Koch, & Olami, 1994). But suppose that we are willing to grant that the power spectrum of single cell spike trains show no signs of oscillation: how then do robust oscillations arise in the local field variables? The answer lies in the correlations in the spike trains *between* cortical neurons, correlations that are imposed by the local network of feedback connections. As first pointed out by Moore, Segundo, Perkel, and Levitan (1970), the cortical architecture dictates the structure of the cross-correlation between any two neurons. We here extend this analysis to the summed activity over many neurons.

Specifically, we explore the dynamics of leaky integrate-and-fire units embedded into a simple neuronal network with local excitation and surround inhibition. Starting from first principles, we explain the origin of partial synchronization between units in such a network. Subsequently, we turn to a phenomenological, model-independent approach that links the oscillations in the local field potential to the sum of cross-correlations over a neuronal population.

2. SPONTANEOUS SYMMETRY BREAKING AND THE ORIGIN OF SYNCHRONIZATION

The model consists of a cyclic 100 × 100 lattice of modified leaky integrate-and-fire units, each characterized by a voltage variable V_i. The leaky integrate-and-fire unit models a nerve cell as a simple RC circuit (with a time constant of τ = 20 ms) subject to a reset mechanism: once a unit reaches a threshold voltage V_{th}, it emits a pulse that is transmitted with a delay of one millisecond to connected neighboring units, and the potential is reset by subtracting the voltage threshold. The discretized dynamics are given by

$$V_i(t+1) = e^{-\frac{1}{\tau}} V_i(t) + I_i(t);\ V(t) < V_{th} \tag{1}$$

$$V_i(t+1) = V_i(t) - v_{th};\ V(t) > V_{th}. \tag{2}$$

The current represents the coupling of the unit to excitatory (inhibitory) pulses of nearby units through the synaptic conductance matrix $\mathbf{W}^E_{ij}$ ($\mathbf{W}^I_{ij}$) and to an independent external current I_i^{ext}:

$$I_i(t) = \sum_j W_{ij}^E \Theta[V_j(t) - V_{th}](E_{rev}^{exc} - V_i(t)) - \sum_j W_{ij}^E \Theta[V_j(t) - V_{th}](V_i(t) - E_{rev}^{inh}) + I_i^{ext}$$

The terms E^{e}_{r} and E^{i}_{r} represent reversal potentials, which are multiplicative factors that model the saturation of excitatory and inhibitory current, respectively. Such a model, known as an integrate-and-fire model (Knight, 1972), is similar to a recently studied self-organized criticality model for earthquakes (Olami, Feder, & Christensen, 1992): in a spring-block model, an earthquake is represented by an avalanche of threshold topplings transmitted from one spring-block to the next. This model is equivalent to an integrate-and-fire model with nearest-neighbor coupling, but without the exponential voltage decay term. The dynamics of Equations (1) and (2) have been shown to mimic reasonably well the discharge patterns of cortical neurons (Softky & Koch, 1993).

Mirollo and Strogatz (1990) first proved that globally coupled and identical leaky integrate-and-fire units will synchronize the timing of output spikes when driven by sufficiently strong external input. Further studies of collective synchronization in networks composed of spiking model neurons have assumed that the coupling is all-to-all (Abbott & van Vreeswijk, 1993; Kuramoto, 1991; Treves, 1993; Tsodyks, Mitkov, & Sompolinsky, 1993), random (Niebur, Schuster, Kammen, & Koch, 1991), or nearest-neighbor (Herz & Hopfield, 1995).

One conclusion is central to all these studies: As long as the sign of the pulse-coupling is positive (excitatory) and the shape of the pulse input is a square-wave or a decaying exponential, the network will evolve to a state in which all network units fire spikes at one common frequency. When driven by noisy external input, a network with all-to-all, random, or nearest-neighbor coupling will undergo a transition from irregular firing of spikes to regular and phase-locked firing as the external input increases in strength. Simulations of such networks show that this phase transition in the temporal pattern persists in the presence of inhibitory connections W^I_{ij} as long as excitation predominates on average, that is, $\langle \Sigma W^I_{ij} \rangle \ll \langle \Sigma W^E_{ij} \rangle$.

An important distinction must be drawn between inhibitory connections in a network where all units belong to the same class and a network with separate populations of inhibitory and excitatory neurons. Although the latter model is biologically realistic, it is also susceptible to synchronization or oscillation for an entirely different reason: An increase in the activity of the excitatory population will lead to an increased firing in the inhibitory population, which, in turn, will lead to a decrease in the firing of excitatory cells. The alternation in activity profiles of the two populations can be quite dramatic and sharp in time. This oscillation cycle has been described analytically and in computer models (Bush & Douglas, 1991; Wilson & Bower, 1991; Wilson & Cowan, 1972).

Although it is true that the predominant majority of synaptic connections in mammalian cortex are excitatory feedback connections (Douglas, Koch, Mahowald, Martin, & Suarez, 1995), the most common assumption of all-to-all connections is patently unrealistic. Motivated by the columnar organization of neocortex, we explore a network model where the extent of synaptic projections from any particular network unit is limited to a local neighborhood and the inhibitory projections extend further than the excitatory ones. Longer-range excitatory connections linking columns across cortex are not considered here, but are explored in Stemmler, Usher, and Niebur (1995).

The particular geometry of local excitatory and inhibitory connections we use is one called a *center-surround* pattern. Each unit has excitatory connections to $N = 50$ units chosen from a Gaussian probability distribution of $\sigma = 2.5$ lattice constants, centered at the unit's position. $N = 50$ inhibitory connections per unit are chosen from a uniform probability distribution on a ring eight to nine lattice constants away. The weight of the excitation and inhibition, in units of voltage threshold, is $W^E = \alpha/N$ and $W^I = \beta W^E$, where $\alpha \geq 1$. We typically choose the inhibition ratio to be $\beta = 2/3$. The external input is modeled independently for each cell as a Poisson process of excitatory pulses of magnitude $1/N$, arriving at a mean rate λ_{ext}.

Scaling the relative degree of inhibition β while keeping the sum of excitation and inhibition constant leads to a transition from a spatially homogeneous state to a clustered activity state. This transition can be understood using a mean-field description of the dynamics, where we write the continuous pulse rate f_i as a function of the averaged currents I_i: $f(I) = \{T_{ref} - \tau \ln [1 - 1/(I\tau)]\}^{-1}$ (Amit & Tsodyks, 1991), where T_{ref} is the refractory period (minimum dead time) between pulses. In this approximation, the dynamics associated with Equations (1) and (2) simplify to

$$\frac{dI_i}{dt} = -I_i + \sum_j W_{ij} f(I_j) + I_i^{ext}. \tag{3}$$

In the mean-field description, the dynamics of Equation (3) will be subject to the Lyapunov potential function (Hopfield, 1984):

$$L = -\frac{1}{2}\sum_{i,j} W_{ij} f_i f_j + \sum_i \left(\int_0^{f_i} I(f)\,df - I^{ext} f_i \right),$$

which exists as long as the following conditions are met:

(1) The coupling matrix $\mathbf{W}_{ij}$ is (statistically) symmetric.
(2) Pulse rates f_i are never zero, which will be true if there is a source of noise.
(3) The external current I^{ext} is spatially homogeneous.

If the Lyapunov function exists (as it does in our case), then the system must relax to a stable state — persistent dynamics are ruled out.

However, pulse-coupled networks are not completely described by the mean-field equations, and can, in fact, show persistent dynamics. For instance, the clusters of high activity that develop will not remain fixed, but instead will diffuse across the network grid. We do not explore the origin of this form of diffusion here, referring the interested reader to the article by Usher, Stemmler, and Olami (1995). Instead, we use the mean-field approximation to study the overall geometrical pattern of activity that develops.

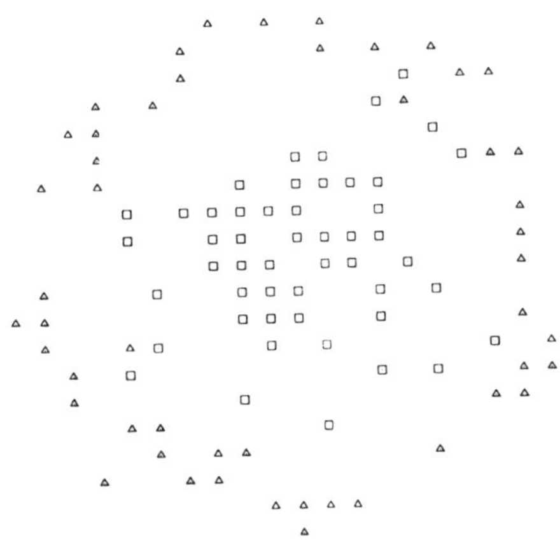

Fig. 4.1. Basic Gaussian connectivity pattern for the standard model. The cell (not shown) at the center of the rectangular array is connected in a probabilistic manner to units within a given distance determined by a Gaussian distribution with $\sigma = 2.5$ lattice constants. These short-range connections are excitatory (squares). The center cell also inhibits a fixed fraction of cells on an annulus 8 and 9 lattice constants away (triangles). During a particular simulation, the connectivity pattern is fixed, although the exact synaptic weight varies stochastically.

The dynamics have a homogeneous solution if the input current remains equal for all units: $I_i = \mathrm{I}$ for all i. Here we assume that the external input I^{ext} itself is spatially homogeneous. In the homogeneous state, all units fire at the same rate, without any spatial variation across the network. I is given by

$$\bar{I} = \tilde{W}(0) f(\bar{I}) + I^{ext}, \tag{4}$$

where $\tilde{W}(0) = \langle \Sigma_j W_{ij} \rangle_i$, and we use the fact that the matrix $\mathbf{W}_{ij}$ is statistically isotropic (i.e., isotropic on average). The homogeneous solution $I_i = \mathrm{I}$ for all i is stable only if the Fourier transform of $\langle \mathbf{W}_{ij} \rangle_i$ satisfies $\tilde{W}(k)\, f'(\mathrm{I}) - 1 < 0$ for the entire (discrete) set of $k >$ 0.

As one increases the relative strength of inhibition, clusters of high firing activity develop. These are the result of spontaneous symmetry breaking: a nonzero wavelength mode becomes unstable as the inhibition parameter β becomes larger. The exponential growth rate $\tilde{W}(k) f'(\bar{I}) - 1$ is illustrated in Fig. 4.2.

The wave number q_0 that is the first to become unstable is the dominant mode and will set the length scale of the hexagonal pattern of clusters. The transition from a homogeneous state to a hexagonal structure is generic to many nonequilibrium systems in fluid mechanics, nonlinear optics, reaction-diffusion systems, and biology (Cowan, 1982; Cross & Hohenberg, 1993; Ermentrout & Cowan, 1979; Newell & Whitehead, 1969). We can use multiple scale perturbation theory to ask how a small-amplitude fluctuation $\exp(i\mathbf{q}_0\mathbf{x})$ on the dominant length scale will evolve. This fluctuation constitutes a plane wave disturbance in an arbitrarily selected direction $\mathbf{x}$. Set

$$\tilde{W}(q_0) = \alpha + \epsilon$$

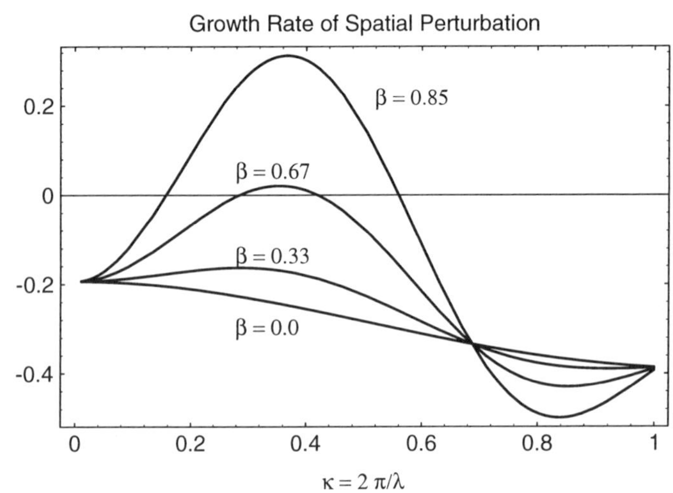

Fig. 4.2. The exponential growth rate behaves as $\tilde{W}(k)\, f'(\bar{I}) - 1$, where $\tilde{W}(k)$ is the Fourier transform of the coupling matrix $\mathbf{W}_{ij}$. As a simple tractable model consistent with the connection scheme used in the model, we take the excitatory couplings to be uniform within a radius r_e = 4.5 lattice units, and the inhibitory couplings on a ring r_i = 9.0 lattice units. Taking the continuous Fourier transform, we have $= (2\pi\alpha/k)\,(r_e J_1(r_e k) - \beta k r_i J_0(r_i k))$, J_1 and J_0 are Bessel functions. As the inhibition ratio β increases, the maximum of $\tilde{W}(k)$ becomes greater than zero, indicating the presence of an unstable mode. Spatial structure will develop at the wavelength given by the maximum $\tilde{W}(k)$. (Note: in the graph above, we have applied a correction factor arising from the use of discrete time-step equations instead of differential equations).

where α is defined such that $\alpha f'(\bar{I}) - 1 = 0$, and we assume that $\epsilon \ll \alpha$. Define a slow time scale $T = \epsilon t$, and denote the amplitude of the fluctuation by $A(T)$. ($A(T)$ is complex so that we can represent spatially translation invariant solutions.) We treat the fluctuation $\delta\tilde{I}(q_0)$ as a power series in $\epsilon^{1/2}$:

$$\delta\tilde{I} = \epsilon^{\frac{1}{2}}\left[A(T)e^{iq_0\cdot x} + A^{\dagger}(T)e^{-iq_0\cdot x}\right] + \epsilon\psi_1(q_0 x) + \epsilon^{\frac{3}{2}}\psi_2(q_0 x) \quad (5)$$

in which Ψ_1 and Ψ_2 represent perturbations of the "ground-state" $\exp(i\mathbf{q}_0\mathbf{x})$ in the higher harmonics of the fundamental spatial frequency. To find a self-consistent solution, we must insist that the perturbations are orthogonal to $\exp(i\mathbf{q}_0\mathbf{x})$. Perturbation theory couples Ψ_1 and Ψ_2 to $A(T)$, allowing us to deduce the so-called "amplitude equation" $A(T)$ must obey to satisfy the orthogonality condition.

In two dimensions, symmetry will allow the superposition of fluctuations along wave vectors $\mathbf{q}_1$, $\mathbf{q}_2$, and $\mathbf{q}_3$ spaced $2\pi/3$ apart. Expanding $f(I)$ in a Taylor series around $\bar{I}$, we can solve for the complex amplitudes A_1, A_2, A_3, using secular (multiple-scale) perturbation theory (for a readable tutorial on these perturbation methods, see Cross & Hohenberg, 1993):

$$\frac{\partial\bar{A}_1}{\partial T} = \beta\bar{A}_1 + \gamma\bar{A}^{\dagger}{}_2\bar{A}^{\dagger}{}_3 - \delta\left(|\bar{A}_1|^2 + 2(|\bar{A}_2|^2 + |\bar{A}_3|^2)\right)\bar{A}_1 \quad (6)$$

$$\frac{\partial\bar{A}_2}{\partial T} = \beta\bar{A}_2 + \gamma\bar{A}^{\dagger}{}_1\bar{A}^{\dagger}{}_3 - \delta\left(|\bar{A}_2|^2 + 2(|\bar{A}_1|^2 + |\bar{A}_3|^2)\right)\bar{A}_2 \quad (7)$$

$$\frac{\partial\bar{A}_3}{\partial T} = \beta\bar{A}_3 + \gamma\bar{A}^{\dagger}{}_1\bar{A}^{\dagger}{}_2 - \delta\left(|\bar{A}_3|^2 + 2(|\bar{A}_1|^2 + |\bar{A}_2|^2)\right)\bar{A}_3 \quad (8)$$

with $\bar{A} = \epsilon^{1/2} A$, $\beta = f'(\bar{I})$, $\gamma = 2\alpha f''(\bar{I})$, and $\delta = -3\alpha\epsilon f^{(3)}(\bar{I})$. These equations fall under the universal class of Ginzburg-Landau equations (Ciliberto et al., 1990). Note that we must include higher order terms if $f^{(3)}(\bar{I}) \geq 0$.

If $f''(\bar{I}) > 0$, the pattern of activity will undergo a transition from the homogeneous state to a non-zero amplitude hexagonal pattern at $\epsilon = 0$:

$$|\bar{A}_1| = |\bar{A}_2| = |\bar{A}_3| = \frac{2}{3}\gamma\sqrt{\delta}f''(\bar{I}).$$

This hexagonal pattern is stable as long as $-(1/12)\gamma^2\delta < \beta < 3\gamma^2\delta$ (Ciliberto et al., 1990). The hexagonal grid of clusters across the network of integrate-and-fire units is illustrated in Fig. 4.3.

In a spiking network, global synchronization and pattern formation will have opposing effects: Synchronization will enforce one unitary firing rate for all neuronal units, while symmetry breaking pushes firing rates of different units apart. The interplay

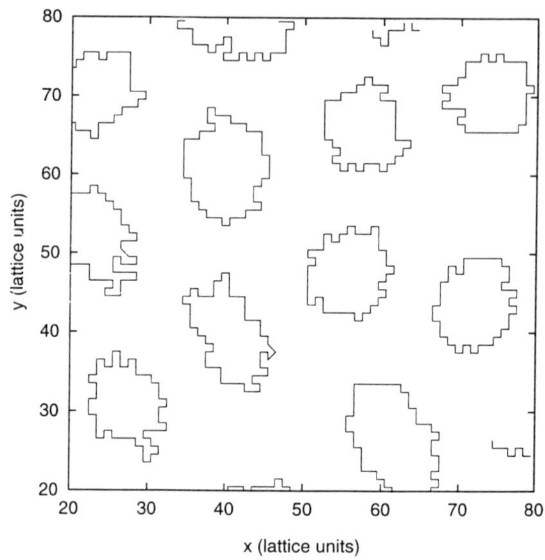

Fig. 4.3. The summed activity for the network over any 50 ms of simulation reveals a nearly hexagonal pattern of clusters of high activity. Solid lines indicate the border of clusters, defined as those units which fired two spikes within a 50-ms time period. Modified from Usher et al., 1995.

of synchronization and pattern formation leads to the phenomenon of partial or intermittent synchronization, in which individual units do not fire in fixed phase to the collective oscillation of a group of units. Note that noise is *not* a necessary ingredient in this phenomenon. Deterministic simulations starting with random initial conditions reveal that partial synchronization is a feature of the inherently chaotic dynamics.

Conversely, the tendency of nearby units to synchronize will seed the formation of clusters of high activity and predispose the system to breaking the symmetry of the homogeneous state. Consequently, the transition from the homogeneous state to the hexagonal state occurs for a lower inhibition ratio β than predicted by the mean-field description (cf. Fig. 4.2).

Let us remark that a unified theoretical description of spatial and synchronization effects can be obtained in the limit where the number of units within the local geometry given by W_{ij} is large (by combining the foregoing approach above with an analysis of the type proposed by Treves, 1993). We do not address this theoretical description here, but instead focus on measures to quantify the oscillatory characteristic of populations or single units, which are introduced in the next section.

3. MEASURING THE LOCAL FIELD POTENTIAL

For mathematical reasons, we define the local field potential (LFP) to be the total spiking activity of all units within a circle of radius r around any particular unit. In general, we use $r = 10$, which encompasses an area large enough to include the inhibitory interactions occurring on a ring 8 and 9 lattice constants away. We will contrast this with the spiking activity from a single unit (single-unit activity or SUA).

Our definition of the LFP is a crude approximation of the signal recorded by low-pass filtering the electrical signal from a low-impedance microelectrode inserted under the skull and does not include any dendritic or synaptic component. Common consensus holds that the actually measured LFP represents the summed dendritic current, which is not necessarily equivalent to spiking activity in all cases of physiological interest. Based on anatomical estimates, however, most of the input to a neuron is excitatory feedback from the local cortical network (Douglas et al., 1995). In this case, the summed spike output constitutes a large fraction of the dendritic input; both the summed spike activity or summed input current accurately reflect the LFP. Grinvald, Lieke, Frostig, and Hildesheim (1994) noted that peaks in the optical signal or LFP and spikes in the SUA typically coincide in time, supporting the notion of strong feedback.

We used the following parameters in the model:

For the weight of each excitatory synapse, $W^{e}_{ij} = \alpha/N$, α is drawn from a uniform probability distribution between 1.15 and 1.4 and allowed to vary for each time the synapse is activated. The weight of inhibitory synapses W^{I}_{ij} is treated similarly, but re-scaled by $\beta = 0.5$. That is, the average inhibitory synapse had half the weight of an average excitatory synapse. The external input I_i^{ext}, which can be thought of a visual input, is modeled independently for each cell as a Poisson process of excitatory pulses of magnitude $1/N$, arriving at a mean rate λ^{ext}. All cells receive the same rate of external input. With λ^{ext} set to 2.3 kHz, the firing of individual cells replicates the known firing properties of single neurons in monkey visual cortex (Usher et al., 1994). Power spectra and correlation functions are computed over 32 sec long trials.

Figure 4.4A shows the LFP, together with the spike train from one of the units within the "recorded" area, during a typical simulation run. The field potential's strongly fluctuating signal has a broad peak (25-45 Hz) in the power spectrum (Fig. 4.4B). This implies that the cells that contribute to the LFP are partially synchronized (at most only about 25 out of the 400 cells fire together), leading to broad oscillatory characteristics. The SUA shows no significant evidence of periodic firing; the associated single-cell power spectrum (Fig. 4.4C) is flat except for a dip at low frequencies introduced by the refractory period.

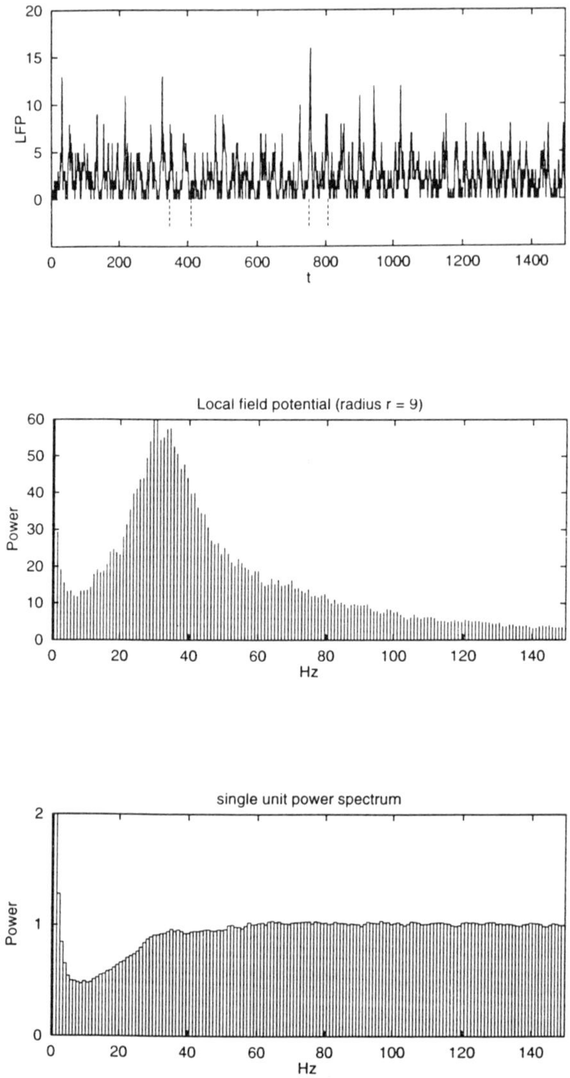

Fig. 4.4. The top graph shows the local field potential (LFP), computed by summing the spiking activity of all leaky integrate-and-fire units within a disk of radius $r = 9$, as a function of time during a typical simulation. We superimposed (dashed line) the spikes from a representative unit in the same part of the network. The power spectrum of the LFP, shown in the center panel, shows a clear peak around 30 Hz. This strong peak disappears nearly completely in the power spectrum of the average single unit activity (SUA); instead, the SUA spectrum is similar to that of a Poisson process with a refractory period. The absence of a peak in the spectrum indicates that the interspike interval is fairly broad, in accordance with experimental data.

To test whether this behavior is a trivial outcome for any model of spiking cells with feedback connectivity, we performed simulations using the same neural model, except for one change: each cell had N_{con} excitatory and N_{con} inhibitory synapses onto units chosen at *random* (independent of distance) on the lattice. The power spectra of the SUA and LFP are displayed in Fig. 4.5. The single cell power spectrum now has a large peak, implying that the discharge pattern of single cells is periodic. Such power spectra are in general not found in spike trains of non-bursting cells (Bair et al., 1994). Furthermore, the interspike interval variability under this condition is much lower than observed experimentally (Usher et al., 1994) in cells firing at medium or large rates. Because of the lack of spatial structure the system is ergodic; that is, the population average (the LFP in Fig. 4.5) has essentially the same structure as the temporal average over a single unit (the SUA in Fig. 4.5). For very low firing rates (less than 5 Hz) we can obtain irregular single cell spike trains that are almost Poisson, but without prominent oscillations in the local field potential.

The oscillations in the LFP depend most strongly on the amount of lateral inhibition β and the rate of external input λ^{ext} in the model. Increasing β leads to a much sharper spectral peak (especially for $0.5 < \beta < 0.7$) and to a small increase in the location of the peak. Increasing the input rate λ^{ext} has a more pronounced effect, leading simultaneously to broadening of the peak and to an increase in the mean frequency.

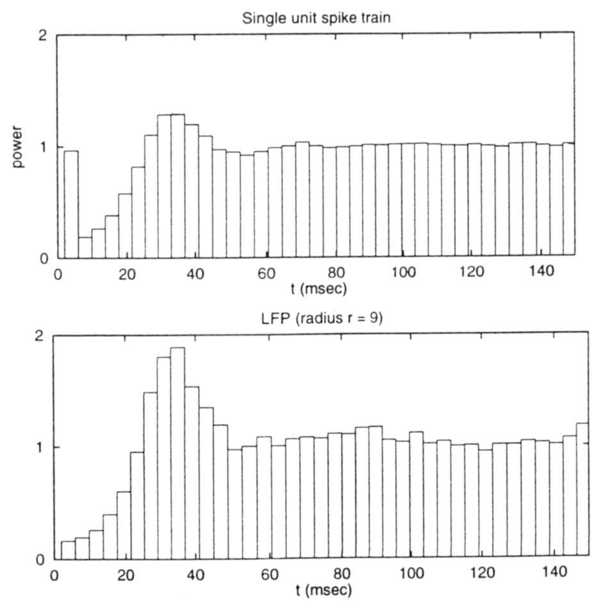

Fig. 4.5. The power spectrum of individual cells (upper panel) versus the spectrum of the LFP (lower panel) in a network with non-local random connectivity with both excitation and inhibition (everything else is identical to the previous figure). Here, both signals display a strong oscillatory component. The interspike interval variability is much lower under these conditions than observed empirically.

4. CORRELATION ANALYSIS

The large, broadly periodic fluctuations in the LFP reflect partial synchronized and correlated discharge patterns of cells in a local population. We can explain the properties of the local field signal by analyzing the correlations between its components. Since we define the LFP to be the sum of all N single-unit spiking activity within a circle of radius r, the autocorrelation function of the LFP will be the sum of N autocorrelation functions $A_{ii}(t)$ of the individual cells and $N \times (N\text{-}1)$ cross-correlation functions $C_{ij}(t)$ among individual cells within the circle,

$$A_{LFP}(t) = \sum_{i=1}^{N} A_{ii}(t) + \sum_{i=1}^{N} \sum_{j=1, j \neq i}^{N} C_{ij}(t). \qquad (9).$$

In general, the autocorrelation of the LFP will be dominated by the cross-correlation functions among individual units and the power spectrum of the LFP — identical to the Fourier transform of the correlation function (Wiener-Khintchine theorem) — will in turn be dominated by the sum of the Fourier transforms of the individual cross-correlation functions. In order to characterize the power spectrum of the LFP, we now describe the characteristics of the cross-correlations and their Fourier transforms.

For mutually excitatory pairs of cells, the cross-correlation terms $C_{ij}(t)$ display a structure called a "castle on a hill" in the neurophysiological literature (Nelson et al., 1992), that is, a 10- to 20-ms wide peak centered at zero (Fig. 4.6) followed by a slower decay to the asymptotic level of chance coincidences for long time lags. The peak of $C_{ij}(t)$ is always around zero and is generated by recurrent excitation. At higher values of inhibition β, a small but significant secondary peak in the cross-correlation appears between the "castle" and the slower decline. For cell pairs that are 8 or 9 units distant, the interaction will be (on average) mutually inhibitory and the associated correlation function is characterized by a gentle trough that rises slowly to the background level of chance coincidences at longer times. As discussed in Usher et al. (1994), the process governing the slow decay in the excitatory and the slow rise in the inhibitory correlation functions is the same.

The principal factor leading to a power spectrum peak in the 30-70-Hz range is the relative width of the excitatory cross-correlation peaks to the inhibitory troughs. In general, the excitatory "castles" are sharp relative to the broad dip in the cross-correlation due to inhibition. In Fourier space, these relationships are reversed: broader Fourier transforms of excitatory cross-correlations are paired with narrower Fourier transforms of inhibitory cross-correlations. Superposition of such transforms leads to a peak in the 30-50-Hz range. A less important factor is the existence (at higher values of inhibition) of a secondary peak around 20 to 30 ms in the excitatory cross-correlations.

The principle behind the formation of the power spectrum peak can be captured in the following simplified but generic example, which assumes that the excitatory and inhibitory correlation functions qualitatively behave as:

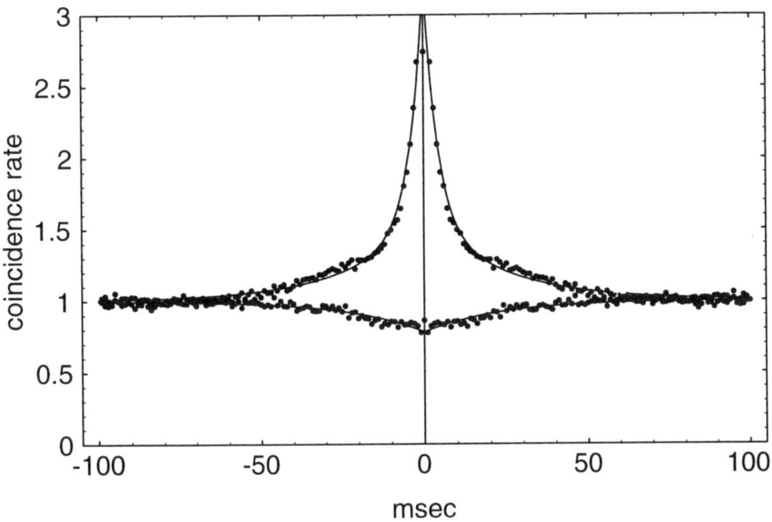

Fig. 4.6. Typical cross-correlation functions between neighboring pairs of mutually excitatory cells (top graph) and mutually inhibitory pairs separated by 9 lattice units. The solid lines indicate the best least square fit of equations 5 and 6 to the data, with the fast initial decay (the "tower") in $C_+(t)$ fitted by an exponential with $\tau_1 = 4$ ms and the slower decay in both $C_+(t)$ and $C_-(t)$ fitted by another exponential with $\tau_2 = 22$ ms.

$$C_+(t) = A\exp(-|t|/\tau_1) + B\exp(-|t|/\tau_2) + 1 \qquad (10)$$

$$C_-(t) = C\exp(-|t|/\tau_2) + 1, \qquad (11)$$

where the baseline of coincidence is normalized to 1. In Fig. 4.6, we fitted these equations against two particular cross-correlation functions from our network using $\tau_1 = 4$ and $\tau_2 = 22$ ms.

The power spectrum of the LFP, $F(\omega)$, will be dominated by the Fourier transforms of many such correlation functions, with

$$F(\omega) = \frac{a}{1+\omega^2\tau_1^2} - \frac{b}{1+\omega^2\tau_2^2}, \qquad (12)$$

for $\omega \neq 0$. The terms a and b account for the strength and the number of excitatory and inhibitory cell pairs within the circle (with $a \geq b$).

Consider now the simple case of $a \approx b$, which will occur in our scenario if the LFP is taken over a circle with $r > 9$. In this case the spectrum increases from low frequencies, reaches a maximum at $\omega_{max} = \sqrt{\frac{1}{\tau_1 \tau_2}}$, and decays back to zero for large frequencies. The superposition of two representative cross-correlation transforms yielding the desired peak is shown in Fig. 4.7.

The predicted strong dependency of the peak in the spectrum of the LFP on the size of the area over which the neuronal activity is summed is illustrated in Fig. 4.8. If only spiking activity within a circle of $r = 8$ units contributes towards the LFP, its spectrum is more-or-less monotonic decaying in frequency. As soon as r is large enough to include significant number of pair-wise inhibitory interactions (here for $r = 10$) the peak appears and remains essentially unchanged for larger areas ($r = 12$ in Fig. 4.8).

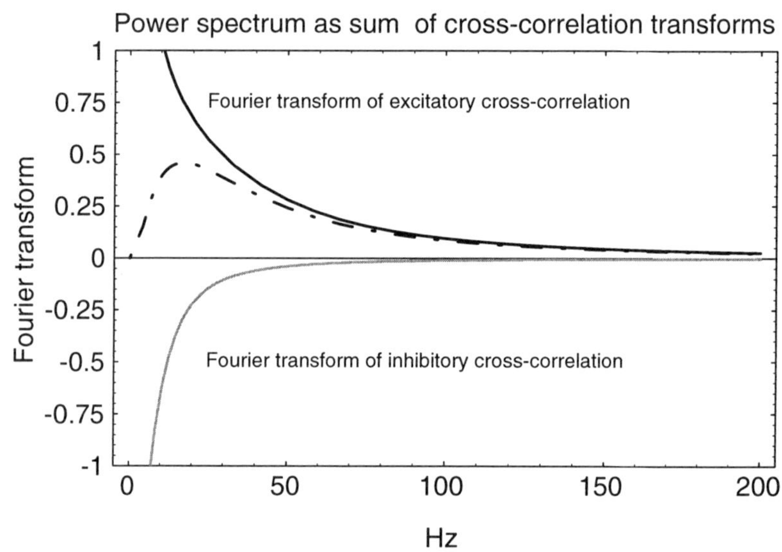

Fig. 4.7. Schematic of how the oscillatory peak in the LFP can be caused by a sharply tuned excitatory cross-correlation function $C_+(t)$ superimposed onto a much broader inhibitory cross-correlation function $C_-(t)$ (Equations (5) and (6) and the previous figure). If the two are subtracted, the low frequency components cancel, leaving a peak at a non-zero frequency.

5. DISCUSSION

We demonstrated how a simple neural network of spiking units can explain one of the more puzzling aspects of neurophysiological recordings, the discrepancy between irregular spike trains and oscillatory local field potentials (Eckhorn et al., 1993).

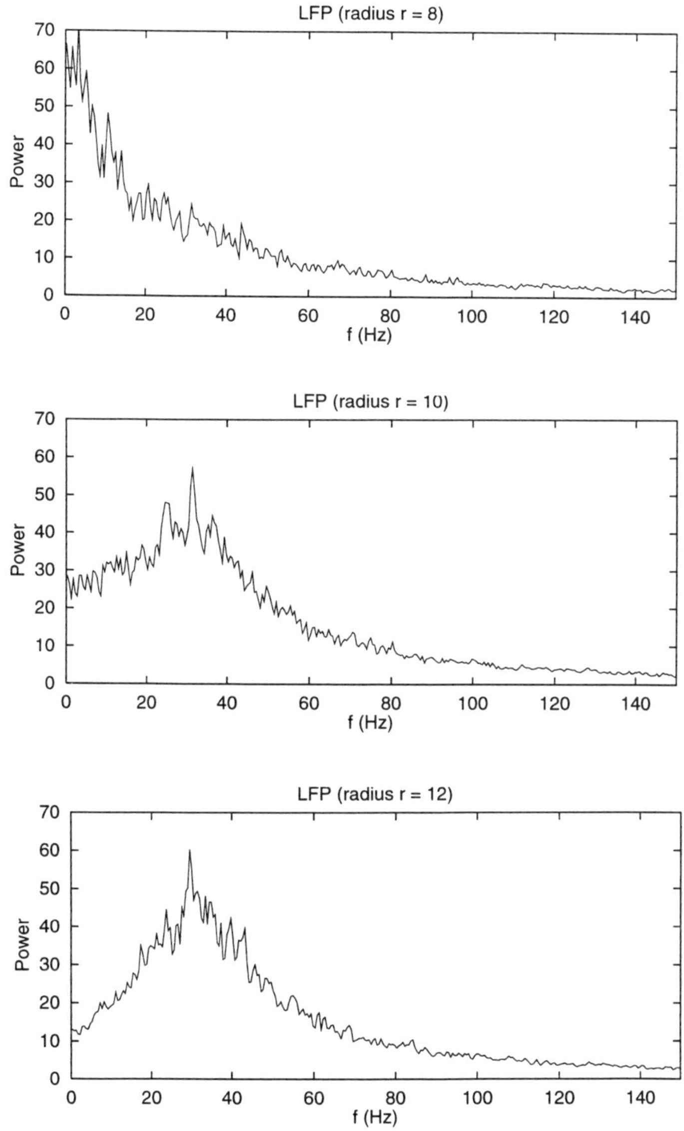

Fig. 4.8. Since the cross-correlations between cells in the model are a function of distance, oscillations in the LFP will depend on the size of the area over which cells contribute to the LFP. If only cells in the near vicinity contribute to the LFP, the power spectrum of the LFP will consist of the superposition of excitatory cross-correlation Fourier transforms and show no oscillatory character. As the radius increases over which single-cell spiking is averaged, the LFP evolves an oscillatory peak.

Although our model is a mere cartoon version of events occurring in cortex (we do not consider, e.g., dendrites and dendritic nonlinearities, Hodgkin-Huxley channel kinetics, or the segregation of neurons into different cell types), it allows us to explain a number of features of neural firing patterns. Our model is a simplification of events occurring in cortex, since we do not consider, for example, dendrites and dendritic nonlinearities, Hodgkin-Huxley channel kinetics, or the segregation of neurons into different cell types. Nonetheless, the model can explain a number of features of real neural firing patterns.

The connectivity scheme used in our model is a reasonable first approximation for connectivity in sensory cortical areas, such as primary visual cortex (Lund, Takashi, & Levitt, 1993; Malach, Amir, Harel, & Grinvald, 1993), where pyramidal cells directly excite nearby cells within the same orientation column and inhibit (indirectly) cells in neighboring columns of different orientations. A more elaborate scheme taking into account the patchy longer-range excitatory connections found in biocytin-tracer studies is investigated in Stemmler et al. (1995). At present, it is not known whether the center-surround connectivity is the only scenario leading to the structure of the cross-correlation functions shown in Fig. 4.6.

We speculate that the length scale of the center-surround connectivity scheme is matched to the underlying columnar structure of mammalian neocortex. Because cortical columns are repeating structures tuned to particular features, such as the angular orientation of a visual stimulus, the structured pattern of activity induced by the lateral connections could serve the purpose of pattern completion: In this computational scheme, a weak or incomplete signal is reinforced by the lateral (feedback) connections (Douglas et al., 1995). The spatial pattern of activity in this case reflects the tuning profile of the neuronal population to the stimulus. At least two models (Somers, Nelson, & Sur, 1995; Wörgötter, Niebur, & Koch, 1991) have proposed a center-surround connectivity scheme similar to ours in which the lateral connections sharpen the tuning of the neuronal response to visual stimuli. Such a role for the lateral connections could be important when the external input is poorly tuned, as may be the case when the stimulus is weak.

The local geometry of connections will lead to stereotypical spatial patterns of activity across the network as long as the external input (signal) is strong enough. The oscillatory behavior in the local neuronal populations is the result of the interaction between the spatial pattern of firing rates and the tendency of pulse-coupled nonlinear oscillators to synchronize. Because partial synchronization assists the formation of spatial patterns of activity, oscillatory behavior in the local field potential (LFP) could be an epiphenomenon of a mechanism for pattern completion.

The frequency of oscillations in the LFP depends on the cross-correlations between units in the ensemble. Independent of the exact time-course of the cross-correlation functions and the details of the network under study, our analysis predicts the emergence of oscillatory LFP's even in the absence of regular periodic spike trains whenever:

(i) the cross-correlation "castles" of mutual excitatory cell pairs have a faster time course than the troughs in the $C_{ij}(t)$'s associated with mutually inhibitory cell pairs, and

(ii) a sufficient number of inhibitory cross-correlations of the type shown in Fig. 4.6 contribute to the LFP. For a model with a connection geometry such as ours, this implies that the area over which cells contribute toward the LFP must be large enough.

A further condition is that the amplitude of the C_{ij}'s must be strong enough to have a significant effect on the power spectrum. Not all connectivity patterns, however, generate strong cross-correlations. If, for instance, the coupling within the network is reduced, that is, $\alpha \rightarrow 0$, $C_{ij}(t) \rightarrow 1$ and the oscillations will disappear.

Ginzburg and Sompolinsky (1994) showed that neural systems with random connections have very weak cross-correlation functions compared to the autocorrelation functions (unless the system is specifically tuned to the vicinity of a dynamical bifurcation point). Simulations of our spiking model with random connectivity confirm this fact, yielding very small, almost flat cross-correlations; therefore, for such a random connectivity scheme, the power of the local field is dominated by the A_{ii}'s and shows the same characteristics as the power spectrum of single cells. The neurobiological evidence (Toyama, Kimura, & Tanaka, 1981), however, points to strong cross-correlations between cortical neurons of the type we achieve in this model.

The segregation of neurons into different cell types has not been considered here. Networks with separate populations of inhibitory and excitatory neurons allow for more complex dynamic behavior than the simple model we have presented. In particular, the LFP in such a biologically more realistic model can be oscillatory for an entirely different reason: Any increase in the activity of the excitatory population will lead to an increased firing in the inhibitory population, which, in turn, will lead to a decrease in the firing of excitatory cells.

Intrinsically oscillating or bursting cells have been observed in cortex (Agmon & Connors, 1991; Llinas, Grace, & Yarom, 1991). A subset of these within the larger population of neurons could also cause the LFP to exhibit oscillations; we have, however, not considered the more complex single cell models required to model such a phenomenon.

The alternation in activity profiles of the two populations can be self-sustained and quite dramatic and sharp in time. This oscillation cycle has been described analytically and in computer models (Bush & Douglas, 1991; Koch & Schuster, 1992; Wilson & Bower, 1991; Wilson & Cowan, 1972). It is not clear whether this mechanism alone can lead to oscillations in the LFP with no oscillations in the single cell spike trains.

Oscillations in the LFP reflecting partial synchronization of local neuronal populations has several implications. First, synaptic input converging upon a neuron is more effective in enhancing the cell's discharge rate if it is synchronized. Moreover, Bernander, Koch, and Douglas (1994) showed that partial synchronization may be more effective in eliciting postsynaptic spikes than total synchronization depending on the exact biophysical parameters (due to the existence of a refractory period and saturating nonlinearities). Second, states of partial synchrony are more easily modulated than fully synchronized ones, allowing for an implementation of oscillation-based models for selective visual attention, segmentation, and binding (Niebur et al., 1993).

ACKNOWLEDGMENTS

This work was supported by the Howard Hughes Medical Institute, the National Institutes of Mental Health, the Air Force Office of Scientific Research, the National Science Foundation, and the Office of Naval Research.

REFERENCES

Abbott, L. F., & van Vreeswijk, C. (1993). Asynchronous states in networks of pulse-coupled oscillators. *Physical Review E*, *48*, 1483-1490.

Agmon, A., & Connors, B. W. (1991). Thalamocortical responses of mouse somatosensory (barrel) cortex in vitro. *Neuroscience*, *41*, 365-379.

Amit, D. J., & Tsodyks, M. V. (1991). Quantitative study of attractor neural network retrieving at low rates: 1. Substrate spikes, rates and neuronal gain. *Network: Computation in Neural Systems*, *2*, 259-273.

Bair, W., Koch, C., Newsome, W., & Britten, K. (1994). Power spectrum analysis of {MT} neurons in the behaving monkey. *Journal of Neuroscience*, *14*, 2870-2892.

Bernander, Ö., Koch, C., & Douglas, R. J. (1994). Amplification and linearization of distal synaptic input to cortical pyramidal cells. *Journal of Neurophysiology*, *72*, 2743-2753.

Bush, P. C., & Douglas, R. J. (1991). Synchronization of bursting action potential discharge in a model network of neocortical neurons. *Neural Computation*, *3*, 19-30.

Ciliberto, S., Coullet, P., Lega, J., Pampaloni, E., & Perez-Garcia, C. (1990). Defects in roll-hexagon competition. *Physical Review Letters*, *65*, 2370-2373.

Cowan, J. D. (1982). Spontaneous symmetry breaking in large scale nervous activity. *International Journal of Quantitative Chemistry*, *22*, 1059-1082.

Cross, M. C., & Hohenberg, P. C. (1993). Pattern formation outside of equilibrium. *Reviews in Modern Physics*, *65*, 851-1112.

Douglas, R., Koch, C., Mahowald, M., Martin, K., & Suarez, H. (1995). Recurrent excitation in neocortical circuits. *Science, 269*, 981-985.

Eckhorn, R., Bauer, R., Jordan, W., Brosch, M., Kruse, W., Munk, M., & Reitboeck, H. J. (1988). Coherent oscillations — a mechanism of feature linking in the visual cortex — multiple electrode and correlation analyses in the cat. *Biological Cybernetics*, *60*, 121-130.

Eckhorn, R., Frien, A., Bauer, R., Woelbern, T., & Kehr, H. (1993). High frequency (60-90 hz) oscillations in primary visual cortex of awake monkey. *Neuroreport*, *4*, 243-246.

Eeckman, F., & Freeman, W. (1990). Correlations between unit firing and {EEG} in the rat olfactory system. *Brain Research*, *528*, 238-244.

Ermentrout, B., & Cowan, J. (1979). A mathematical theory of visual hallucination patterns. *Biological Cybernetics*, *34*, 137-150.

Freiwald, W. A., Kreiter, A. K., & Singer, W. (1995). Stimulus-dependent intercolumnar synchronization of single-unit responses in cat area 17. *Neuroreport*, *6*, 2348-2352.

Ginzburg, I., & Sompolinsky, H. (1994). Correlation functions in a large stochastic neural network. *Neural Information Processing*, *6*, 3171-3191.

Gray, C. M., König, P., Engel, A. K., & Singer, W. (1989). Oscillatory responses in cat visual-cortex exhibit inter-columnar synchronization which reflects global stimulus properties. *Nature, 338*, 334-337.

Grinvald, A., Lieke, E. E., Frostig, R. D., & Hildesheim, R. (1994). Cortical point-spread function and long-range lateral interactions revealed by real-time optical imaging of macaque monkey primary visual cortex. *Journal of Neuroscience, 14*, 2545-2568.

Herz, A. V. M., & Hopfield, J. J. (1995). Earthquake cycles and neural reverberations — collective oscillations in systems with pulse-coupled threshold elements. *Physical Review Letters, 75*, 1222-1225.

Hopfield, J. J. (1984). Neurons with graded responses have collective computational properties like those of two-state neurons. *Proceedings of the National Academy of Sciences, 81*, 3088-3092.

Jagadeesh, B., Gray, C. M., & Ferster, D. (1992). Visually evoked oscillations of membrane-potential in cells of cat visual-cortex. *Science, 257*, 552-554.

Knight, B. W. (1972). Dynamics of encoding in a population of neurons. *Journal of General Physiology, 59*, 734-766.

Kreiter, A. K., & Singer, W. (1992). Oscillatory neuronal responses in the visual cortex of the awake macaque monkey. *European Journal of Neuroscience, 4*, 369-375.

Kuramoto, Y. (1991). Collective synchronization of pulse-coupled oscillators and excitable units. *Physica D, 50*, 15-30.

Livingstone, M. S. (1996). Oscillatory firing and interneuronal correlations in squirrel-monkey cortex. *Journal of Neurophysiology, 75*, 2467-2485.

Llinas, R. R., Grace, A. A., & Yarom, Y. (1991). In vitro neurons in mammalian cortical layer 4 exhibit intrinsic oscillatory activity in the 10-to 50-Hz frequency range. *Proceedings of the National Academy of Sciences, 88*, 897-901.

Lund, J. S., Takashi, Y., & Levitt, J. B. (1993). Comparison of intrinsic connectivity of macaque monkey cerebral cortex. *Cerebral Cortex, 3*, 148-162.

Malach, R., Amir, Y., Harel, M., & Grinvald, A. (1993). Relationship between intrinsic connections and functional architecture revealed by optical imaging and *in vivo* targeted biocytin injections in the primate striate cortex. *Proceedings of the National Academy of Sciences, 90*, 10469-10473.

Mirollo, R. E., & Strogatz, S. H. (1990). Synchronization of pulse-coupled biological oscillators. *SIAM Journal on Applied Mathematics, 50*, 1645-1662.

Moore, G. P., Segundo, J.-P., Perkel, D. H., & Levitan, H. (1970). Statistical signs of synaptic interaction in neurons. *Biophysical Journal, 10*, 876-900.

Murthy, V. N., & Fetz, E. E. (1992). Coherent 25- to 35-hz oscillation in the sensorimotor cortex of awake behaving monkeys. *Proceedings of the National Academy of Sciences, 89*, 5670-5674.

Nelson, J. I., Salin, P. A., Munk, M. H.-J., Arzi, M., & Bullier, J. (1992). Spatial and temporal coherence in cortico-cortical connections: A cross-correlation study in areas 17 and 18 in the cat. *Visual Neuroscience, 9*, 21-38.

Newell, A. C., & Whitehead, J. A. (1969). Finite bandwidth, finite amplitude convection. *Journal of Fluid Mechanics, 38*, 279-303.

Niebur, E., Schuster, H. G., Kammen, D. M., & Koch, C. (1991). Oscillator-phase coupling for different two-dimensional connectivities. *Physical Review A, 44*, 6895-6904.

Niebur, E., Koch, C., & Rosin, C. (1993). An oscillation-based model for the neuronal basis of attention. *Vision Research, 33*, 2789-2802.

Olami, Z., Feder, H. J. S., & Christensen, K. (1992). Self-organized criticality in a continuous, nonconservative cellular automaton modeling earthquakes. *Physical Review Letters, 68*, 1244-1247.

Sanes, J. N., & Donoghue, J. P. (1993). Oscillations in local-field potentials of the primate motor cortex during voluntary movement. *Proceedings of the National Academy of Sciences, 90,* 4470-4474.

Singer, W., (1993). Synchronization of cortical activity and its putative role in information-processing and learning. *Annual Review of Physiology, 55,* 349-374.

Softky, W. R., & Koch, C. (1993). The highly irregular firing of cortical cells is inconsistent with temporal integration of random EPSPs. *Journal of Neuroscience, 13,* 334-350.

Somers, D. C., Nelson, S. B., & Sur, M. (1995). An emergent model of visual cortical orientation selectivity. *Journal of Neuroscience, 13,* 5448-5465.

Stemmler, M., Usher, M., & Niebur, E. (1995). Lateral interactions in primary visual cortex: A model bridging physiology and psychophysics. *Science, 269,* 1877-1880.

Tovee, M. J., & Rolls, E. T. (1992). Oscillatory activity is not evident in the primate temporal visual-cortex with static stimuli. *Neuroreport, 3,* 369-372.

Toyama, K., Kimura, M., & Tanaka, K. (1981). Organization of cat visual cortex as investigated by cross-correlation technique. *Journal of Neurophysiology, 46,* 202-214.

Treves, A. (1993). Mean-field analysis of neuronal spike dynamics. *Network: Computation in Neural Systems, 4,* 259-284.

Tsodyks, M., Mitkov, I., & Sompolinsky, H. (1993). Pattern of synchrony in inhomogeneous networks of oscillators with pulse interactions. *Physical Review Letters, 71,* 1280-1283.

Usher, M., Stemmler, M., Koch, C., & Olami, Z. (1994). Network amplification of local fluctuations causes high spike rate variability, fractal firing patterns, and oscillatory local field potentials. *Neural Computation, 6,* 795-836.

Usher, M., Stemmler, M., & Olami, Z. (1995). Dynamic pattern formation leads to 1/f noise in neural populations. *Physical Review Letters, 74,* 326-329.

Wilson, H. R., & Cowan, J. D. (1972). Excitatory and inhibitory interactions in localized populations of model neurons. *Biophysical Journal, 12,* 1-24.

Wilson, M. A., & Bower, J. M. (1991). A computer simulation of oscillatory behavior in primary visual cortex. *Neural Computation, 3,* 498-509.

Wörgötter, F., Niebur, E., & Koch, C. (1991). Isotropic connections generate functional asymmetrical behavior in visual cortical cells. *Journal of Neurophysiology, 66,* 444-459.

Young, M. P., Tanaka, K., & Yamane, S. (1992). Oscillatory neuronal responses in the visual cortex of the monkey. *Journal of Neurophysiology, 67,* 1464-1474.

5

Computations Neurons Perform in Networks: Inside Versus Outside and Lessons Learned From a Sixteenth-Century Shoemaker

George J. Mpitsos and John P. Edstrom
Oregon State University

(Originally published in: *International Journal of Computing Anticipatory Systems Vol 2* (1998). Ed. by D. M. Dubois, Published by CHAOS, Liège, Belgium, pp. 327-340. ISSN 1373-5411. ISBN 2-9600179-2-7.)

ABSTRACT

Cognitive and other neural processes emerge from the interactions between neurons. Major advances have been made in studying networks in which the interactions occur instantaneously by means of graded synapses (Guckenheimer & Rowat, 1997). In other networks, the interaction between neurons involve time-delayed signals (action potentials or spikes) that activate synapses on other neurons discontinuously in a pulse-like manner. These interactions can also be treated as being graded if, when appropriate, the information transmitted between neurons can be measured as the average number of spikes per unit time (Freeman, 1992); that is, the amount of information carried by individual spikes is relatively low. We refer to both of these types of interactions as "graded." There is a large armamentarium of mathematical and dynamical systems tools for studying the computations that such neurons perform. There is also a complementary connection between these tools and biological experimentation.

The subject of the present chapter is on networks in which averaging cannot be done. The generation of spikes in these neurons is significantly affected by the temporal order of spikes sent to them by other neurons. Two input spike trains, having the same average spikes per unit time but different temporal spacing between the spikes, produce different outputs in target neurons; that is, the amount of information carried by individual spikes is relatively high. We refer to these networks as "spike-activated." By comparison to graded networks, there is little formal or experimental work on the general principles underlying these networks.

There are many nonlinear physiological processes in spike-activated networks that need to be considered. We have begun by focusing on a single nonlinearity analysis, the threshold transition between spiking and nonspiking behavior, and use linear perturbation to examine it. The findings indicate that there may be an epistemological division between graded networks and spike-activated networks. This is reminiscent of the distinction between endophysics and exophysics whose resolution requires an external observer having information about a system and its external universe (Rössler, 1989). Interestingly, the philosophical roots of our approach and the study of dynamics more generally may be traceable to Jacob Böhme (1575-1624), a mystic and contemporary of Descartes. Böhme influenced many philosophers and scientists, and may have provided Isaac Newton the metaphorical insight into his laws of physics (Mpitsos, 1995; Yates, 1972, 1979).

1. INTRODUCTION: TWO TYPES OF BIOLOGICAL NEURAL NETWORKS

Neural systems are hierarchies of interconnected neurons. A great deal of information exists about the anatomic details of these connections (synapses), about the physiology of single neurons, and the chemistry of the synapses. But these important facts describe how networks are built, not how they behave.

Much of the commerce between neurons occurs by means of electrical signals. In neurons, as in all living cells, an electrical potential difference of roughly -70 mV exists across the membrane between the inside and outside of the cell. In neurons, this potential may be endogenously oscillating or it may be induced to change by means of some external influence, which may be the input from another neuron via a synapse. For the purposes of this discussion, consider that there are two broad categories of networks. In one, the synapses are activated instantaneously by graded voltage changes between the neurons. These changes may be chemical (chemotonic) or electrical (electrotonic); some neurons receive both types. Much of the dynamics of how activity emerges in networks can be analyzed (at least numerically) using similar methods as used to analyze systems of differential equations used to model single neurons (Harris-Warrick, Coniglio, Barazangi, Guckenheimer, & Gueron, 1995; Hodgkin & Huxley, 1952; Rinzel & Ermentrout, 1989; Rowat & Selverston, 1997). We shall refer to these as "graded-synapse networks" or "graded networks." Much of what is known about the dynamics of their activity has come from studying the autonomous activity of single model neurons.

In other types of networks, neurons do not interact by means of graded fluctuations in their membrane potential, but by a rapid, regenerative process that propagates along the length (axon) of the neuron. At each successive region of the cell, the membrane potential first rises toward or above zero (depolarizes) and then recovers (repolarizes) toward its original "resting" potential until perturbed by some extrinsic or intrinsic process. Because of the quickness of the depolarizing and repolarizing phases, the process is often referred to as the neuron "firing" action potentials or spikes. These spikes propagate along the axon until they reach the terminus. At this point, the spike-related voltage initiates a series of events that release a neurotransmitter. The transmitter attaches to receptors sites on the postsynaptic neuron which open or close channels controlling the discharge of ionic batteries across the cell membrane. If the current raises the membrane potential above a threshold, the postsynaptic neuron also fires one or more spikes.

An understanding of the dynamical principles underlying the activity in such networks has been more problematic than in graded systems. One can numerically integrate the model equations that describe each neuron and its synapses to observe the activity in the network. Important phenomenological information has been obtained in this way, and in equivalent experiments in real neurons. Because of the discontinuous, spike-activated nature of the interactions it has been difficult to understand the dynamics analytically or numerically in a way that provides generally applicable principles. An approach, justified by experimental evidence, is to bypass the effects produced by individual spikes by using average firing rates to describe the output firing of neuron with respect to the firing of its input neuron(s). This approach requires that the relative timing of individual events in a train of spikes carries relatively little information. The dynamics of the activity in the network can then be described using similar mathematics and phase-space analyses as in graded networks (Freeman, 1992). Because of this similarity we shall refer to neuronal interactions in both types of networks as being graded.

Our interest is in networks in which individual spikes carry a significant amount of information such that averaging techniques cannot be used. Studies into these networks must consider the synaptic currents activated by individual spikes. We shall refer to such networks as being *spike-activated.*

The possibility that the specific temporal order in a series of spikes carries important information in neural integration was proposed a long time ago by Lord Adrian (1928, 1946). The idea was significantly advanced in the 1960s and 1970s (Bryant & Segundo, 1976; Segundo, Moore, Stensaas, & Bullock, 1963; Segundo & Perkel, 1969), and has received recent attention in studies of biological and artificial systems (e.g., Judd & Aihara, 1993; Segundo, Stiber, & Vibert, 1993). However, work in spike-activated networks has lagged far behind the work on graded systems.

We believe it is necessary to proceed experimentally in order to obtain insight on how to treat spike-activated networks, but the implication of the results must be applicable to many systems, if any formal understanding is to emerge. The simplicity of the model networks (or more appropriately, network fragments) that we employ (Edstrom & Mpitsos, 1998; Mpitsos & Edstrom, 1998) is forced by the multiplicity of nonlinear processes that occur in even small biological networks. The findings, however, are quite similar to those obtained from very complex biological networks (Mpitsos, Wildering, Hermann, Edstrom, & Bulloch, 1998).

2. MODEL NETWORK AND PERTURBATION METHODS

Network Fragment. The network we use in these initial studies is designed to focus on a single nonlinear process; the threshold between the ability of a neuron to fire a spike and the failure to produce a spike. We use linear perturbation analysis to study how the membrane behaves around this threshold.

The network consists of two neurons (Fig. 5.1), each having a membrane model of the squid giant axon (Hodgkin & Huxley, 1952). This model has voltage-activated conductances for sodium and potassium ions, and a leakage conductance for nonspecific cations. The membrane is normally at rest at its single fixed point attractor. Cell 1 is used to drive an excitatory postsynaptic current (EPSC) in Cell 2. The amplitude of the EPSC raises the membrane potential of Cell 2 slightly above the threshold at which it generates a single spike. The cells are spherical so that the neuron is isopotential. The projection (axon) from Cell 1 to Cell 2 is shown to illustrate the connection between the two cells, but no neuron membrane is included whose responses must be simulated. The activation of the synapse is simply a delay parameter that adjusts the time in the simulations when the EPSC is activated. These simulations consist of 40-msec time sweeps. After each sweep the network is set to the same initial conditions, such that there is no memory of effects produced from one sweep to the next.

The final component of the experimental setup consists of brief current impulses that are used to perturb the EPSC-evoked membrane changes. Two types of current impulses were used, ones that depolarize the membrane toward more positive potentials, and ones that hyperpolarize it toward more negative potentials. The duration of the impulses was the same as the 0.01-msec time step used in the digital integrations, but, as shown below in Fig. 5.2, the membrane response to these impulses lasts far longer.

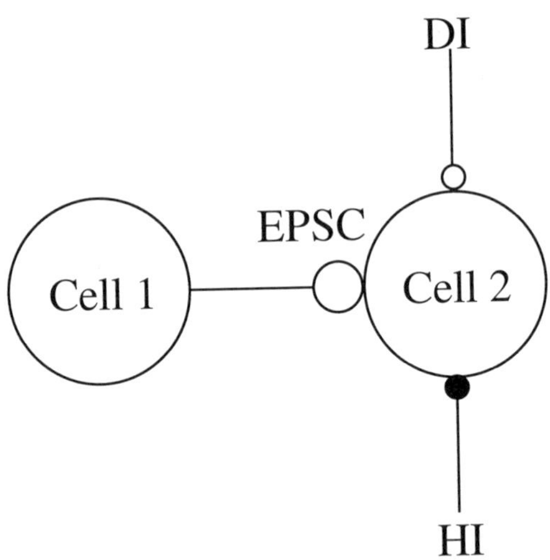

Fig. 5.1. Network fragment.

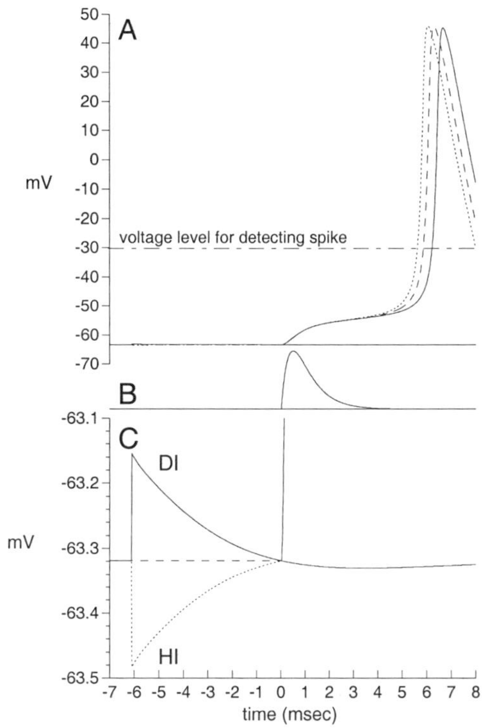

Fig. 5.2. Example perturbations.

We refer to these as depolarizing impulses (DI) and hyperpolarizing impulses (HI), and show them schematically in Fig. 5.1 as small external inputs to Cell 2.

This little network is only a fragment of a network, but it reflects realistic situations where cells are driven by convergent currents of different magnitude. Our approach hinges on the condition that Cell 2 is not autonomously active. It is quiescent until activated by the input currents, and once activated it returns to the resting conditions. The network consists only of feedforward connections because there is no feedback from its output. All we seek to understand here is how the relative timing between the input events (the DI or HI and the temporally fixed EPSC) affect the timing of a spike.

Perturbation of the Spike Threshold Nonlinearity. The perturbation experiments consist of a series of 40-msec simulation sweeps. Three superimposed simulation sweeps are shown in the panels of Fig. 5.2 (15-msec segments are shown to expand the time scale). Panel (B) shows the onset of the EPSC at time zero. The timing of the other events is referenced against the EPSC. Because the EPSC is temporally fixed, all three EPSCs are coincident. Panel (A) shows the three spikes. They are shifted from one another because of differences in the perturbation conditions described next. A quantitative measure of this shift is provided by the spike latency, which we define as the interval between the onset of the EPSC at time zero and the time when the membrane crosses above −30 mV.

Presenting the EPSC by itself produced the spike shown by the long dashes. The other two spikes were obtained by pairing the EPSC with DI (solid trace) or HI (dotted trace). The impulses were presented at about 6 msec before the EPSC. The blow-up in panel C shows the small changes in the membrane potential that the impulses produced. In response to these brief, 0.01-msec impulses, the membrane potential decays slowly. Also shown in the 6 msec preceding the EPSC is the membrane potential when no impulse is presented (horizontal dashed line).

Panel C contains a fourth superimposed trajectory, the membrane potential changes produced by a DI when it was presented in the absence of the EPSC. The initial segment of the trace coincides with the first DI, but extends past time zero, falling below the resting membrane potential and rising again as part of a series of exponentially damped oscillations. Their amplitude depends on the polarization of the membrane and on the amplitude of the perturbing impulse. These oscillations arise from the complex impedance of the squid axon membrane.

Complex Impedance. The complex impedance of the membrane and these oscillations are critical in understanding the computations spike-activated networks perform. There are two conditions that force this requirement: (a) The neuron membrane acts as an electrical circuit composed of resistors, capacitance, and inductance. (b) Such circuits are sensitive to temporally spaced pulses of input currents. As the presentation time of the impulse is varied, the EPSC will encounter different impedances that affect how rapidly the membrane potential crosses the spike-generating threshold, or whether it crosses it at all. Impedance is also important in networks in which neurons communicate by means of chemotonic and electrotonic synapses, but the simplifying factors here are that the communication occurs instantaneously and in a graded fashion. These factors allow for more tractable mathematics and biological experimentation than in spike-activated communication.

3. INPUT-OUTPUT (*I/O*) FUNCTIONS

We can begin to understand how neurons in spike-activated networks respond to and transform their input signals into output spikes by extending the experiments in Fig. 5.2 to obtain a relation between the timing of single input current events and the time (latency) at which the output spike occurs. We refer to these as *i/o functions*.

Figure 5.3 shows the results of four experiments, two in which the EPSC was paired with DI (solid traces) and two in which it was paired with HI (dotted traces). The amplitudes of the two DI were the same as the corresponding two HI impulses. In the region where the dotted curve is broken, the HI completely suppressed spike genesis. The EPSC is included as a reference point to show how the timing of the impulse affects the latency of the spike it produced. The amplitudes of the different phases of the *i/o* functions scale linearly or piecewise linearly with the amplitude of the impulses, and their shape resembles the impulse response function (IRF) that is obtained from the complex impedance (Edstrom & Mpitsos, 1998).

Many-to-One Mapping of the Timing of the Input to the Timing of the Output Spike. It is obvious from the complex shape of the curves that multiple impulse presentation times produce the same output spike latency. A given latency crosses the *i/o* curves at multiple places. However, the uniqueness of the *i/o* mapping in all cases can be shown (and should be expected) by examining the state space of the membrane variables (Edstrom & Mpitsos, 1998; Mpitsos & Edstrom, 1998). The internal state variables are membrane changes relating to the ion conductances. In spike-activated

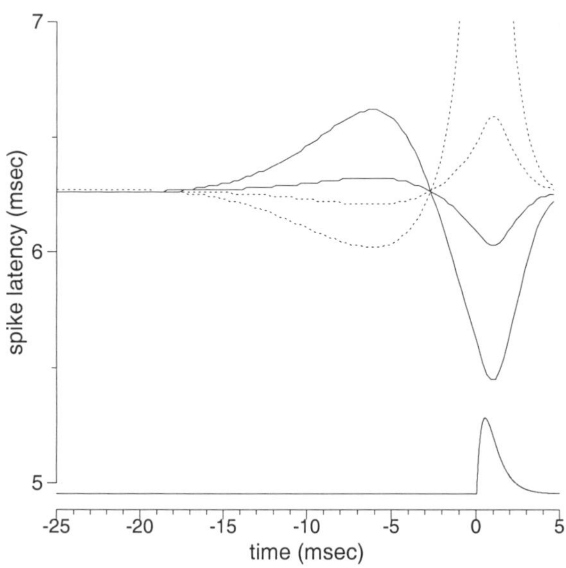

Figure 5.3. Input/output functions.

networks, these internal processes underlie the spikes but their full disclosure remains hidden to other neurons, as shown for example by the fact that different impulse presentation times can lead to the same spike latency. An "all-knowing observer" who has information of the time at which the impulse occurs and of the internal state variables can state precisely when the spike will occur. Conversely, given knowledge of the spike latency and the internal state variables, the observer can state precisely the time at which the impulse was presented. Without information of the internal state variables, such complete *i/o* mapping is not possible. By analogy to the dynamics of quadratic maps, there are multiple temporal preimages for each output spike. Although this is consistent with a deterministic system, it is clear that under the experimental conditions used here, the spike latencies cannot convey information about the exact timing of the events in the input data stream. As all-knowing, external observers, we have the EPSC with which to define absolute time for all events within the system.

Converting Spike Latencies Into "Spike Intervals." As noted earlier, the transfer of information is through the generation of spikes that travel from one neuron to another. An important aspect of this method of communication is presumed to occur by means of the temporal spacing between the spikes. However, our methods involve the generation of only a single spike and the measurement of its latency. The model is not set up to generate trains of spikes in each simulation sweep. We have taken these steps, which initially may seem counterproductive, to create a simplified, controlled environment in which to start the process of resolving the complexity of spike-activated networks. Nonetheless, a type of "spike train sequence" or time series can be constructed from single sweep data. There are two sets of input/output data: (a) The set of times at which the perturbing current impulses are presented in each sweep, and (b) the set of spike latencies that emerge from each sweep. The two sets are in one-to-one registry. We take the impulse presentation series to represent the input spike train and the series of latencies as the output spike train. As in the case of the simplifications used to construct the network in Fig. 5.1, these simplifications yield only a caricature of real spike trains, but we believe that they provide a way to obtain useful information about spike-activated networks that would be difficult to obtain otherwise.

Membrane Filter Properties and the Temporal Order of Input Currents. The shape of the *I/o* functions is independent of the order in which the impulses are presented from one simulation sweep to the next. This is because we reset the membrane to the same initial conditions after each simulation sweep. There is no memory in the membrane of conditions produced by previous simulation sweeps. However, a type of order can be introduced. The experiments are the same as before, except that the signal generator controls the placement of the impulse so that its temporal relation to the EPSC has some order from one simulation sweep to the next. The function we use to generate the placements is the recursive logistic function, $x_{n+1} = k(1-x_n)\,x_n$. The constant can have a value between 0 and 4, and x is between 0 and 1. Setting $k = 3.7$ produces a chaotic regime. The presentation time of the current impulse within the simulation sweep was controlled by scaled values of this function.

Figure 5.4 (A & C) shows the results of two experiments using HI for the perturbations. The same sequence of logistic values (large dots) were used in both. Their presentation times were scaled to fall over different spans of time covered by the fuller *i/o* function (small dots) that was also obtained with the HI. We include the fuller curve only as a landmark to indicate the differences in the placements. It is clear from these curves that the range of output spike latencies is smaller than the range of input times, and because of the differences in the shapes of the *i/o* functions in the two locations, the compression is greater in panel C than in A.

It is not obvious in the *i/o* functions of panels A and C how the membrane impedance affects the dynamics in the long-term correlations of the logistic. These effects can be observed in return maps. These are constructed by the map of one value, x_{n+1}, of the data series against the previous value, x_n, for all values. The results appear in panels B and D for the latencies obtained in A and C, respectively. The return map of the impulse presentation times is the well-known inverted hump or fold of the quadratic map (not shown), but the return map of the spike latencies in panel D has two humps. More interesting is the looped return map in panel B. The overlap is apparent only because the map is a two-dimensional projection of a higher-dimensional map; that is,

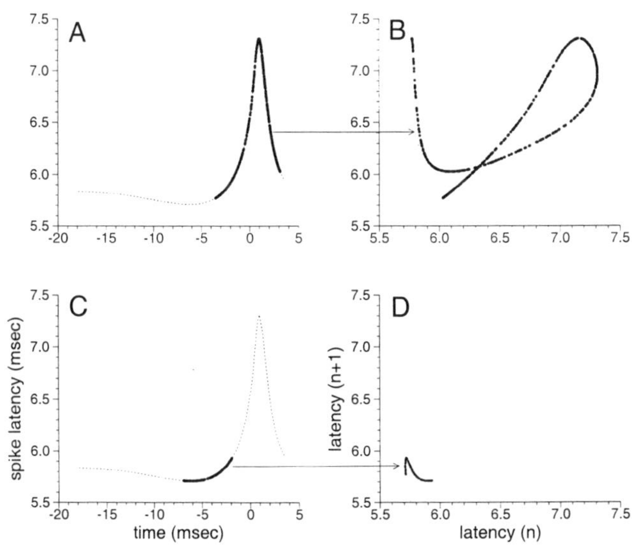

Fig. 5.4. Placement of the same input dynamics on different regions of the *i/o* functions (A & C) induces variable output dynamics (B & D).

there are higher-order (longer-range) correlations in the spike-latency data than are present in the chaotic logistic. The higher-order correlations can be seen in three-dimensional maps, by plotting x_n, x_{n+1}, and x_{n+2} on the three axes shown in Fig. 5.5. Rotating the image uncovers new structure.

Linear low-pass filters, such as the membrane impedance, can increase the dimension of chaotic data by adding the dynamic of the filter to the dynamic of the data (Badii et al., 1988). Here the change is in the embedding dimension; the number of dimensions for viewing the structure of the return map unambiguously. The membrane has not changed the dynamics of the logistic because the logistic receives no feedback from the neuron. The change in the embedding dimension comes from the filter properties of the membrane impedance of Cell 2.

The information Cell 2 adds to the input signal depends on three factors:

(1) The state of the membrane. The *i/o* functions derive from the ion channels whose activation state defines the impedance. For example, by affecting these channels, neuromodulators can affect the membrane impedance and, therefore, change the information that a neuron makes public.

(2) The relative timing of the input signals. The timing of the input is important because the span of time over which an input signal falls within the range of the *i/o* function (Figs. 5.4 A & C) clearly alters the filter information that a neuron adds to the input signal (Figs. 5.4 B & D). By these differences, impedance can be thought of as storing a wide range of information that can be selectively accessed by the timing of the input over the span of time covered by the *i/o* function.

(3) The information of the input signal that a neuron appears to transmit faithfully has to do with the correlations or dynamics in the signal, not absolute times.

Taken together, these factors suggest that the flow of information in spike-activated networks contains information relating directly to neuronal impedance. The neuron broadcasts the details of its impedance not in ohms, of course, but as bits of information in trains of spikes that we can see geometrically in return maps and compute quantitatively using information theory. One might say that the neuron uses its input signal to add its own "two bits" to the public discussion.

Difficulties in Extending the Experiments Beyond Network Fragments. It is easy to generate *i/o* functions. After dealing with them for a while, it is also easy to see what they mean. For example, the change of shape of the *i/o* function with neuromodulation, noted earlier in (1), is easy to understand because of the simplicity of the experiments of pairing a current impulse with a spike-evoking EPSC, and measuring the spike latency. We are encouraged that the *i/o* functions of the simple model neurons used here may have broader applicability since they resemble *i/o* functions obtained from complex biological neurons (Mpitsos et al., 1998).

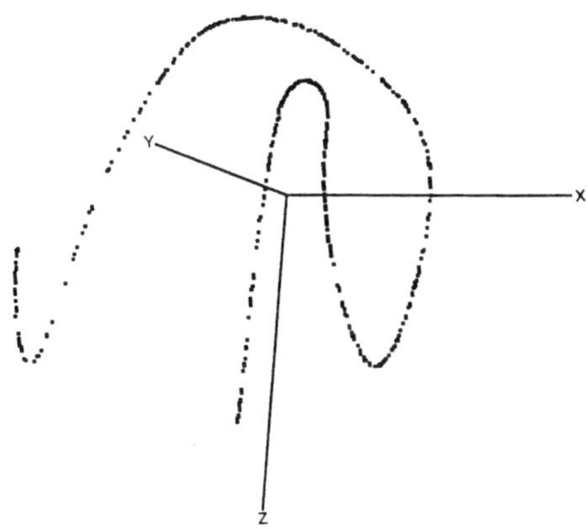

Fig. 5.5. Rotated, 3-D return map of spike latencies shows complex multifolded structure.

Problems arise in extending the approach to more realistic network activity. For example, we refer to the neuron in our simple feedforward network as having filter properties. It does, but they are not the complete filter properties one would expect from a network in which neurons receive feedback of their effect on other neurons. However, within each simulation sweep, the different membrane effects produced by the impulses and the EPSC evoke important features of the membrane filter.

The "relative timing" between input events, noted earlier in (2), is the major culprit behind the problem of implementing the notion of the *i/o* functions in networks with feedback. In our network fragment, the EPSC is the simplifying time mark. We can think of relative timing in a quantitative way, perhaps mathematically, because all else is measured against it. But in a free-running network, events that organize the timing within the network do not necessarily exist. This poses problems in understanding the principles of how even two interconnected neurons work in spike-activated networks. Therefore, our present challenge is to implement the ideas behind the *i/o* functions within a more realistic model involving feedback from temporally unpredictable neurons.

3. DISCUSSION

We have attempted to show how output spike trains that a neuron generates can convey significant but limited information about the temporal structure of input signals. Although the *i/o* transformation is internally completely deterministic, in the absence of information about the internal conductance states the spike latencies appear as degenerate or at least incomplete representations of the signal. Consistent with many other studies, beginning with the seminal work by Segundo and coworkers (Segundo et al., 1963), small input currents can be important to normal function, and in many cases they may be the principal vehicle of information that the system is trying to process. It is clear that a significant feature of the information that is processed has to do with the dynamics of the inputs. Because of the simplifications introduced by the temporally fixed EPSC, it also appears that the specific timing of any event is lost. How this applies to more realistic networks than we have used here is the subject of our present work. Overall, the findings indicate that the membrane is quite sensitive to dynamical structure, the long-term correlations between input events. If this structure exists, it will be transmitted. This agrees with the notion that neurons are analyzers of temporal structure or serial order in spike trains (Segundo & Perkel, 1969). It is interesting that neurons may use (so to speak) the structure of their input dynamics as a carrier of information related to the low-pass filter properties of their membrane impedance.

3.1. Dichotomous Approaches and Concepts: Autonomous Versus *I/o* Functions

We also raised a number of questions or problems relating to the internal-external dichotomy. This dichotomy extends to the way one conceives of neurointegration and the language one uses to describe what neurointegration is. This dichotomy also constrains the types of experiments one performs in search of answers to ultimate questions. In the following subsections, we discuss three issues: mathematics, the observer(s), and the emergence of activity through interactions between internal and external sources in which we give special reference to Jacob Böhme.

Mathematics. In studies of neurointegration, the focus is on the mathematics of differential equations and the dynamics of autonomous systems. When relating neuronal dynamics to single-cell conductances, the attention has been mainly on single unconnected cells or on networks of continuously coupled neurons that share many of the same analytical features of analyses used on single cells. In these cases the neuron is a generator of information. The dynamics are wholly within the system itself and the evolution of the system is specified by its initial conditions. The description involves inspecting the attractor associated with those conditions and using phase spaces constructed strictly from the private, internal parameters. Similar approaches have been applied in networks in which spike firing can be averaged.

In spike-activated systems there is not much of a formal framework, nor even of conceptual constructs, with which to begin to establish experimental hypotheses that might lead to unifying constructs. Mathematics will be important, but whereas growth in continuous systems already has a long period of development, growth in the understanding of spike-activated networks lags far behind. Moreover, the implications of the mathematics may be different. The two approaches are complementary, but where one deals with the mathematics of internal conductances, the other must deal with the biology of how neurons transform the language of the external world. The first has to do with activity, whereas the second has to do with communication, flexible interpretation, and transformation.

In our case, the evolution of the neuron or the network as a whole is not specified by the initial conditions of the neuron nor by the strengths of its synaptic connections to extrinsic influences. The features and contingencies of our system are as follows:

(1) The evolution is contingent on the dynamics of the driving function. Whatever it is, it is not a structural property of the neuron, its afferent synapses, or any part of the local fragment of the network we look at.

(2) In fact, the one structural feature of our neuron is its *i/o* functions. For a given internal state, these are always the same, regardless of the driving function.

(3) The structure of the input signal is encoded by the difference between the time of the impulse and the time of the EPSC. Even here there are contingent aspects of the input that are not fixed locally, such as the temporal scope, the width and offset of the projection onto the *i/o* function (as in Fig. 5.4). These are determined by the correlation of the firing in the two input sources for the impulse and the EPSC, and by the afferent anatomy, such as conduction distances and the relative conduction velocities.

(4) The output has no fixed or single interpretation. It can be read in different ways by different observers. An observer can:

(a) ignore the structure and treat it as a dumb signal; for example, as firing rate, or as a semaphore ("Hey! Something just happened here.")
(b) read the filter function if the input structure is also known to the observer.
(c) recover the input structure, if the filter function is also known.
(d) treat it as a new source of information without caring about the input function or the neuron impedance.

The hallmark of an adaptive system is its ability to cope with or adapt to as many environmental conditions as possible; that is, on its ability to be multifunctional, to *ad lib*, such that a response that might seem "error-prone" in one context becomes adaptive in another (Mpitsos, 1989, 1998; Mpitsos & Cohan, 1986a, 1986b; Mpitsos & Soinila, 1992; Soinila & Mpitsos, 1991). By being transformers of information, spike-activated systems seem to be highly attuned to such flexibility.

Who Is the External Observer? As noted previously, the definition of spike latency, the resolution of the apparent degeneracy in the *i/o* functions and the definition of information require an all-knowing external observer that can see different aspects of the circuit. Individual neurons are internal to the network and cannot make such network-wide distinctions based only on afferent spike trains. The important question is whether evolution has devised network analogs of external observers. This may be the crucial step where "network consciousness" first rears its ugly head.

Jacob Böhme's Hammer and Bell, and Metaphysical Equivalents of Outside and Inside. Dalenoort and de Vries (1994, p. 111) assert "that all properties emerge from interactions." The aim of the work reported here has been to begin the study of what is it that neurons do when they interact; how they respond to and interpret afferent signals through the impedance filter. Neurons are "fair arbiters" because they transmit the dynamics of the extrinsic arguments they receive along with their own internal conductance states. It appears that the inherent separation between opposites, the separation between internal and external sources of information, renders spike-activated systems necessarily flexible. A neuron will express its membrane-stored information differently depending on how the input signals address it (Fig. 5.4).

This flexible interpretive interaction between opposites is what Jacob Böhme saw so clearly. He was neither a mathematician nor an academic philosopher, but it may well be that the development of modern philosophical thought on dynamics can be traced to him, certainly on the inherent dialect in dynamics. He viewed all material and spiritual existence, including ultimate Being, as the manifestation of an unstable dialectic between polar opposites in which the system and its world continually redefine themselves. Böhme deeply understood this movable tension between endo- and exosystems and expressed it metaphorically in theosophic terms that were probably more understandable in his culture than in ours.

Hidden in the density of Böhme's writing, one finds what might be his only humorous, though meaningful, comment: *Understanding occurs when one person has the hammer to ring another person's bell.* In contemporary language, understanding between two people occurs when they both already have similar internal (dynamical) representations of knowledge. We might think of these representations as attractors (Cohen & Grossberg, 1983; Freeman & Skarda, 1990; Mpitsos, Burton, Creech, & Soinila, 1988a; Mpitsos & Cohan, 1986a, 1986b; Mpitsos, Creech, Cohan, & Mendelson, 1988; Skarda & Freeman, 1987).

Böhme's comment has meaning at different levels in the dialectic between internal and external worlds. The hammer (external world) and the bell (internal world) have different intrinsic characteristics. These internal and external representations can never be the same over time. This is also because the result of the interaction has yet another characteristic, sound, the cognitive reply to the source that sent the hammer. Sound introduces qualities that are different from hammer and bell. With each interaction, sound emerges as a new "hammer" to strike the other person's bell, and so forth, as the interaction continues. The transfer of information within this universe is incomplete, unless an all-knowing observer provides the missing elements. Neither person has complete knowledge of the other.

In our open-loop model, the one structural feature or "bell" is the *i/o* function. The "hammer" is the extrinsic input signal provided by the impulses. How the bell responds depends on how and where the hammer hits it (Fig. 5.4). As the membrane changes through learning or neuromodulation, the network gains new dynamics and functional fluidity.

Böhme came from an era foreign to us, but as we strive to understand adaptive systems we begin to understand a little of what he might have experienced. Böhme's vision implicitly included multiple, interdependent layers of dialectic interactions between primordial substances and all creation. This universe is always under perturbation, and the dialectic dynamic is unlikely to resolve into a stable synthesis.

Böhme's impact has been broadly discussed. It may have been Newton's genius to transform Böhme's dense, seminal cogitations into useful mathematical terms and concepts (Yates, 1972, 1979). Our own "byte-size" summary of his ideas is *for every action there is a reaction*, Newton's third law, and the embodiment of dialectic interaction (Mpitsos, 1995). William Law (1686-1761) spoke with more than a little irony when he said, "When Sir Isaac brought forth his laws, he plowed with Böhme's heifer"(see the URL in Mpitsos, 1995).

Four hundred years later, we, too, plow with Böhme's heifer. The self-organization of neural activity has been viewed as a dialectic between neurons and between the animal and its environment, to grasp how error-prone behavior might prove useful in allowing a given network to be adaptively multifunctional and how the vast complexity of neuromodulation takes part in the process (Mpitsos, 1989, 1998; Mpitsos & Cohan, 1986a, 1986b; Mpitsos & Soinila, 1993; Soinila & Mpitsos, 1992).

Physics was not Böhme's goal, nor perhaps Newton's, and, ultimately, the understanding of adaptive behavior of complex systems is probably not ours. One wonders whether Böhme's striving was also an attempt to define himself and to understand his place in the universe. At least in Western minds, there is always the quest for an ultimate observer who can answer our questions. The dichotomy between inside and outside seems inescapable.

'Is my team plowing
    That I used to drive
And hear the harness jingle
    When I was man alive'?

Ay, the horses trample,
    The harness jingles now;
No change though you lie under
    The land you used to plow.

'Is football playing
    Along the river shore
With lads to chase the leather
    Now I stand up no more'?

Ay, the ball is flying,
The lads play heart and soul;
The goal stands up, the keeper
Stands up to keep the goal.

⋮

(A. E. Housman, *Is My Team Plowing?*)

ACKNOWLEDGMENT

This work was supported by ONR Grant N00014-95-1-0681

REFERENCES

Adrian, E. D. (1928). *The Basis of Sensation*. New York: Norton.

Adrian, E. D. (1946). *The Physical Background of Perception*. Oxford: Clarendon Press.

Badii, R., Broggi, G., Derighetti, B., Ravani, M., Ciliberto, A., Politi, A., & Rubio, M. A. (1988). Dimension increase in filtered chaotic signals. *Physical Review Letters*, *60*, 979.

Böhme, J. (1575-1624). *Six Theosophic Points and Other Writings with an Introductory Essay by Nicolas Berdyaev*. Ann Arbor: University of Michigan Press.

Bryant, H. L., & Segundo, J. P. (1976). Spike initiation by transmembrane current: A white-noise analysis. *Journal of Physiology*, *260*, 279-314.

Cohen, M. A., & Grossberg, S. (1983). Absolute stability of global pattern formation and parallel memory storage by competitive neural networks. *IEEE Transactions on Systems, Man, and Cybernetics*, *13*, 815-826.

Dalenoort, G. J., & de Vries, P. H. (1994). Internal and external representations of mental processes. In H. Atmanspacher & G. J. Dalenoort (Eds.), *Inside Versus Outside: Endo- and Exo-Concepts of Observation and Knowledge in Physics, Philosophy, and Cognitive Science*. Berlin: Springer-Verlag.

Edstrom, J. L., & Mpitsos, G. L. (1998). Relating linear membrane impedance to the timing between input currents and output action potentials in a model neuron. Submitted to *Biological Cybernetics*.

Freeman, W. J. (1992). Tutorial on neurobiology: From single neurons to brain chaos. *Journal of Bifurcation and Chaos*, *2*, 451-482.

Freeman, W. J., & Skarda, C. A. (1990). John Searle and his critics. In E. Lepore & R. van Gulick (Eds.), *Mind/Brain Science: Neuroscience on Philosophy of Mind* (pp. 115-127). Oxford: Blackwell.

Guckenheimer, J., & Rowat, P. F. (1997). Dynamical systems analyses of real neuronal networks. In P. S. G. Stein, S. Grillner, A. I. Selverston, & D. G. Stuart (Eds.), *Neurons, Networks, and Motor Behavior* (pp. 151-163).

Harris-Warrick, R., Coniglio, L., Barazangi, N., Guckenheimer, J., & Gueron, S. (1995). Dopamine modulation of transient potassium current evokes shifts in a central pattern generator network. *Journal of Neuroscience*, *15*, 342-358.

Hodgkin, A. L., & Huxley, A. F. (1952). A quantitative description of membrane current and its application to conduction and excitation in nerve. *Journal of Physiology*, *117*, 500-544.

Judd, K. T., & Aihara, K. (1993). Pulse propagation networks: A neural network model that uses temporal coding of action potentials. *Neural Networks*, *6*, 203-216.

Law, W. (1686-1761). *A Serious Call to a Devout and Holy Life — The Spirit of Love*. New York: Paulist Press.

Mpitsos, G. J. (1989). Chaos in brain function and the problem of nonstationarity: A commentary. In E. Basar & T. H. Bullock (Eds.), *Dynamics of Sensory and Cognitive Processing by the Brain* (pp. 521-535). New York: Springer-Verlag.

Mpitsos, G. J. (1995). *Newton's heifer: From metaphor to mechanism*. In the URL http://www.hmsc.orst.edu/~gmpitsos/papers/Böhme_on_Newton/bn.html. From an invited letter to the Society for Chaos Theory in Psychology and the Life Sciences.

Mpitsos, G. J. (1998). Attractor gradients: Architects of network organization. In J. L. Leonard, *Identified Neurons: Twenty-Five Years of Progress*, in press. Cambridge, MA: Harvard University Press.

Mpitsos, G. J., Burton, R. M., Creech, H. C., & Soinila, S. O. (1988). Evidence for chaos in spike trains of neurons that generate rhythmic motor patterns. *Brain Research Bulletin*, *21*, 529-538.

Mpitsos, G. J., & Cohan, C. S. (1986a). Comparison of differential Pavlovian conditioning in whole animals and physiological preparations of *Pleurobranchaea*: Implications of motor pattern variability. *Journal of Neurobiology*, *17*, 498-516.

Mpitsos, G. J., & Cohan, C. S. (1986b). Convergence in a distributed motor system: Parallel processing and self-organization. *Journal of Neurobiology*, *17*, 517-545.

Mpitsos, G. J., Creech, H. C., Cohan, C. S., & Mendelson, M. (1988). Variability and chaos: Neurotransmitter principles in self-organization of motor patterns. In J. A. S. Kelso, A. J. Mandell, & M. F. Shlesinger (Eds.), *Dynamic Patterns in Complex Systems* (pp. 162-190). Singapore: World Scientific.

Mpitsos, G. J., & Edstrom, J. P. (1998). Computations neurons perfrom in networks: Viewing impedance as information in spike-train timing. Submitted to *Biological Cybernetics*.

Mpitsos, G. J., & Soinila, S. (1992). In search of a unified theory of biological organization: What does the motor system of a sea slug tell us about human motor integration. In L. Nadel & D. L. Stein (Eds.), *1991 Lectures in Complex Systes, SFI Studies in the Sciences of Complexity*, Vol. 4 (pp. 67-137). Santa Fe: Addison-Wesley.

Mpitsos, G. J., Wildering, W. C., Hermann, P., Edstrom, J., & Bulloch, A. G. M. (1998). Relating the timing of input currents with the latency of action potentials in cultured neurons of the pond snail *Lymnaea stagnalis*. Submitted to *Biological Cybernetics*.

Rinzel, J., & Ermentrout, B. (1989). Analysis of neural excitability and oscillations. In C. Koch & I. Segev (Eds.), *Methods in Neuronal Modeling* (pp. 135-169). Cambridge, MA: MIT Press.

Rössler, O. E. (1989). Explicit observers. In P. J. Plath (Ed.), *Optimal Structures in Homogeneous Reaction Systems* (pp. 123-138). Berlin: Springer-Verlag.

Rowat, P. F., & Selverston, A. I. (1997). Oscillatory mechanisms in pairs of neurons connected with fast inhibitory synapses. *Journal of Computational Neuroscience*, *4*, 103-127.

Segundo, J. P., Moore, G. P., Stensaas, L. J., & Bullock, T. H. (1963). Sensitivity of neurones in *Aplysia* to temporal pattern of arriving impulses. *Journal of Experimental Biology*, *40*, 643-667.

Segundo, J. P., & Perkel, D. H. (1969). The nerve cell as an analyzer of spike trains. *UCLA Forum in Medical Science*, *11*, 349-389.

Segundo, J. P., Stiber, M., & Vibert, J. F. (1993). *Synaptic coding by spike trains*. Nagoya, Japan: ICNN, 7-21.

Skarda, C., & Freeman, W. J. (1987). How brains make chaos to make sense of the world. *The Behavioral and Brain Sciences*, *10*, 161-195.

Yates, F. A. (1972). *The Rosicrucian Enlightenment*. London: Routledge and Kegan Paul.

Yates, F. A. (1979). *The Occult Philosophy in the Elizabethan Age*. London: Routledge and Kegan Paul.

II

Oscillations in Cortical and Cortical/Subcortical Systems

6

The Interplay of Intrinsic and Synaptic Membrane Currents in Delta, Theta, and 40-Hz Oscillations

Ivan Soltesz
University of California, Irvine

ABSTRACT

The mammalian central nervous system displays several electroencephalographic (EEG) rhythms that differ in their frequencies, behavioral correlates and in the neuronal mechanisms that are responsible for their generation. In this chapter I concentrate on the role of intrinsic properties and synaptic inputs underlying the rich repertoire of electrical behaviors exhibited by neurons in thalamocortical and cortico-hippocampal circuits. It will be shown that although the basic delta oscillation of thalamocortical neurons is generated by the interplay of two intrinsic inward currents, the activity patterns observed in these cells either in wakefulness or in sleep, in physiological states as well as in pathological conditions, are more than the simple expression of the intrinsic membrane conductances of neurons. Indeed, synaptic potentials (either rhythmic or randomly occurring) and different transmitters modulate, abolish, and sometimes are fully responsible for the occurrence of specific electrical activity patterns. In contrast to thalamocortical cells, pharmacologically or physically isolated hippocampal neurons are not capable of exhibiting membrane potential oscillations. In hippocampal principal cells it is the synaptic inputs that play the major role in the generation of electrical rhythms such as the hippocampal theta and 40-Hz oscillations. However, intrinsic currents can modulate the synaptically driven hippocampal theta oscillations. Finally, I discuss some of the available evidence and recent hypotheses for the functional roles of neuronal oscillations, and for the roles of rhythmic as well as random synaptic events which bombard neuronal membranes at particular frequencies.

1. INTRODUCTION

Oscillations in neuronal networks of the mammalian central nervous system occur at frequencies ranging from less then 1 Hz to more than 200 Hz. How are such varied electrical behaviors generated? What is the role of single cells versus connectivity in generating synchronized oscillations in the brain? What is the relative importance of the intrinsic membrane conductances of neurons versus the barrage of rhythmic or nonrhythmic synaptic inputs that neurons receive? To answer these questions we have been conducting intracellular and extracellular electrophysiological recordings from neurons *in vivo* as well as in *in vitro* slices. Two different neuronal systems were investigated, the thalamocortical system, which generates various sleep rhythms including the spindle oscillations and the delta waves, and the hippocampal network, which exhibits the theta rhythm and the fast, 40-Hz oscillations. These neuronal rhythms are all recordable *in vivo* with large extracellular EEG electrodes, reflecting the synchronized activity of a large number of neurons. Detailed intracellular studies revealed that, whereas the low-frequency delta oscillations observable in thalamocortical cells are generated by the interplay of two inward currents (Leresche, Jassik-Gerschenfeld, Haby, Soltesz, & Crunelli, 1990; Leresche, Lightowler, Soltesz, Jassik-Gerschenfeld, & Crunelli, 1991; McCormick & Pape, 1990a; Nuñez, Amzica, & Steriade,1992; Soltesz, Lightowler, Leresche, Jassik-Gerschenfeld, Pollard, & Crunelli, 1991), and are modulated, phase reset and synchronized by synaptic inputs (Nuñez et al., 1992; Soltesz & Crunelli, 1992), the hippocampal theta and 40-Hz oscillations are generated by the rhythmic synaptic inputs themselves, and intrinsic currents play only modulatory roles (Soltesz & Deschênes, 1993; Ylinen et al., 1995). These recent data about the cellular mechanisms underlying neuronal oscillations and the role of synaptic inputs in generating and synchronizing brain waves make it possible to gain a better understanding of the emergence, modulation, and the behavioral state-dependence of neuronal electrical activities in both physiological and pathological conditions.

2. LOW-FREQUENCY OSCILLATIONS OF THALAMOCORTICAL NEURONS

Neurons in the thalamus that project to the cortex (thalamocortical or TC cells) exhibit two basic modes of action potential firing (Andersen & Andersson, 1968; Steriade, Jones, & Llinas, 1990). One occurs most often during wakefulness and rapid-eye-movement (REM) sleep, and is characterized by tonic firing. The other is burst firing, when clusters of high frequency (intraburst frequency: 100 to 450 Hz) discharge of action potentials can be observed. Burst firing predominantly occurs during the deep stages of slow-wave sleep. It is interesting to note that in some pathological states, such as absence epilepsy and Parkinson's disease, burst firing is present during wakefulness also (Buzsáki, Smith, Berger, Fisher, & Gage, 1990; Gloor & Fariello, 1988). In the last few years a large amount of experimental data has been obtained which shed light on the biophysical and synaptic mechanisms underlying the burst firing characteristic of TC cells, and the relative importance of intrinsic membrane conductances versus extrinsic (i.e., synaptic) inputs.

The most commonly observed low-frequency oscillation in TC cells in *in vitro* slices is the pacemaker (also known as the delta) oscillations. The pacemaker oscillations are characterized by the rhythmic occurrence of large-amplitude (10 to 25 mV) low-threshold Ca^{++} spikes at 0.5 to 4 Hz (Leresche et al., 1991; McCormick & Pape, 1990a); (Fig. 6.1(A)). Importantly, each low-threshold Ca^{++} spike (Deschênes, Paradis,

Roy, & Steriade, 1984; Jahnsen & Llinas, 1984a, 1984b) can evoke a burst of action potentials. The low-threshold Ca^{++} spikes appear as large depolarizations, and are mediated by the activation of the low-threshold Ca^{++} current, I_T (Coulter, Huguenard & Prince, 1989; Crunelli, Lightowler, & Pollard, 1989; Suzuki & Rogawski, 1989). Following each low-threshold spike, a hyperpolarization-activated, mixed Na^+/K^+ current, I_H (McCormick & Pape, 1990a, 1990b; Soltesz et al., 1991), generates a slow depolarization, as indicated in Fig. 6.1(A). The slow depolarization serves as the pacemaker potential, which brings the membrane potential back to the threshold for

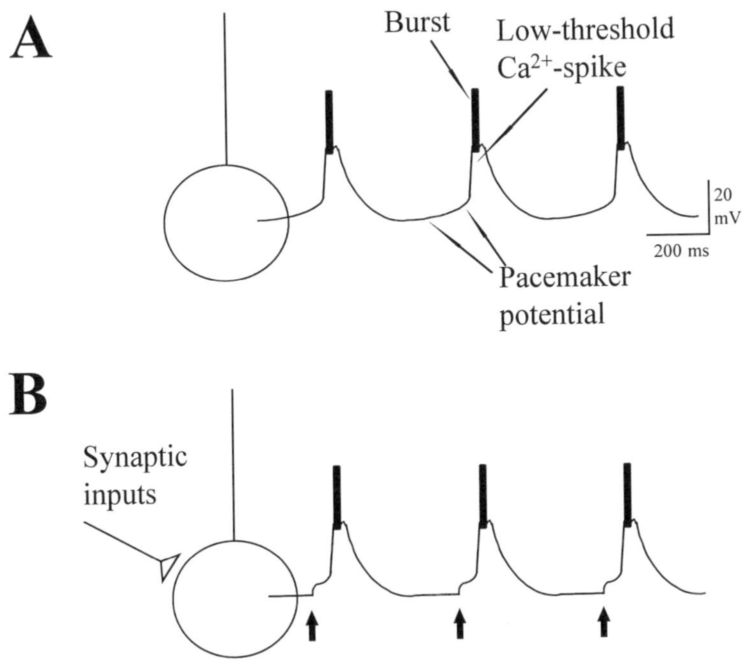

Fig. 6.1. Thalamocortical (TC) cells display two basic forms of low-frequency oscillations. A. The pacemaker oscillations are generated by the interplay of two intrinsic currents, the low-threshold Ca^{++} current I_T and the hyperpolarization-activated depolarizing current I_H. The pacemaker oscillations are present even after pharmacological disconnection of the cells from each other (e.g., in the presence of tetrodotoxin, which blocks the bursts of action potentials but leaves the underlying oscillation intact). Although all TC cells have I_T and I_H, not all can oscillate in the pacemaker mode. In order to illustrate the main points better, in this and all subsequent figures schematic drawings of the neuronal activities are presented. Consequently, the time- and voltage-scales are approximate. For raw data and details, see references in the text. B. Nonoscilllating cells can be driven to oscillate by rhythmic synaptic inputs (Soltesz & Crunelli, 1992). Clearly, these synaptically driven delta oscillations are blocked by tetrodotoxin. Such synaptic synchronizing influence may originate from the cortex, the reticularis thalami, and from those relatively few thalamocortical dLGN neurons which possess local collaterals.

de-inactivation of I_T and brings about the occurrence of the low-threshold spike. Detailed biophysical studies have shown that the pacemaker oscillations can be fully accounted for by the interplay of these two inward currents, I_T and I_H (McCormick & Pape, 1990a; Soltesz et al., 1991). Importantly, delta membrane potential oscillations in single neurons can occur even in the presence of tetrodotoxin, a blocker of Na^+ channels and action potentials, indicating that currents intrinsic to the cell are responsible for these oscillations (Leresche et al., 1991).

However, *in vivo*, as well as *in vitro*, TC cells receive synaptic inputs. These synaptic inputs can be glutamatergic (e.g., sensory and cortical afferents), GABAergic (e.g., from interneurons or from neurons of the nucleus reticularis thalami), and they can also be serotonergic, histaminergic, or noradrenergic. Synaptic inputs influence low-frequency oscillations in a variety of ways. Because a prerequisite of the pacemaker oscillations is that the I_T and I_H are finely tuned in their amplitudes and kinetics (e.g., an excessive I_H would depolarize the cell and bring the membrane potential out of the oscillatory range); (Soltesz et al., 1991), it is not surprising that some of the TC cells do not exhibit pacemaker oscillations. On the other hand, rhythmic synaptic inputs, originating from either the corticothalamic feedback, the nucleus reticularis or from those oscillating TC cells that possess intranuclear axon collaterals, can help nonoscillating TC cells to exhibit pacemaker oscillations (Fig. 6.1(B)); (Nuñez et al., 1992; Soltesz & Crunelli, 1992). Such synaptically driven oscillations require rhythmic input from other neurons, and they can be blocked by tetrodotoxin or antagonists of glutamate receptors, and thus differ fundamentally from the "true" pacemaker oscillations (Soltesz & Crunelli, 1992), which result from the interaction of membrane currents intrinsic to the recorded cell and cannot be blocked by tetrodotoxin or glutamate receptor antagonists. In the cases of driven oscillations, synaptic inputs are actually necessary for the pacemaker oscillations to occur.

Another important example of synaptic inputs to TC cell is the noradrenergic input. Noradrenaline, via the activation of beta adrenergic receptors, increases I_H, and results in the augmentation of the frequency of the pacemaker oscillations (Fig. 6.2(A)). Higher concentration of noradrenaline, however, activates I_H to the point where it can bring the membrane potential out of the oscillatory range by its depolarizing influence, and can stop the pacemaker oscillation (Fig. 6.2(B)); (McCormick & Pape, 1990b; Soltesz et al., 1991). Such a mechanism may be responsible for the arousing action of noradrenaline during the transition from sleep to wakefulness.

Interestingly, synaptic events can also reset the phase of pacemaker oscillations (Soltesz & Crunelli, 1992), in a manner similar to the phase resetting mechanisms described in the heart (Jalife & Antzelevitch, 1979). Moreover, our experiments also demonstrated that an appropriately timed single, relatively small and short intracellular depolarizing current pulse of a critical amplitude and duration, mimicking excitatory postsynaptic potentials, can stop the pacemaker oscillation (Fig. 6.2(C)), provided the current pulse arrives at one sensitive point during the cycle (Soltesz & Crunelli, 1992). Such synaptic events reaching the cell at the sensitive point during the cycle may come into play and contribute to the end of pacemaker oscillations when there is a sudden barrage of synaptic inputs, for example, during increased sensory activity at the transition from sleep to wakefulness.

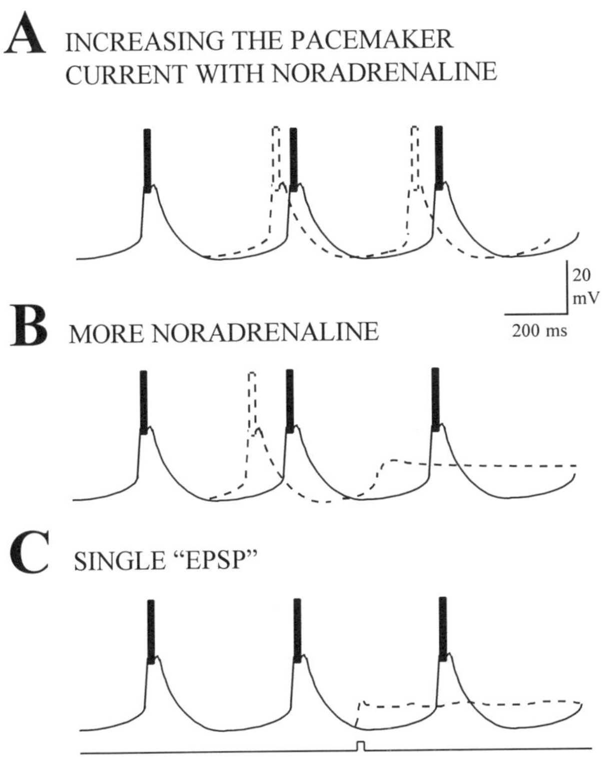

Fig. 6.2. Modulation of pacemaker oscillations. A. Noradrenaline (bath applied, in the presence of α-receptor blockers), potentiates the pacemaker current and increases the frequency of the oscillation (McCormick & Pape, 1990a, 1990b; Soltesz et al., 1991). B. Increasing the dose of noradrenaline blocks the oscillation by bringing the cell's membrane potential out of the oscillatory voltage range. Such mechanisms may come into play during arousal. C. Single, fast EPSPs are capable of resetting the phase of the oscillations (detailed in Soltesz & Crunelli, 1992), and a stimulus of critical amplitude and duration, applied at a particular phase during the cycle, can also abolish the oscillation.

3. THE THETA RHYTHM AND THE 40-HZ OSCILLATIONS IN THE HIPPOCAMPUS

The largest and one of the most regular EEG rhythms of the entire brain is the hippocampal theta oscillation. The theta rhythm occurs at 4-10 Hz, and it has been implicated in sensory processing, memory, and voluntary control of movement (Grastyan, Lissak, Madarasz, & Donhoffer, 1959; Vanderwolf, 1969). The coherent membrane potential fluctuations of the orderly aligned hippocampal pyramidal and granule cells are the main current generators of the extracellularly recorded theta oscillation. Extracellular studies using laminar voltage versus depth and current source density measurements in the behaving animal revealed multiple, phase-shifted theta dipoles along the somatodendritic axis of pyramidal cells (Buzsáki, Leung, & Vanderwolf, 1983). Based on data obtained from such studies, it was suggested that the theta rhythm in the awake animal may be generated by rhythmic somatic hyperpolarizations of the principal cells by GABAergic interneurons, followed by the rhythmic, phase-shifted dendritic excitation provided by the input from the entorhinal cortex (Buzsáki et al., 1983). Although the issue of whether the entorhinal-cortex-to-CA1 input is excitatory or inhibitory is still intensely debated (Soltesz & Jones, 1995), recent intracellular data clearly determined the nature and properties of the somatic inhibitory input (Leung & Yim, 1986; Soltesz & Deschênes, 1993; Ylinen et al., 1995).

Extracellular single unit studies provided evidence indicating that principal cells, such as the CA1 and CA3 pyramidal cells and the granule cells of the dentate gyrus, do not discharge at each cycle (Buzsáki & Eidelberg, 1983; Buzsáki et al., 1983). By contrast, fast-spiking cells, the putative interneurons, were suggested to be true theta cells, that is, neurons that fire rhythmically at most theta cycles. The fact that most pyramidal cells do not fire at each theta wave is a crucial characteristic of hippocampal functions during theta rhythm. For example, the so-called place cells (cells that fire when the animal is in a particular spatial location) are thought to be pyramidal cells. Indeed, such coding by pyramidal cell firing requires that not all pyramidal neurons are brought to firing threshold rhythmically at the theta frequency. Pyramidal cells not only do not fire at each theta cycle, in fact they decrease their firing rates during theta waves. Convincing evidence in favor of the basic theta rhythm's being generated by rhythmic barrages of inhibitory postsynaptic potentials (IPSPs) bombarding the somatic membranes of principal cells came from *in vivo* intracellular studies (Leung & Yim, 1986; Soltesz & Deschênes, 1993; Ylinen et al., 1995). First, intracellular studies showed that principal cells display subthreshold membrane potential oscillations around the resting membrane potential at the theta frequencies, at times when theta waves are recordable with the extracellular EEG electrode. Importantly, intracellular recordings from morphologically identified pyramidal cells unequivocally demonstrated that the phase of the intracellular theta oscillations with respect to the EEG theta is strongly voltage-dependent (Leung & Yim, 1986; Soltesz & Deschênes, 1993; Ylinen et al., 1995). This observation could be explained by the arrival of synchronized bursts of IPSPs during one half of the theta cycle. Because the $GABA_A$-receptor-mediated IPSPs reverse in sign at the chloride equilibrium potential E_{Cl} (which in these cells is close to the resting membrane potential), hyperpolarization of the membrane from a depolarized potential by current injection through the recording microelectrode would make the initially hyperpolarizing IPSPs depolarizing. Such a reversal of the sign of the IPSPs would thus result in approximately 120°-180° phase-shift of the intracellular theta oscillation in the recorded cell with respect to the EEG theta (which, of course, goes on undisturbed by the manipulation of the membrane potential of a single pyramidal neuron by the experimenter via the intracellular micropipette). When recordings were made with a pipette filled with KCl, which results in the injection of Cl^- ions into the cell and thus in a prominent depolarizing shift in E_{Cl}, all the chloride-dependent, $GABA_A$-receptor-mediated IPSPs became depolarizing even at relatively depolarized membrane potentials, and the voltage dependency of the phase of the intracellular theta with respect to the EEG theta was abolished (Leung & Yim, 1986; Soltesz & Deschênes, 1993). These data strongly suggested the involvement of fast, chloride-dependent, $GABA_A$-receptor-mediated events in the generation of the hippocampal theta rhythm.

Importantly, in addition to the dominant peak of the theta rhythm, the power spectrum of the hippocampal EEG reveals an additional component, the fast oscillations, which occur at 25-70 Hz (the "40-Hz" oscillations); (Bland & Whishaw, 1976; Buzsáki et al., 1983; Leung, 1992; Stumpf, 1965). Stumpf (1965) showed that the hippocampal fast oscillations were frequently phase-locked to the hippocampal theta rhythm. Stumpf's early studies, together with more recent results showing that hippocampal interneurons fire phase-locked to the fast oscillations, suggest a causal relationship between the theta and the 40-Hz oscillations (Buzsáki & Eidelberg, 1983; Buzsáki et al., 1983; Soltesz & Deschênes, 1993) on the one hand, and oscillations and $GABA_A$ IPSPs on the other. Indeed, our recordings from identified pyramidal cells with KCl-filled pipettes demonstrated the appearance of fast oscillations at around 40 Hz on the intracellular trace, phase-locked to the theta oscillations (Soltesz & Deschênes, 1993). These results clearly indicated that the basic theta rhythm was generated by the rhythmic hyperpolarization of the somatic membrane of pyramidal neurons at the theta frequencies. During each hyperpolarizing phase of the theta cycle the cell receives IPSPs which arrive at around 40 Hz (Fig. 6.3). It should be noted here that although synaptic inputs are clearly necessary for the emergence of theta oscillations, intrinsic currents, such as high-threshold Ca^{++} spikes, can modulate the phase of the theta oscillations (Ylinen et al., 1995).

The hippocampal theta rhythm is crucially dependent on the integrity of the septo-hippocampal pathway (Petsche, Stumpf, & Gogolak, 1962). Importantly, this pathway contains both cholinergic and GABAergic components (Freund & Antal, 1988). Recent results provided strong evidence in favor of the scenario where the cholinergic input provides a slow, tonic, depolarizing influence for both the principal as well as the GABAergic hippocampal neurons (Buzsáki et al., 1983; Pitler & Alger, 1992; Soltesz & Deschênes, 1993; Traub & Miles, 1991). Partly as a result of this cholinergic depolarization, hippocampal interneurons augment their firing rate and provide increased inhibition for the postsynaptic principal cells (Fig. 6.3). However, the rhythmic, theta-locked input from the septum provided by the GABAergic septo-hippocampal axons, which terminate exclusively on hippocampal GABAergic neurons, inhibit the firing of these hippocampal interneurons during one half of the theta cycle. During this disinhibitory phase, the firing rate of interneurons decreases and the pyramidal cell membrane starts to return from the hyperpolarization and become depolarized. However, pyramidal cells reach firing threshold only rarely, since their membrane potential is soon hyperpolarized again when the disinhibitory phase ends and interneurons are able to fire at the beginning of the new theta cycle (Fig. 6.3).

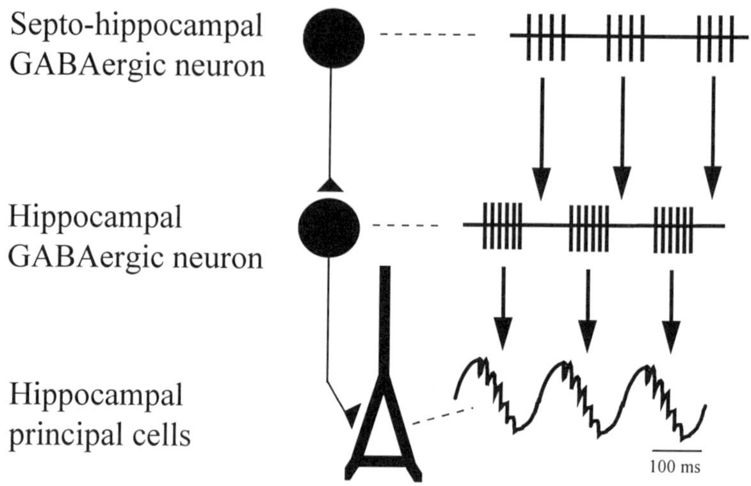

Fig. 6.3. The hippocampal theta rhythm is a synaptically driven oscillation. Septo-hippocampal cholinergic neurons (not shown) depolarize the membrane of both the hippocampal GABAergic cells as well as the pyramidal neurons. Septo-hippocampal GABA neurons, which terminate exclusively on hippocampal GABAergic cells, rhythmically inhibit hippocampal GABAergic neurons. When hippocampal GABAergic cells fire, they cause the synchronized hyperpolarization in large populations of pyramidal somatic membranes. During each hyperpolarizing subcycle, the IPSPs arrive at approximately 40 Hz, corresponding to the firing-patterns of interneurons.

4. FROM HIPPOCAMPAL OSCILLATIONS TO THE 7±2 RULE AND HEBBIAN COACTIVATION OF CELL ASSEMBLIES

What is the relevance of the role of rhythmic synaptic events to our understanding of the psychophysics of memory formation and to the role of oscillations in brain functions? Although we are still far from understanding the neurobiological basis of hippocampal functions, recent work by Lisman and Idiart (1995) provided some intriguing possibilities. These authors suggested that the 7 ± 2 rule of psychophysics regarding short-term memory formation (i.e., that humans can store no more than about seven individual memory items in their short-term memory) may be explained by the presence of about seven 40-Hz oscillatory subcycles during each theta cycle. Computational modeling showed that one can indeed achieve the storage of about seven short-term memory items with a simple pyramidal cell-interneuron network undergoing theta and phase-locked 40-Hz oscillations. Although this bold proposal must be further refined in the future, it shows us the possibility of bridging the gap between basic neuroscientific data and psychophysical observations about higher brain functions.

As described earlier, the basic theta rhythm represents an oscillation between high and low levels of inhibition of pyramidal cells. During the low-level inhibitory phase of the theta cycle, Hebbian mechanisms can come into action. Buzsáki's (1989) two-stage memory model suggests that the theta rhythm plays an important role during the initial phase of memory formation. During exploration by rats, a behavior associated with the presence of theta waves, particular sets of entorhinal cells excite specific groups of granule cells which, in turn, excite particular groups of CA3 neurons. During the exploratory behavior and the associated theta rhythm, CA3 neurons do not fire at high rates. After the end of the exploratory behavior, however, those CA3 pyramidal cells that received inputs from granule cells during the exploratory phase initiate the so-called sharp waves. During sharp waves groups of CA3 cells discharge, which results in the long-term potentiation of the CA3 to CA1 inputs (the Schaffer collateral input). Inasmuch as CA1, subicular, and granule cells all participate in sharp waves, particular cortico-hippocampal loops could be potentiated and selected through Hebbian mechanisms.

Miller (1991) elaborated on the concept of resonance at the theta frequency, which may be a central property of cortico-hippocampal interactions. In Miller's hypothesis, the hippocampus serves as a pointer that selects particular groups of cortical neurons. Hebbian processes of synaptic strengthening via temporally contiguous activity of interconnected neurons would select bidirectional neuronal loops between the hippocampus and the entorhinal cortex. A reference or framework of information ("context") would be represented as patterns of resonance at the theta frequency between specific groups of hippocampal and cortical neurons. Thus, the theta rhythm may play a central role in the generation of Hebbian cell assemblies underlying memory formation. The importance of oscillations may be that Hebbian mechanisms favor the potentiation of neuronal connections that permit resonance. It is also of interest to note that the most efficient frequency of stimulation for LTP is 5 Hz, that is, within the theta range. Thus, it is an exciting possibility that there is likely to be a strong causal connection between the theta rhythm and Hebbian plasticity associated with memory formation.

5. RANDOM VERSUS RHYTHMIC SYNAPTIC INPUTS: ORIGIN AND FUNCTIONS

Transmitter release between neurons in the mammalian CNS occurs when action potentials invade the synaptic terminals. As discussed before, neurons frequently receive rhythmic synaptic inputs from presynaptic neurons that exhibit membrane-potential oscillations resulting in the periodic and/or phase-locked discharge of the cells. However, in addition to action potential-dependent release of neurotransmitters such as GABA and glutamate, terminals are also capable of generating random synaptic events in the absence of action potentials (Alger & Nicoll, 1980; Collingridge, Gage, & Robertson, 1984; Otis, Staley, & Mody, 1991; Scanziani, Capogna, Gahwiler, & Thompson, 1992; Soltesz, Smetters, & Mody, 1995). These events, recordable in the presence of the Na^+ channel blocker tetrodotoxin (TTX) are referred to as "miniature" events, miniature inhibitory postsynaptic potentials (currents) (mIPSP(C)s), or excitatory postsynaptic potentials (currents) (mEPSP(C)s). For example, mIPSCs occur in most neurons at relatively high frequencies (1-50 Hz) (Otis et al., 1991). Importantly, the interevent intervals of mIPSCs are exponentially distributed, indicating their random occurrence. The exact function of miniature events is not known, but it is likely that they exert a strong influence on the output of the neuron. In a recent study (Soltesz et al., 1995), it was shown that the random, tonic, action potential-independent release of GABA takes place mostly at sites close to the action potential initiation site in hippocampal neurons. Because distinct subclasses of inhibitory cells innervate spatially segregated parts of neurons (Halasy & Somogyi, 1993), these results suggest that a functional division of labor may exist between proximal versus distal terminals belonging to different interneuron classes. Specifically, these data (Soltesz et al., 1995) suggest that, in contrast to terminals innervating distal dendritic sites, proximal inhibitory terminals (i.e., those at the axon initial segment, soma and proximal dendrites) release GABA not only when excitatory inputs bring the interneuron to firing threshold, but also in the absence of such excitatory inputs to interneurons, which may provide an independent safety mechanism against failure of inhibitory control due to a drop in the excitatory drive onto inhibitory cells. Whether such division of labor exists between proximal versus distal excitatory inputs is not known. Similarly, how the random release of excitatory and inhibitory neurotransmitters from presynaptic terminals may influence neuronal oscillations remains to be studied in the future. Interestingly, theoretical studies indicate that some level of noise improves signal-to-noise ratios and may also help to achieve synchrony (Bezrukov & Vodyanoy, 1995; Bulsara & Gammaitoni, 1996). It is also an intriguing possibility that the frequency of the random barrage of synaptic events ("synaptic noise") may be dependent on the behavioral state of the animal.

6. CONCLUSIONS

The mammalian brain can display a vast repertoire of eletrical behaviors, including rhythmic waves originating from the synchronized membrane potential oscillations of a large number of neurons. Some oscillatory patterns emerge from the intricate interplay of intrinsic currents, and are phase-reset, modulated and abolished by synaptic inputs. Other rhythms result from the rhythmic bombardment of cells by synaptically released neurontransmitters, however, such oscillations can be modulated by the intrinsic currents of the neuron undergoing membrane potential oscillations.

Intriguingly, rhythmic brain activity may subserve the formation of self-organized Hebbian cell assemblies, information storage, and the retrieval of memory traces from neuronal circuits.

ACKNOWLEDGMENTS

This chapter was supported by a UCI Young Investigator Award. I thank Mr. Scott Talkovic for his assistance.

REFERENCES

Alger, B. E., & Nicoll, R. A. (1980). Spontaneous inhibitory post-synaptic potentials in hippocampus: Mechanism for tonic inhibition. *Brain Research, 200*, 195-200.

Andersen, P., & Andersson, S. A. (1968). *Physiological Basis of Alpha Rhythm*. New York: Appleton-Century-Crofts.

Bezrukov, S. M., & Vodyanoy, I. (1995). Noise-induced enhancement of signal transduction across voltage-dependent ion channels. *Nature, 378*, 362-364.

Bland, B. H., & Whishaw, I. Q. (1967). Generators and topography of hippocampal theta (RSA) in the anaesthetized and freely moving rat. *Brain Research*, 118, 259-280.

Bulsara, A. R., & Gammaitoni, L. (1996). Tuning in to noise. *Physics Today, 49*, 39-45.

Buzsáki, G. (1989). Two-stage model of memory trace formation: a role for "noisy" brain states. *Neuroscience, 31*, 551-570.

Buzsáki, G., & Eidelberg, E. (1983). Phase relations of hippocampal projection cells and interneurons to theta activity in the anesthetized rat. *Brain Research, 266*, 334-339.

Buzsáki, G., Leung, L. W., & Vanderwolf, C.H.(1983). Cellular bases of hippocampal EEG in the behaving rat. *Brain Research, 287*,139-171.

Buzsáki, G., Smith, A., Berger, S., Fisher, L. J., & Gage, F. H. (1990). Petit mal epilepsy and parkinsonian tremor: hypothesis of a common pacemaker. *Neuroscience, 36*, 1-14.

Collingridge, G. L., Gage, P. W., & Robertson, B. (1984). Inhibitory post-synaptic currents in rat hippocampal CA1 neurones. *Journal of Physiology (London), 356*, 551-564.

Coulter, D. A., Huguenard, J. R. & Prince, D. A. (1989). Calcium currents in rat thalamocortical relay neurones: Kinetic properties of the transient, low-threshold current. *Journal of Physiology (London), 414*, 587-604.

Crunelli, V., Lightowler, S., & Pollard, C. E. (1989). A T-type Ca^{2+} current underlies low-threshold Ca^{2+} potentials in cells of the cat and rat lateral geniculate nucleus. *Journal of Physiology (London), 413*, 543-561.

Deschênes, M., Paradis, M., Roy, J. P., & Steriade, M. (1984). Electrophysiology of neurons of lateral thalamic nuclei in cat: resting properties and burst discharges. *Journal of Neurophysiology, 51*, 1196-1219.

Freund, T. F., & Antal, M. (1988). GABA-containing neurons in the septum control inhibitory interneurons in the hippocampus. *Nature, 336*, 170-173.

Gloor, P., & Fariello, R. G. (1988). Generalized epilepsy: some of its cellular mechanisms differ from those of focal epilepsy. *Trends in Neuroscience, 11*, 63-68.

Grastyan, E., Lissak, K., Madarasz, I., & Donhoffer, H. (1959). Hippocampal electrical activity during the development of conditioned reflexes. *Electroencephalography and Clinical Neurophysiology, 11*, 409-430.

Halasy, K., & Somogyi, P. (1993). Subdivisions in the multiple GABAergic innervation of granule cells in the dentate gyrus of the rat hippocampus. *European Journal of Neuroscience, 5*, 411-429.

Jahnsen, H., & Llinas, R. (1984a). Electrophysiological properties of guinea-pig thalamic neurones: an in vitro study. *Journal of Physiology (London)*, *349*, 205-226.

Jahnsen, H., & Llinas, R. (1984b). Ionic basis for the electro-responsiveness and oscillatory properties of guinea-pig thalamic neurones in vitro. *Journal of Physiology (London)*, *349*, 227-247.

Jalife, J., & Antzelevitch, C. (1979). Phase resetting and annihilation of pacemaker activity in cardiac tissue. *Science*, *206*, 695-697.

Leresche, N., Jassik-Gerschenfeld, D., Haby, M., Soltesz, I., & Crunelli, V. (1990). Pacemaker-like and other types of spontaneous membrane potential oscillations of thalamocortical cells. *Neuroscience Letters*, *113*, 72-77.

Leresche, N., Lightowler, S., Soltesz, I., Jassik-Gerschenfeld, D., & Crunelli, V. (1991). Low-frequency oscillatory activities intrinsic to rat and cat thalamocortical cells. *Journal of Physiology (London)*, *441*, 155-174.

Leung, L. S. (1992). Fast (beta) rhythms in the hippocampus: A review. *Hippocampus*, *2*, 93-98.

Leung, L. S., & Yim, C. Y. (1986). Intracellular records of theta rhythm in hippocampal CA1 cells of the rat. *Brain Research*, *367*, 323-327.

Lisman, J. E., & Idiart, M. A. (1995). Storage of 7 +/- 2 short-term memories in oscillatory subcycles. *Science*, *267*,1512-1515.

McCormick, D. A., & Pape, H. C. (1990a). Properties of a hyperpolarization-activated cation current and its role in rhythmic oscillation in thalamic relay neurones. *Journal of Physiology (London)*, *431*, 291-318.

McCormick, D. A., & Pape, H. C. (1990b). Noradrenergic and serotonergic modulation of a hyperpolarization-activated cation current in thalamic relay neurones. *Journal of Physiology (London)*, *431*, 319-342.

Miller, R. (1991). *Cortico-Hippocampal Interplay*. Berlin: Springer-Verlag.

Nuñez, A., Amzica, F., & Steriade, M. (1992). Intrinsic and synaptically generated delta (1-4 Hz) rhythms in dorsal lateral geniculate neurons and their modulation by light-induced fast (30-70- Hz) events. *Neuroscience*, *51*, 269-284.

Otis, T. S., Staley, K. J., & Mody, I. (1991). Perpetual inhibitory activity in mammalian brain slices generated by spontaneous GABA release. *Brain Research*, *545*, 142-150.

Petsche, H., Stumpf, C., & Gogolak, G. (1962). The significance of the rabbit's septum as a relay station between the midbrain and the hippocampus. I. The control of hippocampus arousal activity by septal cells. *Electroencephalography and Clinical Neurophysiology*, *14*, 202-211.

Pitler, T. A., & Alger, B. E. (1992). Cholinergic excitation of GABAergic interneurons in the rat hippocampal slice. *Journal of Physiology (London)*, *450*, 127-142.

Scanziani, M., Capogna, M., Gahwiler, B. H., & Thompson, S. M. (1992). Presynaptic inhibition of miniature excitatory synaptic currents by baclofen and adenosine in the hippocampus. *Neuron*, *9*, 919-927.

Soltesz, I., Lightowler, S., Leresche, N., Jassik-Gerschenfeld, D., Pollard, C. E., & Crunelli V. (1991). Two inward currents and the transformation of low-frequency oscillations of rat and cat thalamocortical cells. *Journal of Physiology (London)*, *441*, 175-197.

Soltesz, I., & Crunelli, V. (1992). A role for low-frequency, rhythmic synaptic potentials in the synchronization of cat thalamocortical cells. *Journal of Physiology (London)*, *457*, 257-276.

Soltesz, I., & Deschênes, M. (1993). Low- and high-frequency membrane potential oscillations during theta activity in CA1 and CA3 pyramidal neurons of the rat hippocampus under ketamine-xylazine anesthesia. *Journal of Neurophysiology*, *70*, 97-116.

Soltesz, I., & Jones, R. S. (1995). The direct perforant path input to CA1: excitatory or inhibitory? *Hippocampus*, *5*, 101-103.

Soltesz, I., Smetters, D. K., & Mody, I. (1995). Tonic inhibition originates from synapses close to the soma. *Neuron*, *14*, 1273-1283.

Steriade, M., Jones, E. G., & Llinas, R. R. (1990). *Thalamic Oscillation and Signalling*. New York: Wiley.

Stumpf, C. (1965). The fast component in the electrical activity of rabbit's hippocampus. *Electroencephalography and Clinical Neurophysiology*, *18*, 477-486.

Suzuki, S., & Rogawski, M. A. (1989). T-type calcium channels mediate the transition between tonic and phasic firing in thalamic neurons. *Proceedings of the National Academy of Sciences*, *86*, 7228-7232.

Traub, R. D., & Miles, R. (1991). *Neuronal Networks of the Hippocampus*. Cambridge, UK: Cambridge University Press.

Vanderwolf, C. H. (1969). Hippocampal electrical activity and voluntary movement in the rat. *Electroencephalography and Clinical Neurophysiology*, *26*, 407-418.

Ylinen, A., Soltesz, I., Bragin, A., Penttonen, M., Sik, A., & Buzsáki, G. (1995). Intracellular correlates of hippocampal theta rhythm in identified pyramidal cells, granule cells, and basket cells. *Hippocampus*, *5*, 78-90.

7

Dynamics of Low-Frequency Oscillations in a Model Thalamocortical Network

Elizabeth Thomas
University of Liège

ABSTRACT

A model of the thalamocortical system was constructed for the purpose of a computational analysis of low-frequency oscillations that take place in the system. Experimental values were used to guide the parameters used in the model. Both the thalamic reticular and relay nuclei were represented in the model. The thalamic cells were capable of undergoing a low-threshold Ca^{2+}-mediated spike. The values of parameters were varied across the neuronal population in order to ensure that synchrony did not arise due to a false uniformity in the properties of the neurons. Many neurons in the network were not directly connected. The simulation was used to investigate the plausibility and ramifications of certain proposals that have been put forward for the production of synchronous, rhythmic activity in the thalamocortical system. An initial stimulus to the model reticular thalamic layer was found to give rise to rhythmic synchronous activity in the entire system. The production of this activity was found to depend on the presence of connections between the reticular thalamic neurons as well as on the generation of an average inhibitory postsynaptic potential on each reticular thalamic neuron that was similar for all of them. The frequency of thalamic oscillations was found to decrease with increase in the durations of inhibitory postsynaptic potentials as well as the time it took the neurons to rebound once they were released from inhibition. Cortical feedback to the pacemaking reticular thalamic layer was found capable of increasing the amplitude of the oscillations.

1. INTRODUCTION

The neurons of the thalamocortical system (Fig. 7.1) undergo low-frequency synchronous rhythmic oscillations between 3 and 14 Hz during several states. Many of these states occur during sleep. One of them is spindle sleep, an early stage of sleep during the transition from wake to sleep. Another occurrence of synchronous, rhythmic activity takes place during delta sleep, a stage of deep non-REM sleep. The incidence of synchronous, rhythmic activity in the thalamocortical system not only takes place during normal states such as sleep but also during abnormal states such as epilepsy

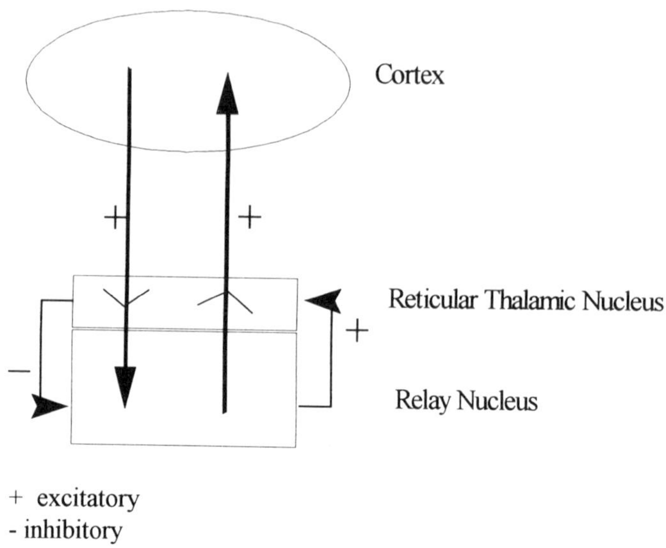

Fig. 7.1. Highly schematic diagram of thalamocortical system. Arrows indicate the presence of connections between two areas. Signals are carried in the same direction as the arrows. See Fig. 7.2 for the connectivity within each individual area of the thalamocortical model.

(Hobson & Steriade, 1986; Steriade, 1991; Steriade, Jones, & Llinas, 1989; Steriade & Llinas, 1988).

Studies have shown that these low-frequency oscillations could still be recorded in the isolated thalamus, that had been dissociated from the cortex (Steriade et al., 1989). Many attempts to understand the production of rhythmic activity in the thalamocortical system have therefore focused on the production of rhythmic activity in the isolated thalamus. Further attempts to isolate the source of rhythmic activity within the thalamus have led to the reticular thalamic (RE) nucleus. Experiments show that synchronous, rhythmic activity is preserved in the RE nucleus that has been disconnected by transection from all other thalamic nuclei. Lesions of the RE nucleus however, were found to abolish such oscillations in the thalamus (Steriade, Domich, Oakson, & Deschênes, 1987). These findings led to the idea that the RE nucleus could play a pacemaker role in the generation of rhythmic activity in the thalamocortical system. Other experiments on the production of oscillatory activity in the thalamocortical system have uncovered more distributed mechanisms in which the dorsal thalamus plays a more crucial role (Buszáki, 1991; Von Krosigk, Bal, & McCormick, 1993). This work does not address the latter mechanisms but only investigates the plausibility and ramifications of a mechanism in which the RE nucleus plays the primary role in the production of network oscillations.

On the cellular level, an intrinsic capability of the thalamic cells to undergo a Ca^{2+}-mediated low-threshold spike (LTS) is thought to underlie the population oscillations (Jahnsen & Llinas, 1984a, 1984b; Mulle, Madariaga, & Deschênes, 1986; Steriade & Llinas, 1988). This burst mode has been found to operate mainly during states of non-REM sleep, whereas the tonic mode of cell discharge dominates the behavioral states of wake and REM sleep (Domich et al., 1986; Steriade et al., 1988). Although the intrinsic burst properties of the thalamic cells is thought to underlie the synchronous, rhythmic activity, it is uncertain if it is sufficient to explain the entire thalamocortical rhythmic behavior (Lopes da Silva, 1991).

In this study we investigated if the Ca^{2+}-mediated low-threshold spike in the RE nucleus is capable of maintaining synchronous, rhythmic activity in the thalamocortical system. The simplified low-threshold spike in the model consisted of an all or nothing burst that occurred once a low threshold was reached after hyperpolarization of sufficient amplitude and duration. The values of parameters were varied across the population in order to ensure that synchrony could arise in a realistically heterogeneous population. The connectivity and number of neurons used were such that many of the neurons in the network were not directly coupled. The conditions essential for the maintenance of synchrony in such a network were investigated. The manner in which neuronal parameters affected network frequency was studied. The role of cortical feedback in the oscillations was investigated. Delays in signal arrival times were computed from experimentally measured axonal conduction velocities. This was done in order to ensure a biologically realistic phase relationship between the signals of the cortex and thalamus. More recent studies on the production of synchronous activity in the thalamic system have also been carried out on more detailed models of the isolated thalamus (Lytton & Thomas, 1997).

2. METHOD

2.1. Overall Geometry of the Model

A model was developed of the RE nucleus, dorsal thalamus, and cortex. Each of the model sections could be viewed as an infinitely thin, vertical slice having a height and a length, but no thickness. Most of the information used to create the dorsal thalamus came from the vast literature available on the lateral geniculate (LG) nucleus. We therefore in future references to the dorsal thalamus, use the term LG nucleus. Cells of an appropriate type were assigned to each of these layers. Each cell was represented anatomically by an x and y coordinate for its somatic location and two rectangular boxes to represent the axonic and dendritic arbors. The axonic and dendritic boxes were included in order to compute the connections between the model neurons rather than imposing it through an assumed function. There was only one cell class represented in the RE layer. It was thought unnecessary for the purpose of this study, to include both the X and Y relay cells of the LG nucleus. Therefore, we only represented the dendritic and axonic boxes of the Y cells. The LG interneuron was not represented in this study. It is inhibition from the RE neurons that is thought to play a crucial role in the generation of synchronized oscillations in the system. The LG interneurons have been observed to be inhibited during several states of synchronized oscillations in the thalamocortical system (Steriade, 1991). Only one class of excitatory and inhibitory cells was represented in the cortical layer. The pyramidal cells, as the predominant excitatory cells of the neocortex (Lund, Henry, MacQueen, & Harvey, 1979), were chosen to represent the excitatory cells, while the basket cell represented the cortical inhibitory interneurons.

As mentioned earlier, connections between the model neurons were computed based on cell morphologies and positions. A connection between a pair of neurons was based on whether there was an overlap between their arbors. Figure 7.2 provides a summary of the connections made in the model. Note that there are no connections between the LG relay neurons. A good summary of the connectivity between these systems is available in a review by Sherman and Koch (1990). Many neurons in the model network were not directly coupled in this scheme of connectivity.

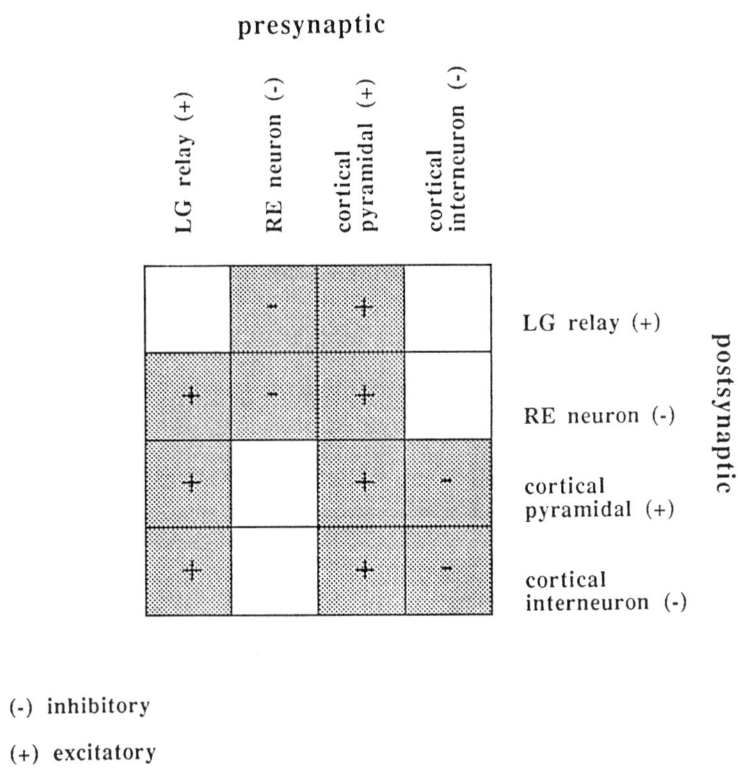

Fig. 7.2. Connection matrix for the model. Presynaptic cells are labeled on the top and postsynaptic cells on the right. A shaded box indicates the possibility of connections from the cell class on the top to the cell class on the right.

2.2. Subthreshold Activity

A description of the physiology of the model neurons can be divided into two sections. The first is concerned with the cell's subthreshold mode and the other with its firing activity. The simulation began with all neurons in the subthreshold mode. They were all assigned initial activities corresponding to the range of resting potentials that have been measured in the cortex and thalamus. Significant deviations from cell rest activity arose upon the arrival of input from other cells. The firing of an LG relay neuron or cortical pyramidal cell generally depolarized the postsynaptic cell while input from cortical interneurons or RE neurons brought about inhibition (Friedlander, 1981; Ide, 1982; Sherman & Koch, 1990). All inhibition in the model was treated as being mediated by GABA (Douglas & Martin, 1990; Sherman & Koch, 1990). Both the short-time-scale acting $GABA_A$, as well as long-time-scale acting $GABA_B$, inhibitions are known to exist both in the thalamus (Crunelli & Leresche, 1991) and cortex (Douglas & Martin, 1990). We, however, used only one idealized inhibition in the model. Excitation from glutamatergic input to the thalamus and cortex can be mediated by both NMDA and non-NMDA receptors (Douglas & Martin, 1990; Sherman & Koch, 1990). All synaptic excitation present in the model represents only the simpler non-NMDA mediated excitation. It therefore acted only on a shorter time scale. Different types of excitatory and inhibitory conductances were not represented in order to obtain an understanding of a general, relatively simple model before moving on to a more complicated one. This approach has been useful in uncovering some of the more prominent conditions necessary for the existence of the population oscillations and the parameters that influence it most. Delays in the arrival of the excitatory and inhibitory signals at the postsynaptic cell were incorporated in the model. These were due both to synaptic delays and the time taken for a signal to propagate along the presynaptic axonal arbor. Other than synaptic inputs, the model neurons had certain intrinsic properties that could bring about changes in their activity. One of these is the tendency to rebound after hyperpolarization. Another intrinsic property represented is the occurrence of an afterhyperpolarization (AHP) following an action potential. The AHP is thought to play a role in the deinactivation of the Ca^{2+}-dependent low threshold spike (LTS).

Subthreshold activity of a neuron V_i at each time step was computed by summing over all excitatory and inhibitory inputs, as well as by taking into account changes to cell activity mediated by the rebound and AHP terms. The change in the activity of a neuron V_i could be described using the following equation:

$$\frac{dV_i}{dt} = G(V_i)\frac{(V_r - V_i)}{\tau r} + (P_E - V_i)\sum^{(+)}(t) - (V_i - P_I)\sum^{(-)}(t) - T(t-\alpha_j)\frac{(V_i - V_k)}{\tau k}.$$

$G(V_i)(V_r - V_i)/\tau r$ is the rebound term. $G(V_i)$ is a sigmoid function that describes the current-voltage relationship of the persistent sodium current (French, Sah, Buckett, &

Gage, 1990). Its importance lies in bringing a cell from hyperpolarized potentials to the low threshold values necessary for the LTS. $\sum^{(+)}$ is the total excitatory input, and $\sum^{(-)}$ is the total inhibitory input. An alpha function was used to describe the change in postsynaptic potentials with time. The duration of inhibitory and excitatory PSPs was determined by the time constants τ_I and τ_E respectively. $(P_E - V_i)$ gates the excitatory term. For a given input the magnitude of postsynaptic excitation decreases as V_i approaches P_E. A value of 0 mV was assigned to P_E. This is the reversal potential for non-NMDA-mediated excitation in the cortex (Brown & Johnston, 1983). $(V_i - P_I)$ gates the inhibitory term. The magnitude of inhibition due to a given input decreases as V_i approaches P_I. The value assigned P_I was −90 mV, the reversal potential for K^+. $T(t - a_j)(V_i - v_k)/\tau k$ is responsible for the AHP of a cell after an action potential. The function $T(t - a_j)$ acts like a switch to limit the action of an AHP to a specified duration following an action potential. A more complete description of the model can be found in a previous study of other aspects of these oscillations (Thomas & Wyatt, 1995).

2.3. Suprathreshold Activity

Once a model neuron reached threshold, it fired an action potential. As mentioned earlier, the thalamic neurons could either fire a Na^+-mediated single action potential or a Ca^{2+} -dependent low-threshold spike. The cortical neurons in the model could only fire a Na^+-mediated single action potential and not the Ca^{2+}-dependent low-threshold spike.

In order to fire the single Na^+ action potential, the cell had to be depolarized until it reached a threshold value of −35 +/− 5 mV. The conditions necessary for LTS were obtained from the experiments of Jahnsen and Llinas (1984a). They demonstrated that the process is both a voltage- and time-dependent one. In the model, a thalamic neuron had to be hyperpolarized below -65 mV for a duration randomly assigned between 100 and 120 ms. Experimentally it has been found that the amplitude and duration of the LTS for a cell can vary depending on the extent and duration of the hyperpolarization used to activate it (Jahnsen & Llinas, 1984a). In the model, however, once all the conditions necessary to evoke the spike were met, the spike was "pasted" on. All neurons were treated as refractory during the action potentials and unable to receive input.

2.4. Computing Multiunit Frequency

We used an autocorrelogram in order to compute the frequency of the population firing (Glaser & Ruchkin, 1976). A filter was used so that the computed frequencies would reflect interevent rather than intraevent firing frequencies. The event being referred to is an occurrence of synchronous, rhythmic firing in the network. The filter was used because each incident of population synchrony was accompanied by a high frequency of single neuron firing that did not reflect the low frequency of population events (Thomas & Wyatt, 1995).

3. RESULTS

The first section reports the outcome of tests done in order to determine if the model is capable of developing synchronized, rhythmic firing. In Section 3.2 the conditions necessary for the maintenance of this activity are examined. We study the network parameters that alter the frequency of the population oscillations in Section 3.3. Finally, in Section 3.4 we report on our investigation of the role of excitatory input to the pacemaking RE layer, both from the LG neurons and cortex.

3.1. Tests for Synchronous Rhythmic Firing

The first test was performed to see if the coupled nets described before could develop synchronous, rhythmic activity. In order to carry out the test, an initial stimulus was delivered to the RE layer. This stimulus comprised a small, random number of RE neurons that burst fired at random times within the first 80 ms of the simulation. The results of this test are presented in Fig. 7.3. Figures 7.3(a), (b), and (c) are plots of the number of cells firing in 5-ms bins for the RE, LG, and cortical layers, respectively.

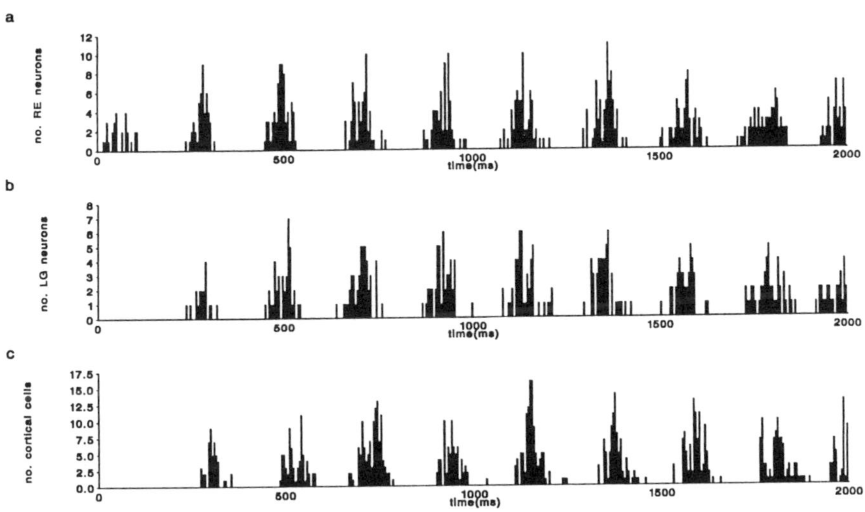

Fig. 7.3. (a) The number of RE neurons that fire after an initial stimulus to the RE layer. The simulation was run for 200 ms. Time was divided into 5 ms bins Each cell was counted as having fired when it reached the crown portion of the Ca^{2+}-mediated low threshold spike where the Na^{+} spikes began. (b) The number of LG neurons firing after the initial stimulus to the RE layer. Cells were counted as having fired in the same manner as the RE cells. (c) The number of cortical that fire as the result of the same stimulus as in (a). durations was increased beyond a certain limit, desynchronized activity resulted. One parameter that determines IPSP durations is τ_I

Figure 7.3 shows that synchronized, oscillatory firing develops in the RE, LG, and cortical layers. An initial stimulus to the RE layer therefore demonstrates that a network of thalamic cells, capable of firing the Ca^{2+}-mediated low-threshold spike, is able to lead to the production of synchronous, rhythmic activity in the system. An autocorrelogram of the activity in the RE layer, as described in Section 2.4 was carried out. It showed a peak at around 4.8 Hz.

3.2. Conditions for Synchrony

A comparison of the activity in Figs.7.3(a), (b) and (c) show that the activities in the RE, LG, and cortical layers are phase-locked. Steriade and Llinas (1988) supplied a number of references in their review article that point to a good correlation between cortical spindles and thalamic spindles from an area where the thalamic cells project to the cortex. Buszaki (1991) also took recordings that show multiunit activity recorded in the thalamus to be phase-locked to the neocortical spindle EEG. An observation of the manner in which single cells of the network fired displayed that although they fired at a lower frequency than the population, the spikes were always phase-locked with population firing.

Tests in this section were done in order to determine the conditions necessary for synchronous firing among the model neurons. Two such conditions were found. One of them was the necessity for a degree of uniformity in the properties of the RE neurons and the input they received so that many of them would undergo inhibition of a similar duration and rebound together. The other was the presence of synaptic inhibition in order to restrict activity to certain "windows." Both these conditions were mentioned by Andersen and Andersson (1968) as part of their inhibitory phasing theory for the development of synchronous, rhythmic activity in the thalamus.

We focus in this section on the requirement for similar IPSP durations. Recall from Section 2 that each model neuronal parameter was not assigned a single value but rather, was assigned by randomly choosing from an appropriate range of values. We found, however, that if the range of IPSP durations was increased beyond a certain limit, desynchronized activity resulted. One parameter that determines IPSP durations is τ_I which was introduced in Section 2. By increasing the range of τ_I values from 5-10 ms to 5-20 ms we found that the same initial stimulus described in Section 3.1 failed to cause synchronous firing in the network (figure not included). Synchronous firing in the RE layer with the wider range of τ_I was still found to develop however once the number of RE neurons was increased from 150 to 1000. This shows that a wide range of τ_I can still yield synchronized population oscillations provided there are sufficient cell numbers.

The requirement that each neuron should experience similar lasting inhibition does not, however, imply that all neurons have to produce single IPSPs of similar durations in a neuron. The resultant IPSP for any neuron is the result of input from a large number of surrounding neurons. This being the case, even when a single IPSP produced by a presynaptic neuron in the model can vary by as much as 50-200 ms, many of the neurons undergo summated IPSPs of similar duration. We ran a test to support this idea. This time the resultant IPSP of each neuron was assigned a value in the range 50-200 ms rather than computing it as a result of many single IPSPs lying in the same range. All input to the neuron resulted in single IPSPs of this assigned duration. The result of this test was desynchronized activity as shown in Fig. 7.4. Synchronized activity could not develop when a range of single IPSP values were used unless the IPSP of each neuron was the result of summation of the many single IPSPs over this range.

The other condition necessary for the development of synchrony in the model was inhibitory coupling between the RE neurons. It has been proposed that dendrodendritic interactions between the RE neurons play an important role in synchronization (Deschênes et al., 1985; Mulle et al., 1986). That inhibitory coupling is a key element in the development of synchrony, was also demonstrated in the model. We ran a test with a net of RE units capable of self-inhibition but with all coupling disabled. The network developed desynchronized activity (figure not included). An examination of events on the cellular level in the model indicates that the inhibitory coupling produces synchronous firing by acting as a clamp to restrict firing to certain windows. Due to the reasons mentioned in the previous paragraph, a number of neurons experience IPSPs of a similar duration and are able to fire together. However, differences in intrinsic properties and input would have led many neurons to fire outside of this group. Inhibition from the neurons that fired together earlier, however, are able to inhibit and prevent any further firing from the surrounding neurons. This clamp on firing continues until the inhibition decays away. At this point, a few cells fire together once again and send an inhibitory input to surrounding neurons. Activity is therefore restricted to certain windows and inhibition controls "stray" firing.

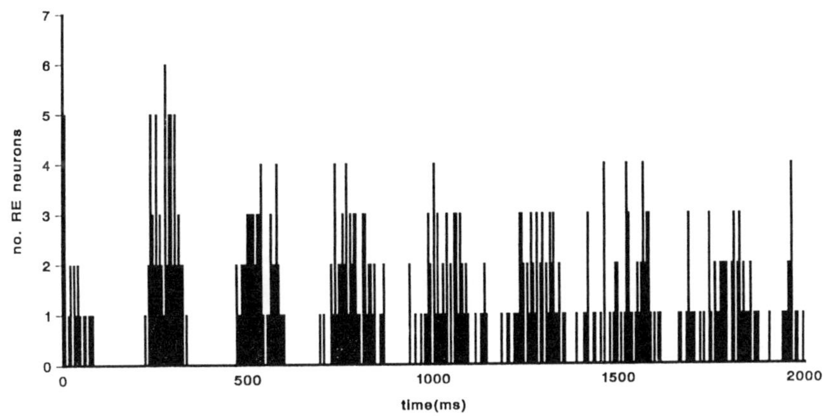

Fig. 7.4. The number of RE neurons that fire after an initial stimulus to a modified RE layer. The RE layer was exactly the same as the one that had generated Fig. 7.3(a) except that each RE neuron was assigned a fixed IPSP duration (fixed τ_I) instead of having one that resulted from the input of cells producing a variety of IPSP durations.

3.3. Parameters That Determine Frequency

In this section, we describe the tests that were done in order to determine how network parameters affect the frequency of population oscillations. Changes in IPSP durations and rebound times were found to alter the network oscillation frequency.

Changes in IPSP durations were made by increasing the maximum τ_I possible. Fig. 7.5 shows that the computed firing frequency decreased as the maximum τ_I increased. The frequency of firing with each increment of τ_I was computed as described in Section 2.4.

Another factor playing a role in the frequency of the oscillations was the time taken by the cells to rebound from hyperpolarized potentials to threshold values for the LTS. Rather than changing τ_r, the parameter that determines the rate at which rebound takes place for the RE neurons, we disabled the rebound capacity of the model RE neurons and instead varied the connection strength from the excitatory LG relay neurons to the RE neurons. Because in this case, the excitation from the LG layer to the RE layer would be providing the excitation necessary for rebound, varying the excitatory connection strength would indicate how frequency depends on rebound durations. The frequency of population firing was determined by using the autocorrelogram as described in Section 2.4. As Fig. 7.6 shows, the frequency of population firing decreased as the excitatory connection strength was decreased. This is because the time taken for

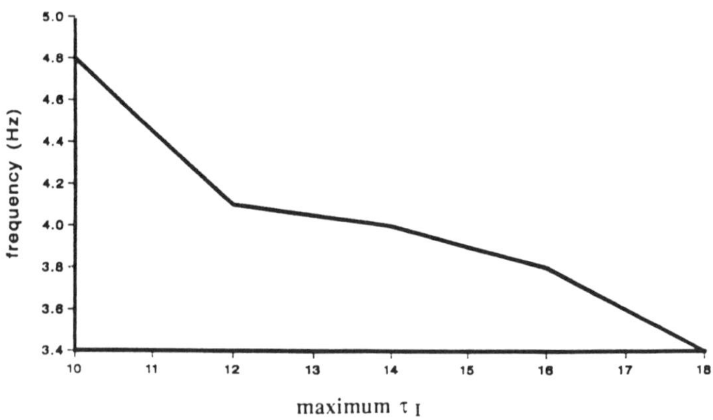

Fig. 7.5. The frequency of multiunit firing in the RE layer as τ_I is varied. The frequency in each case was computed as described in Section 2.4.

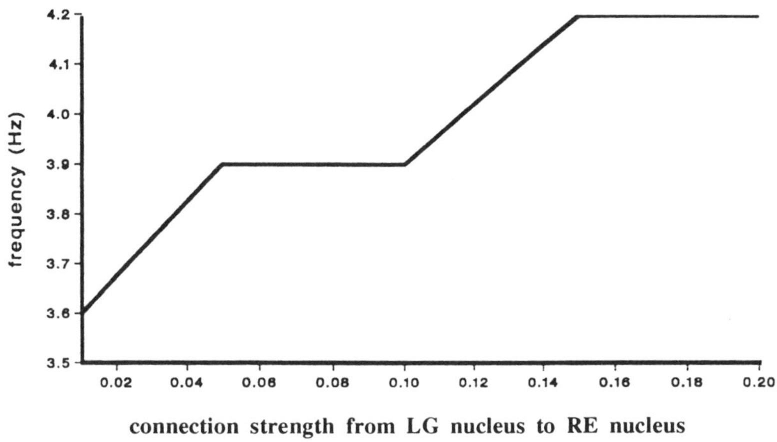

Fig. 7.6. The frequency of multiunit firing in the RE layer as the strength of the excitatory connection strength from the LG to RE layer is varied. The frequency of multiunit firing in the case of each run was computed as described in Section 2.4.

rebound increases as the excitatory connection strength is decreased. In the tests conducted, the number of RE neurons firing at the lowered excitatory strength was also found to decrease. The inspiration for this test came from experiments by Buszaki (1991) in which he obtained a decrease in spindle frequency and amplitude as a result of an injection of NMDA blockers in the thalamus.

3.4. Excitatory Input to the RE Layer

We next conducted tests in order to determine the role of excitatory input to the pacemaking RE layer. Critical to the effect of any excitatory input to the RE layer would be the phase at which this excitatory input arrived. The RE neurons could be undergoing the inhibition that would deinactivate the Ca^{2+}-channels, could be rebounding to threshold, or could be firing an LTS. The distance from the cortical layer to the RE layer is about 21 mm. The computed delays in cortical feedback to the thalamic layer, lie in a range from 5 to 80 ms. Figure 7.7 displays the phase of RE firing at which the cortical feedback arrives. In Fig. 7.7(a), all the model RE neurons firing are counted within 5-ms bins. In this case, an RE neuron was counted as having fired at a different point than before. While previously the point at which the cell was marked as having fired was where the crowning Na^+ spikes began, this time, we used the threshold for LTS. This was in order to determine if excitation from the cortex arrived in time to contribute to the rebound of the RE neurons to threshold. In order to plot Fig. 7.7(b), excitation arriving to all RE cells was summed. All input from the LG layer to the RE neurons had been disabled for this test. Figure 7.7(b) shows that in most cases, the excitation arrives after most of the RE neurons have already reached threshold. A comparison of the cell numbers firing with and without cortical feedback, however, shows that there is an increase in the number of RE neurons firing with cortical feedback. The frequency of firing was the same in each case. All these tests were done at excitatory connection strengths that were insufficient to cause single Na^+ spikes in the RE layer since the LTS is supposed to dominate this mode. Investigations also showed that excitatory input from the LG neurons arrived in the RE layer at about the same phase of RE neuronal activity as cortical input.

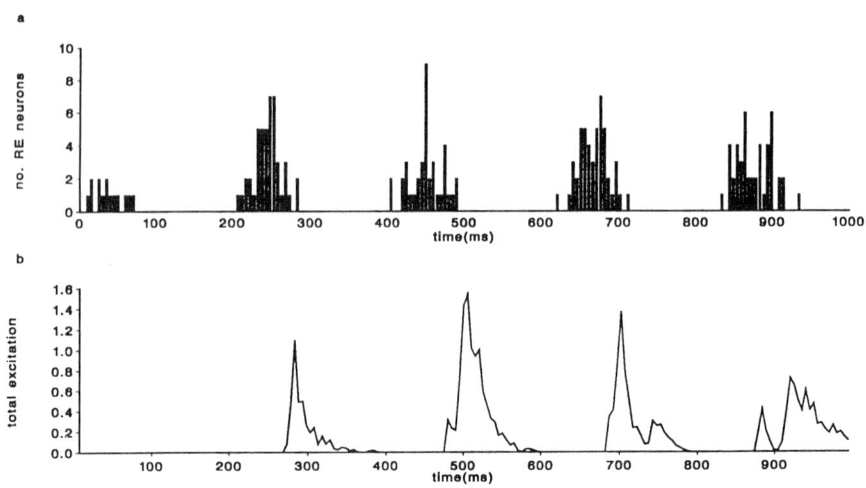

Fig. 7.7. (a) The number of RE neurons firing. LG layer excitatory input to the RE layer was disabled. The only excitatory input to the layer came from the cortex. Unlike the case for Fig. 7.3(a), RE neurons were counted as having fired when they reached threshold for the Ca^{2+}-mediated low threshold spike. This was done in order for comparison with Fig. 7.7(b) to determine whether excitatory input from cortical feedback arrived after or before most RE neurons had already fired an LTS. (b) The total excitatory input from the cortex to the RE neurons at each time step.

Based on the reported electrophysiological similarity of thalamic neurons in different parts of the thalamus (Jahnsen & Llinas, 1984a), we assigned the RE units in the model the capability to rebound from hyperpolarized potentials. For want of more exact data, the rebound times assigned the RE neurons were the same as for the LG neurons. We found, however, that the resulting synchrony was much more robust if the rebound times of the RE cells were made longer than that of the LG cells. This is demonstrated by comparing Figs. 7.8 and 7.9. As had been the case in all other tests, the RE cells in Fig. 7.8 were able to rebound as fast as the LG cells. In Fig. 7.9 however, the capacity of RE cells to rebound was slower than that of LG cells. The activity here is of higher amplitude than that of the RE layer in Fig. 7.8. At these longer rebound times for RE cells, we found that cortical feedback was also capable of bringing about a significant increase in the amplitude of the population oscillations. This was found in tests in which LG feedback had been disabled. An examination at the cellular level yields a reason for the lower synchrony when the RE cells can rebound to threshold as fast as the LG cells. As inhibition decays away on the RE cells, some reach threshold faster than the others, and fire. This then inhibits other RE cells and LG cells from reaching the threshold for LTS. In the case where the RE cells have a rebound time slower than that of the LG cells, excitatory input (either from the LG layer or cortex) simultaneously excites many of the RE cells to threshold for LTS.

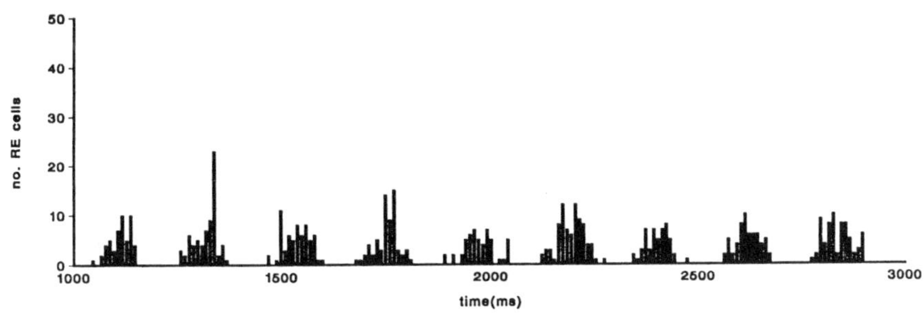

Fig. 7.8. Activity in the RE layer 2000-3000 ms after an initial stimulus to the RE layer. This figure is to be used for comparison with Fig. 7.9 where the rebound time of the RE neurons was slower than that of the LG neurons. For the RE neurons used to generate Fig. 7.8, rebound durations are similar to those of the LG neurons.

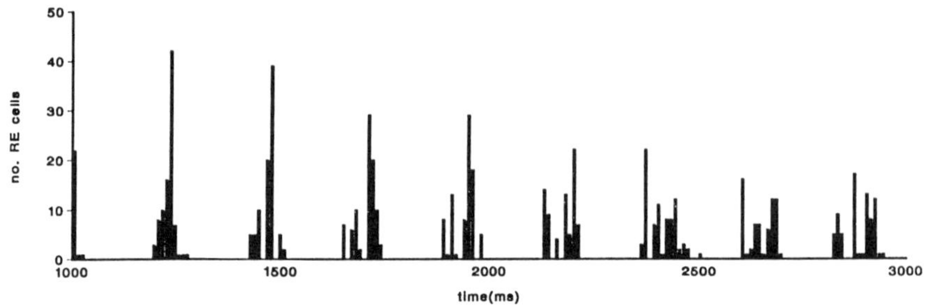

Fig. 7.9. Increased synchrony in RE layer where rebound durations of RE neurons is assigned to be slower than that of LG neurons.

4. DISCUSSION

We mentioned in the result section that synchrony required many cells to decay out of inhibition and to reach threshold at similar times. This however does not mean that all single GABA IPSPs have to be of a similar duration. The IPSP in any cell is the result of input from a large number of cells. Even if we have a range of IPSPs in the model, we would expect a large number of cells to experience a similar IPSP. Figure 7.4 demonstrates how a situation in which the IPSPs are not the result of such an overlap leads to desynchronized activity. The development of a similar resultant IPSP on each neuron despite a range of individual IPSPs may probably be explained using the Central Limit Theorem. The Central Limit Theorem deals with the probability distribution of the means of samples drawn from populations that have both normal and nonnormal probability distributions. Consider $\bar{x}$, the random variable denoting the sample mean calculated from samples of size n drawn from a population x. According to the Central Limit Theorem, if x has any nonnormal probability distribution, then the distribution of $\bar{x}$ approaches the normal distribution as the sample size n increases (Eason, Coles, & Gettinby, 1980). Pedley, Traub, and Goldensohn (1982) mentioned how the difficulty with a theory of inhibitory phasing is that it seems to require that the recurrent IPSPs have similar time constants, and that any type of "jitter" in the system would lead to temporal dispersion of the crucial phasing event. We argue that similar resultant IPSPs can occur in the neurons without requiring that single IPSPs be of similar durations because they are the result of overlap from a large number of neurons. In Section 3.2, we describe how the network activity can become desynchronized when the range of individual IPSPs becomes too large. The fact that synchrony became reestablished when a larger number of neurons were used with the larger range of individual IPSPs is further proof that the Central Limit Theorem is involved in the establishment of synchrony.

Following the decay of inhibition, the RE neurons have to reach a low threshold value before the occurrence of LTS. Co-activity of the RE neurons therefore requires that these neurons not only undergo inhibition of similar durations, but that they are then also able to rebound to threshold for LTS within similar times. Only one type of RE cell was represented in the model. It has been reported that although the RE neurons appear to be a homogenous set, they do display certain differences in electrophysiological properties. The potential that this variation in intrinsic properties has for disrupting the synchrony of RE firing can probably be offset by a common source of excitation for many RE neurons. This can be excitation from the LG and cortical layers. As Fig. 7.9 shows, excitatory input does have the potential to increase the degree of synchrony among the RE neurons.

ACKNOWLEDGMENTS

We would like to thank Paul Patton, Vinod Menon, and Tai-Guang Wei for their helpful suggestions and comments. We would also like to thank the Center for High Performance Computing for providing access to the Cray Y-MP8/864.

REFERENCES

Andersen, P., & Andersson, S. A. (1968). *Physiological Basis for the Alpha Rhythm.* New York: Appleton-Century-Crofts.

Brown, T. H., & Johnston, D. (1983). Voltage-clamp analysis of mossy fiber synaptic input to hippocampal neurons. *Journal of Neurophysiology, 50,* 487-507.

Buzsáki, G. (1991). The thalamic clock: Emergent network properties. *Neuroscience, 41,* 351-364.

Crunelli, V., & Leresche, N. (1991). A role for $GABA_B$ receptors in excitation and inhibition of thalamocortical cells. *Trends in Neuroscience, 14,* 16-21.

Deschênes, M., Madariaga-Domich, A., & Steriade, M. (1985). Dendrodentritic synapses in the cat reticularis thalami nucleus: a structural basis for thalamic spindle synchronization. *Brain Research, 334,* 165-168.

Domich, L., Oakson, G., & Steriade, M. (1986). Thalamic burst patterns in the naturally sleeping cat: A comparison between cortically projecting and reticularis neurons. *Journal of Physiology, 379,* 429-449.

Douglas, R. J., & Martin, K. A. C. (1990). Neocortex. In G. M. Sheperd (Ed.), *The Synaptic Organization of the Brain* (pp. 389-438). New York: Oxford University Press.

Eason, G., Coles, C. W., & Gettinby, G. (1980). *Mathematics and Statistics for the Bio-Sciences,* New York: Halsted Press.

French, C., Sah, P., Buckett, K., & Gage, P. (1990). A voltage-dependent persistent sodium current in mammalian hippocampal neurons. *Journal of General Physiology, 95,* 1139-1157.

Friedlander, M. J., Lin, C. S., Stanford, L. R., & Sherman, S. M. (1981). Morphology of functionally identified neurons in lateral geniculate nucleus of the cat. *Journal of Neurophysiology, 46,* 80-129.

Glaser, E. M., & Ruchkin, D. S. (1976). *Principles of Neurobiological Signal Analysis*. New York: Academic Press.

Hobson, J. A., & Steriade, M. (1986). The neuronal basis of behavioral state control. In V. B. Mountcastle & F. E. Bloom (Eds.), *Handbook of Physiology* (Vol. 4, pp. 701-802). Bethesda, MD: American Physiological Society.

Ide, L. S. (1982). The fine structure of the perigeniculate nucleus in the cat. *Journal of Comparative Neurology, 210,* 317-334.

Jahnsen, H., & Llinas, R. (1984a). Electrophysiological properties of guinea-pig thalamic neurons — an in vitro study. *Journal of Physiology, 349,* 205-226.

Jahnsen, H., & Llinas, R. (1984b). Ionic basis for the electroresponsiveness and oscillatory properties of guinea-pig thalamic neurons in vitro. *Journal of Physiology, 349,* 227-247.

Lopes da Silva , F. H. (1991). Neural mechanisms underlying brain waves: from neural membranes to networks. *Electroencephalographic and Clinical Neurophysiology, 79,* 81-93.

Lund, J. S., Henry, G. H., MacQueen, C. L., & Harvey, A. R. (1979). Anatomical organization of the primary visual cortex (Area 17) of the cat: A comparison with area 17 of the macaque monkey. *Journal of Comparative Neurology, 184,* 599-617.

Lytton, W., & Thomas, E. (1997). Modeling thalamocortical oscillations. In P. S. Ulinski & E. G. Jones (Eds.), *Cerebral Cortex, Vol. 13: Models of Cortical Circuity*. New York: Plenum.

Mulle, C., Madariaga, A., & Deschênes, M. (1986). Morphology and electrophysiological properties of reticularis thalami neurons in cat: In vivo study of a thalamic pacemaker. *Journal of Neuroscience, 6.* 2134-2145.

Pedley, T. A., Traub, R., & Goldensohn, E. S. (1982). *Cellular Pacemakers I.* New York: Wiley.

Sherman, S. M., & Koch, C. (1990). Thalamus. In G. M. Sheperd (Ed.), *The Synaptic Organization of the Brain* (pp 246-278). New York: Oxford University Press.

Steriade, M. (1991). Alertness, quiet sleep, dreaming. In A. Peters & E. G. Jones (Eds.), *Cerebral Cortex* (Vol. 9, pp. 279-357). New York: Plenum.

Steriade, M., Domich, L., Oakson, G., & Deschênes, M. (1987). The deafferented reticular thalamic thalamic nucleus generates spindle rhythmicity. *Journal of Neurophysiology, 57,* 260-273.

Steriade, M., Jones, E. G., & Llinas, R. R. (1989). *Thalamic Oscillations and Signalling*. New York: Wiley.

Steriade, M., & Llinas, R. R. (1988). The functional states of the thalamus and the associated neuronal interplay. *Physiological Review, 68,* 649-738..

Thomas, E., & Wyatt R. (1995). A computational model of spindle oscillations. *Mathematics and Computers in Simulation, 40,* 35-69.

Von Krosigk, M., Bal, T., & McCormick, D. A. (1993). Cellular mechanisms of a synchronized oscillation in the thalamus. *Science, 261,* 361-364.

8

Toward the Function of Reciprocal Corticocortical Connections: Computational Modeling and Electrophysiological Studies

Mark E. Jackson
State University of New York at Stony Brook

Larry J. Cauller
University of Texas at Dallas

ABSTRACT

We have studied some of the functional aspects of reciprocally connected neural elements using both computer simulations and in vivo studies. Computer simulations were conducted using the general purpose neural simulation package GENESIS. Two biologically realistic network models were constructed; the first consisted of a pair of interconnected excitatory and inhibitory neurons, and the second model extended the first to include long-range corticocortical connections. Both of these models exhibited chaotic dynamics that depended on the strength of the reciprocal connections. The behavior of these networks were explored using the methods of bifurcation diagrams, phase plots, and Fano-factor analysis, which revealed the fractal nature of the simulated spike trains. The chaotic dynamics of the real brain were studied by recording field potentials from the cortex of chronically implanted rats during anesthetized and awake states. The correlation dimension of the field potentials was found to decrease under the effects of anesthesia, possibly because of decreases in the strength of reciprocal connections.

1. TOWARD THE FUNCTION OF RECIPROCAL CORTICOCORTICAL CONNECTIONS

A common feature of the organization of the mammalian brain is the extensive connectivity between neural structures. In the sensory system, information about the environment travels from the peripheral sensory system to structures in the central nervous system. The bottom-up flow of information leads from the sensory receptor cells, to brainstem structures, to the sensory thalamus, and finally to the cerebral cortex. In the cortex, cells in the primary sensory cortex then project to higher order cortical areas, functionally characterized by the cell's response to specific features of the sensory environment. This bottom-up view of the organization of the brain, influenced by the serial description of visual perception by Marr (1982), dominated neuroscience research for years, but the accumulation of anatomical evidence has revealed that this view of neural connectivity is too simplistic. Many of the bottom-up projections are reciprocated by "top-down" projections, and in many cases the top-down projections outnumber the bottom-up projections. For example, while the thalamus projects to the cortex, there is an even greater projection from the cortex to the thalamus. The cortex also makes direct projections to sensory structures in the brainstem, including the superior colliculus and the inferior colliculus (Arnault & Roger, 1990; Clancy, 1996; Herbert, Aschoff, & Ostwald, 1991; Hubener, Schwarz, & Bolz, 1990). Similarly, each of the bottom-up projections from primary to secondary areas in auditory, somatosensory, and visual cortex is reciprocated by top-down projections from the secondary area back to the corresponding primary area (Carvell & Simons, 1987; Coogan & Burkhalter, 1990; Fabri & Burton, 1991; Koralek, Olavarria, & Killackey, 1990; Schwark, Esteky, & Jones, 1992). At the neural level, there are examples of neurons that have functional reciprocal connections with each other (Nicoll & Blakemore, 1993). It is clear from the anatomy that the nervous system is not organized as a series of serial projections from the periphery to the central nervous system, but instead is organized as loops within loops where the distinction between bottom-up and top-down quickly becomes muddied.

Reciprocal connectivity is also common within the cerebral cortex, the center for cognitive and perceptual experience. In the rat, reciprocal cortical connections are known to exist between primary somatosensory cortex (SI), ipsilateral homotopic secondary somatosensory cortex (SII), ipsilateral homotopic motor cortex (MI), and contralateral homotopic SI (Fabri & Burton, 1991; Koralek et al., 1990). Reciprocal connections also exist between the rat primary (Te1) and secondary auditory cortex areas (Te2 and Te3); (Arnault & Roger, 1990; Clancy, 1996). Considering these and other examples, the reciprocal nature of corticocortical connections has been recognized by many authors as a general principle of cortical organization (Felleman & van Essen, 1991; Pandya & Yeterian, 1985; Zeki & Shipp, 1988).

An important aspect of corticocortical connectivity that bears mentioning is the unique pattern of termination depending on the direction of the projection. The bottom-up projections from primary to higher cortical areas terminate primarily in middle cortical layer IV in dense clusters that preserve topographic information from the sensory environment, much like the bottom-up thalamic projection to the primary sensory cortex. In contrast, the top-down projections avoid middle cortical layers, ascending to the outermost layer of the cortex where the axons turn and travel long horizontal distances across the surface of the cortex (Fleischhauer & Laube, 1977; Jones & Powell, 1968). The significance of this asymmetric pattern of projections is that the top-down projection selectively activates a particular subset of cortical neurons. Only two groups of neurons have dendrites that reach the outermost layer of the cortex and are therefore recipients of top-down projections: layer II/III regular-spiking (adapting) pyramidal neurons that project to other cortical areas and layer V bursting pyramidal neurons that project out of the cortex to the superior colliculus, pons, and spinal cord (Hubener et al.,

1990; Jones, 1981; Larkman & Mason, 1990; Miller, Chiaia, & Rhoades, 1990; Pockberger, 1991). In higher cortical areas, this same group of neurons is the origin of the top-down projections to lower sensory areas (Clancy, 1996).

Although the existence of some of these top-down projections has actually been known for some time, the functional significance of this massive projection to layer I has often been discounted because it was assumed that synapses on the distal apical dendrites of large pyramidal cells would be insignificant due to the electrotonic decay of synaptic potential along the long apical trunk of these cells. However, physiological studies in vitro have demonstrated that excitation of horizontal layer I fibers generate significant somatic potentials and action potentials in all pyramidal neurons whose apical dendrites extend to layer I (Cauller & Connors, 1994). This finding suggests that the layer I inputs mediate more than a simple, tonic modulatory interaction between cortical areas, it may be possible to activate primary sensory neurons via this top-down pathway. It is not certain what affect the extensive yet distributed reciprocal inputs to layer I have on the activity of neurons in the primary sensory cortex in vivo, although there is evidence that these projections contribute to active sensory perception (Cauller, 1995). In one experiment that required monkeys to perform a tactile discrimination task, a strong excitatory potential was identified in layer I of SI that reliably predicted performance (Cauller & Kulics, 1991). This input was presumably the result of backward corticocortical projections and was not present during periods of inattention or under anesthesia (Cauller & Kulics, 1988). Other studies have also suggested important roles for the backward connections on visual perception in the primary visual cortex (Bullier, McCourt, & Henry, 1988; Bullier & Nowak, 1995; Sandell & Schiller, 1982), and the importance of reciprocal connectivity has also been stressed in many theoretical models of neural processing (Cauller, 1995; Koch & Crick, 1994; Rolls, 1989; Squire & Zola-Morgan, 1991; Ullman, 1994). The reciprocal nature of corticocortical, as well as the reciprocal nature of cortical connections with other brain structures, opens up the possibility of very complex interactions between bottom-up and top-down pathways. In conjunction with thalamic inputs via the bottom-up pathway, the layer I inputs might have a dramatic effect on the excitability of the primary sensory neuron or on the temporal pattern of the resulting spike train.

Considering this evidence of the abundance and possible functional significance of reciprocal corticocortical connections, we designed a set of experiments to gain an increased understanding of the functional significance of reciprocal connections between neural elements. We designed our experiments to take advantage of two complementary methods of research, computational modeling and electrophysiology. One of the difficulties of any neuroscience research is the difficulty of controlling the number of variables in something as complex as the brain so that the experimenter can be reasonably confident that the results of an experiment reflect the experimental manipulation. The most common way to eliminate many of the possible variables is to perform the experiment on anesthetized animals. The obvious difficulty with this is that the findings obtained in anesthetized animals may not be relevant to the way the system functions in the awake, behaving animal, or at the very least it is only part of the substrate of the function of the complete system in the awake state. Experiments can be performed in awake, behaving animals, but the experimenter usually has to sacrifice control over many variables, and the results of such experiments are sometimes difficult to interpret. In contrast, computational models give the experimenter complete control over all parameters, which is also the most serious limitation of such models because many of the parameters are not known and few unique solutions exist. For this reason we combine our modeling studies with physiological experiments that help to constrain and validate the performance of the models. We begin with a biologically realistic model from which some conclusions or observations about the physiological system can be postulated, and then use the model results to plan physiological experiments to validate some aspect of the model. As these two processes evolve into a more sophisticated model, it is hoped that an increased understanding of the neural system will result.

2. MODELING EXPERIMENTS

Because our modeling studies are based on the tenet that they can help us to understand the processes occurring in the brain, it is important for our model to have a sufficient amount of biophysical realism. The basic components of our models are compartmental neuron models based on real neurons recorded and stained in slices of rat somatosensory cortex. Compartmental neuron models closely simulate the essential aspects of real neurons, including dendritic integration of synaptic currents and the realistic effect of complex voltage-gated and ion-gated active channels on the input-output functions of the neuron. These models are constructed by representing small sections of each dendrite by equivalent electric circuits, which are then linked together to represent the electrotonic structure of the neuron. These simulated electric circuits account for the capacitance and resistance of the nerve membrane, as well as the resistance to current flow along the length of the dendrite (Rall, 1959; Rall, Burke, Holmes, Jack, & Redman, 1992). By this means, compartmental neuron models simulate both the temporal and the spatial flow of current throughout the dendritic tree, and the action of active conductances can be superimposed on this passive structure by adding differential equations which model the physiologically measured kinetics of specific ion channels. Thus compartmental models provide a realistic platform on which to explore synaptic and dendritic integration and also the contributions of the many varieties of sodium, calcium, and potassium channels.

The first step in constructing our compartmental neuron models was to fill real neurons in slices of rat somatosensory cortex with dye so that their complete dendritic morphology could be visualized. Neurons were impaled by sharp microelectrodes in vitro, electrophysiological measurements taken to characterize the input-output function of the cell, and biocytin injected into the cell so that the complex dendritic structure could be visualized under the microscope after histological processing (Cauller & Connors, 1992). The diameter and length of each dendritic segment were measured under an optical microscope and these dimensions were translated into cell description data files that could be read by the public-domain neural simulation package GENESIS, available by ftp from Caltech (Bower & Beeman, 1995). GENESIS provides a user-friendly graphical interface that allows users to model detailed neural structures, incorporating detailed morphology, active channels, and synaptic channels and also to easily create large biologically realistic networks using these detailed neuron models.

Although detailed compartmental models have obvious biological advantages over less detailed point-process neuron models often used in connectionist networks, the use of such detailed models have two related disadvantages. For most neurons, and for the type of neocortical neuron we are interested in, the dendritic tree is very large and has many branches. A detailed compartmental model of such a neuron could contain thousands of compartments, each of which must be modeled by a differential equation. The solving of thousands of differential equations for every simulation time step places a great computational burden on even the fastest computer. Having to deal with thousands of individual compartments also places a great burden on the modeler, who must keep track of synaptic inputs and ion channel parameters for each compartment, as well as interpret the resulting data. For this reason it is often useful to reduce the detailed model to a simplified model that is more computationally efficient yet retains many of the essential properties of the detailed neuron model. Fortunately, methods have been developed to accomplish this feat by reducing sections of several compartments into equivalent single compartments (Bush & Sejnowski, 1993; Jackson & Cauller, 1997; Stratford, Mason, Larkman, Major, & Jack, 1989). These methods can reduce a detailed cell model containing thousands of compartments into one containing less than 50, with obvious increases in computational efficiency and ease of use. Although reducing the number of dendritic compartments imposes obvious limitations on the realism of synaptic inputs into the dendrites, a certain amount of dendritic structure still exists that does allow for realistic passive and active propagation of dendritic synaptic currents (Jackson & Cauller, 1997). We constructed our network models using compartmental models based on two types of neurons: layer III pyramidal neurons that are involved in reciprocal corticocortical projections, and smooth stellate cells that are involved in local inhibitory circuits (Fig. 8.1). The complex morphologies of these detailed compartmental models were then reduced to simplified models that retained many of the electrotonic properties of the detailed model as well as the gross morphological characteristics of the real neuron (Jackson & Cauller, 1997).

2.1. Model 1: Reciprocally Connected Excitatory/Inhibitory Network

The first type of reciprocally connected network we examined was a very simple model of an excitatory and an inhibitory cell reciprocally connected (Fig. 8.1). This is a very common type of neural circuit in which an excitatory neuron is inhibited by a cell which it excites (feedback inhibition) (Douglas & Martin, 1992; Shepherd & Koch, 1990). We used the previously described reduced layer III pyramidal cell model as the excitatory cell (E1) and the reduced stellate cell model as the inhibitory cell (I1). Hodgkin-Huxley type sodium and potassium channels, standard components of GENESIS, were added to the soma of each model so that they produced a periodic pattern of action potentials when a simulated current input was applied to the soma. This is not the normal spike pattern of layer III pyramidal cells, which typically produce an adapting spike train in response to constant current stimulation. This adapting spike train

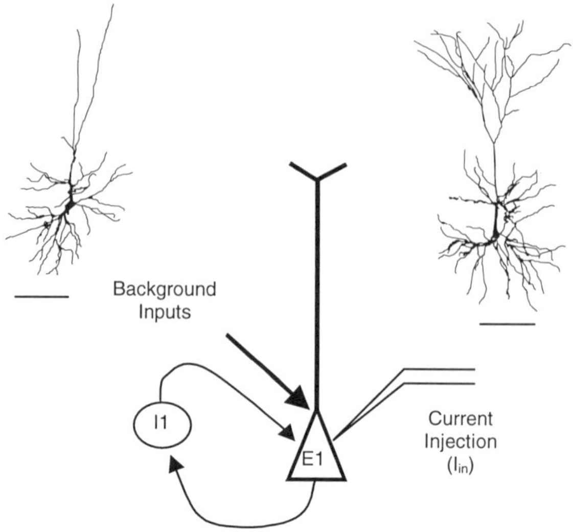

Fig. 8.1. Schematic diagram of computational model of reciprocally connected excitatory inhibitory network. The pyramidal cell model (E1) represents a primary sensory cortex neuron that projects to an inhibitory interneuron (I1) which in turn inhibits E1. Each model neuron receives random background synaptic inputs to simulate the inputs the cells would receive if they were embedded in a large network. The E1 cell model is driven by a constant current injection. In the upper right is the camera-Lucida drawing of the pyramidal neuron upon which the electrotonic properties of the pyramidal cell model were based. In the upper left is the camera-Lucida drawing of the stellate cell upon which the inhibitory interneuron cell model was based.

is mediated by calcium-dependent potassium channels that were not included in this simple model because we did not wish to introduce the additional complexities of calcium dynamics at this early stage. For this same reason, no active channels were simulated in the dendrites of either cell model. The two cells were connected to each other with appropriate synaptic currents, modeled as alpha functions that approximate the smooth shape of the experimentally observed synaptic conductance change (Jack, Noble, & Tsien, 1975), with a synaptic delay time appropriate to a local circuit between two neighboring neurons (≈ 2 ms). The strength of the excitatory synaptic connection on I1 was set to be suprathreshold, so that every action potential in E1 caused an action potential in I1. The strength of the inhibitory synaptic connection on E1 was set so as to produce a 5-mV inhibitory postsynaptic potential (IPSP), which is within a biologically realistic range of synaptic inhibition. Because in the real brain a neuron is always receiving a large number of synaptic inputs at any one time, we applied a random background synaptic current (normal probability distribution with a mean frequency of 400 Hz and mean EPSP amplitude of 0.1 mV) to each cell to simulate the noisy environment of the real brain. The strength of this random input was set to be subthreshold for each cell, but strong enough to provide some variation in the membrane potential that was qualitatively similar to what is seen in vivo.

A constant current injection (I_{in}), sufficient to cause a steady train of action potentials, was applied to the soma of E1. This current injection is an unnatural input into the cell, but can be abstractly considered to be a thalamocortical driving input. The reason for using an artificial current injection to drive the model is because it is a constant input, and in an isolated neuron model it would cause a periodic spike train. Therefore, any nonperiodicity in the network can be more easily analyzed knowing that the driving input was constant. The magnitude of I_{in} was the major parameter that was varied during the series of simulations.

2.2. Model 1: Results

We found that increasing the strength of I_{in}, while keeping all other variables constant, caused a very interesting change in the spiking pattern of E1 (Fig. 8.2). At low I_{in} the spike train consisted of very regular spikes, but as I_{in} was increased the spike train

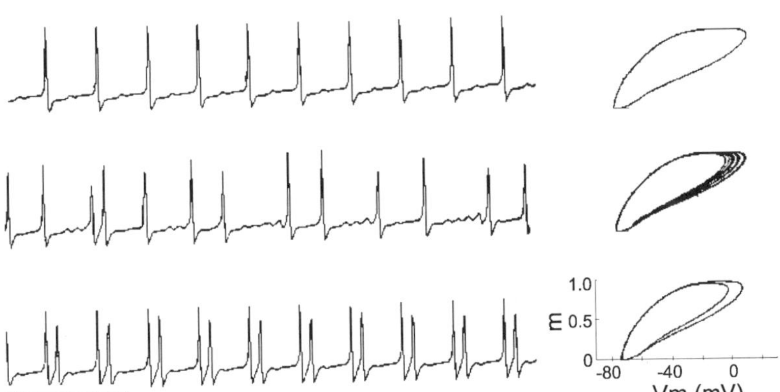

Fig. 8.2. Example of spike trains from the model of excitatory/inhibitory reciprocal connections. At the top is a periodic spike train produced when $I_{in} = 4.0$ nA. In the middle row is a complex spike train produced when $I_{in} = 5.0$ nA. At the bottom is a doublet pattern of spikes produced when $I_{in} = 8.0$ nA. To the right of each spike train is the corresponding phase plot produced by plotting the activation gate variable of the EI cell Hodgkin-Huxley Na channel (m) versus membrane voltage (V_m). The top and bottom phase plots show single and double periodic patterns, respectively. The phase plot in the middle, corresponding to the complex spike pattern to its left, is suggestive of chaos. The scale bar is 100 ms.

became very irregular, and at high I_{in} the spike train shifted into a regular pattern of doublet spikes. We looked at phase plane projections of these spike train patterns by plotting the activation variable of the Hodgkin-Huxley sodium channel (m) of the E1 cell model, which varies from 0 to 1 and represents the percentage of open sodium channel gates, versus the membrane potential (Fig. 8.2, right side). At low I_{in} the phase plot is a single orbit, corresponding to a periodic oscillation with only one phase. At very high I_{in} levels the phase plot is a double orbit, corresponding to a periodic oscillation with two phases. In between, however, intermediate I_{in} levels produce phase plots with multiple orbits and no distinguishable pattern of oscillation can be observed.

We noted that this type of phase plot is reminiscent of what is seen when a system enters a chaotic state (Canavier, Baxter, Clark, & Byrne, 1993; King, 1991; Pritchard & Duke, 1995). If our network is indeed chaotic, we can use methods of nonlinear dynamics to describe the network activity. The advantage of chaos is that activity that appears to be random is actually deterministic. Therefore, it is often possible to quantitatively describe the activity by such quantities as the Lyapunov exponent, which measures how rapidly the system deviates when perturbed, or by estimating the fractal dimension, which measures the amount of symmetry or correlation in the system.

One method to observe possibly chaotic behavior is to produce a bifurcation diagram of some observable parameter (Guckenheimer, Gueron, & Harris-Warrick, 1993; King, 1991). We measured the interspike intervals (ISI) between spikes recorded from E1 for several levels of sustained I_{in}. The reciprocal of each ISI (instantaneous frequency) was then plotted against the level of current injection (Fig. 8.3) and the resulting bifurcation diagram is typical of chaotic activity (Guckenheimer et al., 1993). At low I_{in} levels, the instantaneous frequency is constant at around 22 Hz. Then a critical threshold is crossed, at which point a very complex pattern of spikes emerges. Although the pattern of spikes appears to be almost random, closer observation reveals bands of points, starting left to right as four prominent bands that break into many more bands, eventually form two prominent bands, which finally stabilize to a constant pattern of spikes at around 22 Hz but this time with a second, higher frequency component at around 100 Hz. It is important to note that this pattern is not seen if the two cells are not reciprocally connected, in which case the spike pattern is completely regular and increases linearly with an increase in I_{in} (thin dotted line, see Fig. 8.3). This complex pattern of spikes is the result of the dynamic interaction between the two neural elements and demonstrates the complex activity that can be produced by very simple neural elements. At low I_{in} the action of the inhibitory cell governs a constant, low spike rate in the excitatory cell for a certain range of I_{in}, whereas without the reciprocal inhibition the spike rate increases for increasing I_{in}. At a certain point however, the dynamics of the spike rate of the excitatory cell conflicts with the dynamics of the reciprocal inhibitory influence, leading to what appears to be a chaotic attractor. A stable condition returns as I_{in} continues to increase, although with the addition of a doublet spike. Of significance is the fact that a very regular, periodic spike train was changed into a very complex spike pattern and eventually into a doubled periodic pattern without changing any local variables in the network, but by just changing the magnitude of current input injected into the network.

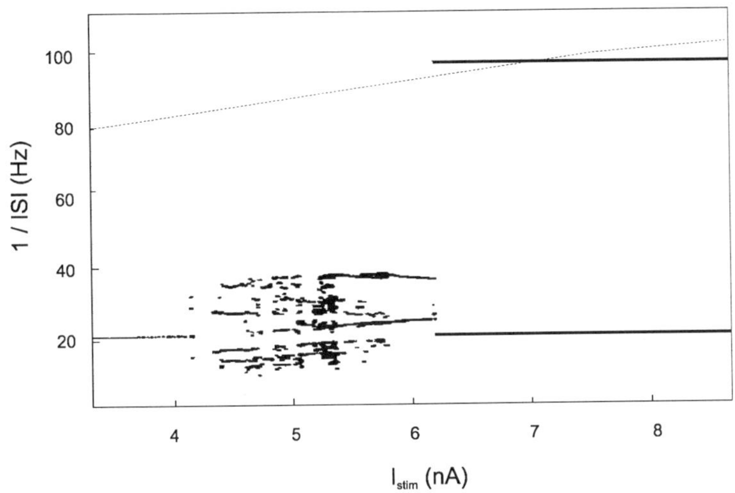

Fig. 8.3. Bifurcation diagram of interspike intervals (ISI) using I_{in} as the control parameter. Each dark point on the graph represents one ISI from a 5 second spike train at different levels of I_{in}. There are two stable state conditions, a single periodic condition for $I_{in} < 4.2$ and a double periodic condition for $I_{in} > 6.1$. The pattern of ISI's bifurcate between $4.2 < I_{in} < 6.1$ in a manner similar to that produced by a chaotic attractor, where only a few points appear to form the attractor and a banded appearance is apparent. The thin dotted line shows the result of removing the reciprocal connection between the neural elements but with all other parameters unchanged. In this condition there is no bifurcation and the response of the model linearly follows the increase in I_{in}.

2.3. Model 2: Asymmetric Corticocortical Connections

After seeing the rich dynamics that a simple excitatory-inhibitory network could produce, we wanted to see if a simple oscillatory model of excitatory reciprocal connections would produce similar dynamics. Our second model (Fig. 8.4) used two local excitatory-inhibitory networks: one local network (E1 and I1) represented a lower-order cortical sensory area and the second local network (E2 and I2) represented a higher-order cortical sensory area. The excitatory cell models of the two local networks were connected in anatomically appropriate ways, E1 projecting to the basal dendrites of E2, and the reciprocal projection from E2 projecting to the distal apical dendrites of E1. The strength of the synaptic connection from E1 to E2 cell model was adjusted to be suprathreshold (10 mV EPSP measure from rest = −70 mV).

The excitatory cell models (E1 and E2) differed from those in the first experiment, however, in that they contained a greater variety of active channels to make them

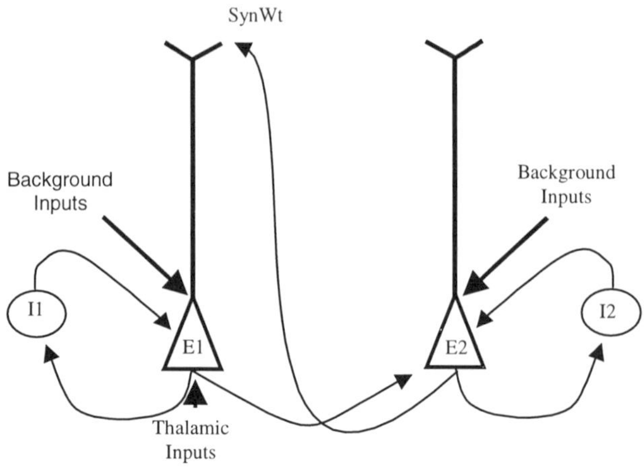

Fig. 8.4. Schematic diagram of model of reciprocally connected corticocortical oscillators. Excitatory (E1) and inhibitory (I1) neuron models are reciprocally connected to represent a local circuit in the primary sensory cortex. The second pair of cells (E2 and I2) are also reciprocally interconnected and represent a local circuit in the secondary sensory cortex. The two excitatory cells are reciprocally connected to each other to represent a corticocortical circuit, with E1 projecting to the soma of E2 and E2 projecting to the distal apical dendrites of E1. All cells receive subthreshold random synaptic inputs that simulate the normal background activity of the cortex. E1 is driven by suprathreshold synaptic currents that represent thalamic inputs to the primary sensory cortex.

respond like typical layer III pyramidal neurons as seen in vitro (Agmon & Connors, 1992). These cells are characterized by an adapting spike train (regular-spiking) in response to a constant current stimulus, and this adaptation of the spike frequency is known to be related to the presence of calcium channels and after-hyperpolarizing potassium channels (Hille, 1984). We used standard prototype channels from the Traub91 (Traub, Wong, Miles, & Michelson, 1991) channel libraries included with the GENESIS distribution, adding to the soma of the E1 and E2 fast sodium (Na), delayed rectifier (K_{DR}), transient potassium (K_A), voltage dependent calcium (Ca), voltage and calcium dependent potassium (K_{Ca}), and calcium dependent after-hyperpolarizing potassium (K_{AHP}) channels. Active channels were also added to the apical trunk (Na, Ca, K_{DR}, and K_{Ca}) to provide the efficient propagation of layer I inputs reported by Cauller and Connors (1994). The inhibitory cell models (I1 and I2) were unchanged from the first experiment, using Na and K_{DR} active channels in the soma to produce the fast, nonadapting spike train typical of inhibitory stellate cells seen in vitro.

This network model simulated a typical network of corticocortical connections, where sensory input from the thalamus excites the cells in the primary sensory cortex, which then project to and excite neurons in the secondary sensory area, which in turn reciprocally project back to the primary sensory area. All cells in the network received subthreshold random synaptic inputs (normal probability distribution with a mean frequency of 400 Hz and mean EPSP amplitude of 0.1 mV), simulating background activity. Instead of driving the network with a constant current injection, as we did in the first experiment, a more realistic condition was simulated by driving E1 with suprathreshold random synaptic inputs with an average frequency of 40 Hz. This input simulated the thalamic input into the primary sensory area. Because physiological evidence suggests that the strength of the projection of SII to SI is a major factor in conscious sensory perception (Cauller & Kulics, 1991), the main parameter that was explored in this model was the strength of the synaptic connection from E2 to E1 (SynWt). SynWt was scaled from 0 to 1, with 1 being the weight that produces somatic EPSP's typical of those produced by strong stimulation of isolated layer I fibers recorded in layer III pyramidal cells in vitro (Cauller & Connors, 1994).

2.4. Model 2: Results

The simulation was started with SynWt set to zero, meaning that there was no reciprocal connectivity between the two local networks, while E1 was driven by random synaptic thalamic input. As expected, the model produced spike trains that appeared to be random (Fig. 8.5(A)). As SynWt was increased, however, clusters of spikes became more pronounced, although the spike train still appeared to be random (Fig. 8.5, (B)-(C)). By visual inspection we could see that the strength of the reciprocal connection had a dramatic effect on the input/output function of E1, but we needed some method to quantify the observed changes in the spike train. The clustering of spikes was reminiscent of the type of clustering often seen in fractal spike trains (Lowen & Teich, 1992; Teich, 1989). If the spike train could be characterized as fractal, we should be able to quantify changes in the spike train and possibly relate such changes to the strength of the reciprocal connection. Thus, we examined the spike trains using Fano-factor analysis that had previously been used to reveal fractal spike trains in the auditory nerve vivo (Lowen & Teich, 1992; Teich, 1989).

The *Fano-factor time curve* (FFC) provides a useful statistic to describe any fractal point process, such as a sequence of action potentials. It is simply the variance of the number of counts in a specified time window divided by the mean number of counts for different counting times. If the signal is fractal, the FFC grows in a power-law fashion for long counting times, and the slope of the powerlaw growth portion provides an estimate of the fractal dimension of the point process, which falls between the integer values of 0 and 1. The FFC also provides useful information if the signal is not fractal. If the signal is a Poisson process, then the FFC approaches unity as T is increased; this is because the standard deviation of a single exponential density function (the square root of its second moment) is equal to its mean (its first moment; Bassingthwaighte, Liebovitch, & West, 1994). If the signal is periodic, however, the FFC will tend toward zero because the variance will decrease as T is increased (for a complete description and mathematical proof see Teich, 1989). The FFC is quite easy to calculate and can tell us not only that the spike train is random, fractal, or periodic, but also gives us a quantitative measure of the amount of correlation between spikes if the spike train is

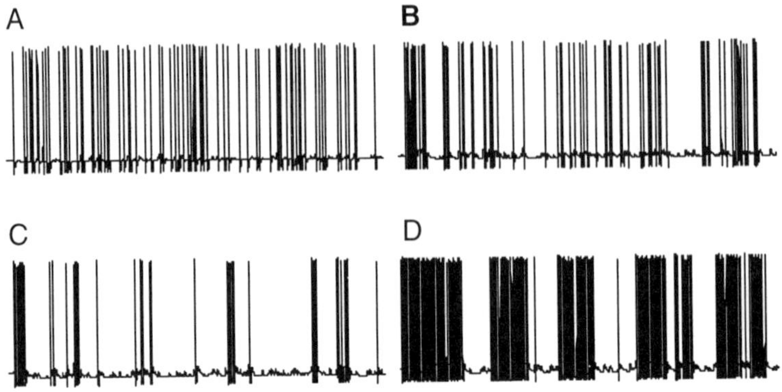

Fig. 8.5. Simulated spike trains from model of corticocortical connections with (A) SynWt = 0, (B) SynWt = 0.3, (C) SynWt = 0.5, and (D) SynWt = 1.0. Fano-factor analysis revealed that the spike train in (A) was random but (B), (C), and (D) were fractal spike trains.

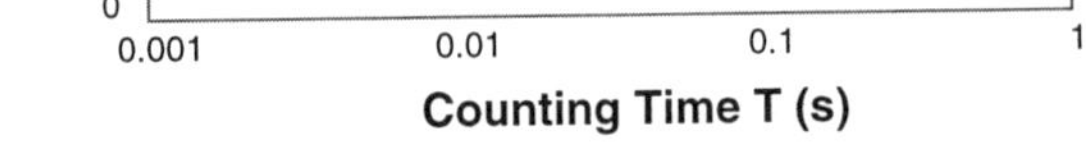

Fig. 8.6. Log-log plot of Fano-factor time curves (FFC) for examples of fractal (solid line, solid square markers) and Poisson (dotted line, open triangle markers) spike trains. The fractal data exhibits characteristic power-law growth for long counting times. The slope of this line, calculated by linear regression, provides an estimate of the Fano exponent. The random data has no such power-law growth. Modified from Jackson, Patterson, and Cauller, 1996).

fractal. Calculation of FFCs for spike trains produced by our model revealed both random and fractal spike trains (Fig. 8.6). The fractal spike train shows the characteristic power-law growth and is similar to the curve produced from spike trains of real neurons vivo (Lowen & Teich, 1992; Teich, 1989), while the random data shows no power-law growth trend and fluctuates around unity. The *Fano exponent* was estimated by linear regression of the log-log plot of $F(T)$ vs. T for an appropriate scaling range of T, typically 10 ms to 500 ms. Limiting the estimate of the power-law growth to less than one tenth of the length of the data segment helps to minimize errors in estimating the variance (Lowen & Teich, 1995).

Fano exponents were estimated from E1 spike trains during 30-second simulations for different levels of SynWt from 0 to 1 in steps of 0.02. Plotting the Fano exponents versus SynWt revealed a very interesting pattern (Fig. 8.7). For the range $0 < \text{SynWt} < 0.2$, the spike train was random. However, as SynWt was increased to greater than 0.2, the spike train became fractal. The Fano exponent increased as SynWt increased until it reached a plateau between 0.8 and 0.9. This formed a scaling region where, for a range of SynWt, an increase in SynWt was reflected by an increase in the Fano-factor exponent. The implication of this scaling region is that, in this region, it is possible to detect changes in SynWt by estimating the Fano exponent from the spike train for a range of SynWt. In the real nervous system it is very difficult, if not impossible, to detect changes in the synaptic strength of corticocortical connections, but it is possible to record spike trains from individual neurons. If the spike train in vivo is fractal, the Fano-factor exponent may prove to be a very useful measure of changes in the strength of neural connections.

Although the Fano-factor suggests that the spike train is fractal and that the system is chaotic, the most reliable indicator of chaos is the Lyapunov exponent. The calculation of the Lyapunov exponent is based on the fundamental characteristic of chaos that small perturbations of a parameter can lead to large deviations from predicted behavior, and it quantifies the rate at which the system diverges, with positive values of divergence indicating chaos. Lyapunov exponents were calculated by directly manipulating single parameters of the model during two identical runs, and positive Lyapunov exponents were obtained for each set of parameters that had produced fractal spike trains (Paul & Cauller, 1995). This provided strong evidence of chaotic activity

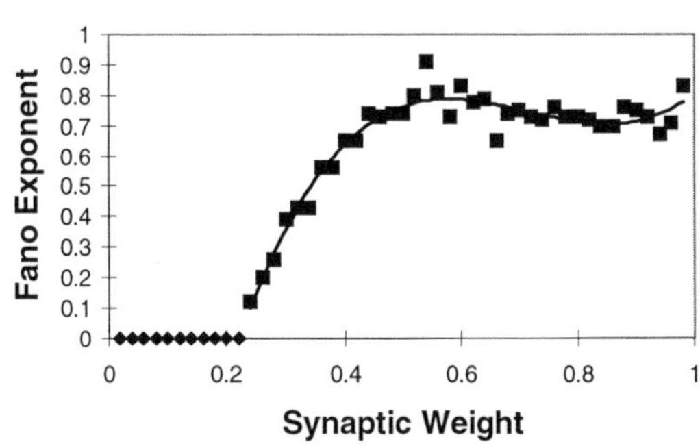

Fig. 8.7. Scatter plot of Fano exponents for different levels of SynWt. The zero points represent random spike trains. As SynWt is increased > 0.22 the spike train becomes fractal. A third degree polynomial function is fit to the fractal data to highlight the general trend of the Fano exponents as SynWt was increased.

and prompted us to call this model of oscillatory reciprocally connected neural elements a "chaoscillator" (Jackson et al., 1996).

2.5. Conclusions From Modeling Studies

We made several important observations about reciprocally connected neural elements based on these models. Most interesting is the fact that very simple oscillatory neural circuits can produce very complex spike trains if the elements are reciprocally connected. The output of the first model of reciprocally connected excitatory-inhibitory cells changed from periodic (with a single period), to chaotic, and back to periodic (with two periods), depending on the strength of a single parameter. Without the reciprocal connection the spike train is periodic at all levels of the current stimulus input. Increasing the strength of the reciprocal connection in the second model of corticocortical connections changed a random spike train into a fractal spike train. In the first case, the reciprocal connection allows the output of the E1 cell to depend in a very complex way on the level of input into the system, giving the neural network a much wider range of response. In the second case, the output of the system depends on the strength of the reciprocal connection. In both cases the reciprocal connection has the effect of qualitatively altering the output of the network, perhaps increasing the computational ability of the network.

A second important observation is the fact that both models lead to chaotic activity. Several other neural models have also exhibited chaotic activity, and a common thread between each chaotic model in the literature is reciprocal (feedback) connections between elements (Babloyantz & Lourenco, 1994; Hoppensteadt, 1989; Lopes da Silva, Pijn, & Wadman, 1994). In general, one of the most efficient ways to get chaos is to have oscillatory nonlinear elements coupled with feedback, which describes the pattern of reciprocal connectivity common in the brain. If this is the case, then chaos should be a common phenomena in the brain and there is ample evidence that this is indeed the case (Birbaumer, Flor, Lutzenberger, & Elbert, 1995; King, 1991; Molnar & Skinner, 1992; Pijn, Van Neerven, Noest, & Lopes da Silva, 1991). If the nervous system is chaotic, advantage can be made of the methods of nonlinear dynamics to quantify the level of chaos or fractal activity, and possibly correlate this measurement with the physiological influence of an important control variable. Our chaoscillator model demonstrates that changes in the Fano exponent can be correlated with such an important control variable, the strength of the reciprocal corticocortical projection. This would be a very valuable tool for exploring reciprocal corticocortical connections in the real nervous system, as it is difficult if not impossible to directly measure the strength of corticocortical connections, but it is easy to record spike trains from a single neuron. If real neurons exhibit similar behavior, it might be possible to detect subtle changes in the strength of corticocortical connections by changes in the Fano-factor exponent.

However, our enthusiasm must be tempered by the fact that we have only simulated very simple neural networks, and we do not know if many of the parameters we used in the model are valid assumptions or adequately represent the behavior of real neural networks. However, our models do give us a starting point from which we can plan our physiological studies and they prompted us to ask two questions. First, can we record chaotic neural activity from the sensory cortex of rats using some of the methods of nonlinear dynamics? If so, can we manipulate the activity of the cortex to cause measurable changes in the chaotic activity that can be related to putative changes in the strength of reciprocal corticocortical projections? We designed a physiological study to help answer these questions.

3. ELECTROPHYSIOLOGICAL STUDIES

In order to answer the second question, we needed a preparation in which we could change the efficacy of the reciprocal corticocortical projection. Fortunately, a simple preparation does exist which is suspected of eliminating the effects of the top-down projection to layer I of the primary sensory cortex. Previous experiments had shown that barbiturate anesthesia blocks the layer I response in primary sensory areas (Cauller & Kulics, 1988; Jackson & Cauller, 1994), putatively mediated by corticocortical connections. Of course, this is not the only effect of barbiturate anesthesia, which is also known to generally increase the effect of inhibition in the cortex among other things, but we felt it would serve as a means to manipulate cortical activity in a semi-known way. A simple experiment would be to measure cortical activity under barbiturate anesthesia and again without anesthesia. This could be accomplished by chronically implanting electrodes into the cortex and attaching an electrical connector to the skull of a rat so that cortical activity could be recorded through a small wire tether while the animal is awake and moving around. This is a common procedure and the animals show no sign of distress over either the presence of the surgically implanted electrodes, the presence of the electrical connector attached to the skull, or to being tethered to the recording equipment during the experiment. Although it is possible to record single unit activity in chronically implanted rats, there are technical difficulties associated with such recordings and we chose in this first experiment to record only field potentials. Although this made reliable recordings in the awake animal much easier to obtain, it did impose some limitations on our analysis of the data in that it is difficult to directly compare in vivo field potentials to the individual spike trains we were able to observe in our models. The field potential is the combined activity of large numbers of neurons, both local and distal, and is thus difficult to relate to a model that only consists of four neurons. However, future evolutions of the model will contain many more neurons, so this information will prove useful in developing larger models.

Another ramification of not recording individual spike trains in vivo is that we cannot analyze our data using Fano-factor analysis, which is only defined for point processes. However, other methods of nonlinear dynamics analysis can be used to measure chaotic and fractal properties of field potentials, so we will be able to answer our first question concerning the chaotic nature of neural activity in rat sensory cortex. In our experience, we found that the most straightforward and reliable method of estimating the fractal dimension of the cortical field potential is by estimating the pointwise fractal correlation dimension (D2) (Molnar & Skinner, 1992; Pritchard & Duke, 1995). D2 is similar to the regular correlation dimension, familiar to those with a knowledge of chaotic and fractal dynamics, but instead of averaging the correlation dimension for all points in the time series, the correlation dimension is estimated for individual reference points, and any points that do not fall within established linearity and convergence criteria are discarded. By discarding invalid reference points, D2 avoids the most significant, and most often violated, limitation of the standard correlation dimension that requires that the time series must be recorded during a period of attractor stability (Molnar & Skinner, 1992). Attractor stability is probably never a valid assumption in a system as complicated as the brain, so estimating the fractal dimension using D2 is likely more accurate than the simple correlation dimension (Pritchard & Duke, 1995).

Electrophysiological Methods. Electrodes were implanted in adult rats (Sprague Dawley) using standard sterile stereotaxic surgery procedures. Animals were anesthetized with an intraperitoneal injection of sodium pentobarbital (Nembutal: 50 mg/kg) and supplements were provided as needed to insure deep anesthesia though out the surgical procedure (2-3 hr). Electrodes were Teflon-coated nicrome wire (75 micron) with gold pins soldered to one end that were inserted into a plastic nine-pin connector. In one animal, electrodes were implanted in the primary motor cortex (MI), primary somatosensory cortex (SI), primary auditory cortex (AI), and the medial geniculate body of the thalamus (MG). In the second animal, electrodes were implanted in MI, SI, AI, and also in a polysensory area between SI and AI which is responsive to both somatic and auditory stimuli (PS). Five stainless steel screws were attached to the skull to serve as ground and reference electrodes and also to ensure proper anchoring of the connector to the skull. After the electrodes had been positioned and their pins inserted into the connector, the craniotomy was sealed and the electrode connector firmly attached to the skull with Crainoplastic (Plastic One, Roanoke, VA).

Both rats were allowed 1 week to recover from surgery before any recordings were made. Prior to connection of the wire bundles to the electrode connector on the rats head, each rat was given an intraperitoneal injection of Nembutal (25 mg/kg). A multiple-channel amplifier was used to record from each electrode simultaneously (gain 10K, bandpass 0.1 Hz to 5kHz) and field potentials were sampled on a 486 IBM PC-compatible computer and digitized with an A/D converter at 10 kHz.

Epochs of 3.2768 seconds (32768 points) were collected from each recording channel. Recordings in the anesthetized state were started 30 minutes after injection of Nembutal while the animals were still nonresponsive to tail pinch. Animals typically recovered from the anesthesia after 2 hours, and awake-state recordings were made after the animals had been active for a minimum of 30 minutes (2-3 hours after injection).

3.1. Electrophysiological Results

By visual inspection, obvious differences exist between field potentials in the anesthetized and awake animal (Fig. 8.8). In general, the field potentials in the awake animal are higher frequency and lower amplitude than those in the anesthetized state. In the anesthetized state the Fast Fourier Transform power spectrum (fft power) shows that most of the power is between 5 and 10 Hz, and this was consistent for all anesthetized recordings (top row, Fig. 8.8). D2 was estimated to be 4.31 for this set of data. The field potentials in the awake-state, however, proved to have much more variability in both the visual appearance of the waveform and in the fft power (lower two rows, Fig. 8.8). Although the fft-power of these two recordings were quite different from each other, the D2 estimates were the same for both sets of data (5.53). In other cases (not shown), time series with very similar fft power spectra had very different D2 estimates and in general there was no relation between the fft power and the D2 estimate. This suggests that the fft power and the D2 estimates are measuring different aspects of neural activity. The fft power reflects the frequency components of the slow electrical waves that course through the cortex and are produced by the summed electrical activity of large groups of neurons. D2, on the other hand, may reflect the state of particular parameters involved in the interaction between neural elements, such as the strength of the reciprocal corticocortical connections. If this is indeed an accurate statement, then we might expect that changing such a parameter would be reflected in a change in D2.

The parameter state we were attempting to change in this experiment was the strength of the reciprocal corticocortical connection by blocking the efficacy of this projection with anesthesia. When we compared the D2 estimates for time series obtained in the anesthetized state and the awake state, we found that D2 estimates for the awake state were higher than D2 estimates for the anesthetized state. When we compared mean D2 estimates for the two conditions in each of the four cortical recording locations by a two-tailed t-test for paired means ($p < .05$), we found in all cases significant differences between D2 estimates in the anesthetized and the awake state (Fig. 8.9).

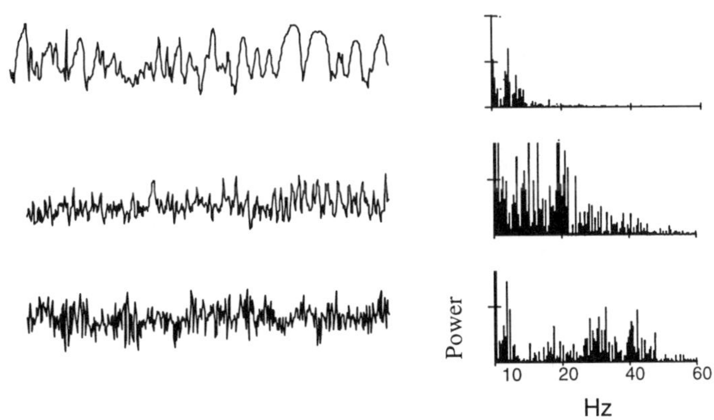

Fig. 8.8. Examples of field potentials recorded in both the anesthetized (top row) and awake (lower two rows) animal and the associated power spectrums. In general, the field potentials in the awake animal are higher frequency and lower amplitude and the power spectrums show broadly spaced peaks, typical of fractal time series. D2 for the anesthetized data was 4.31, and 5.53 for both sets of awake data. The length of each time series is 3.2768 seconds.

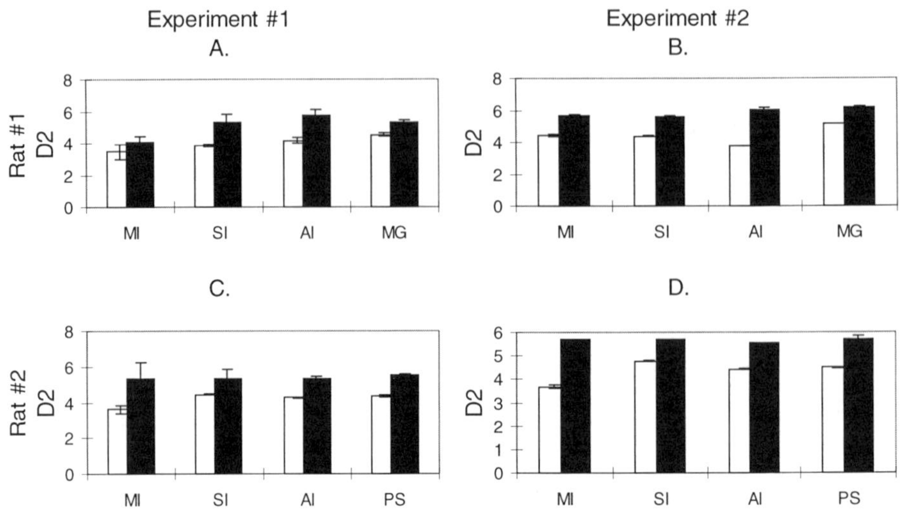

Fig. 8.9. Results from four different experiments with two rats. Mean D2s from four epochs (3.2768 s.) recorded at one minute intervals are shown for each condition and electrode, with the anesthetized data in open bars and the awake data in solid bars. In each case the difference in mean D2 between the anesthetized state and the awake state was significant, as confirmed by a two-tailed t-test for paired means ($p < 0.05$).

3.2. Electrophysiological Conclusion

We are confident that our experiment has provided answers to our two questions. Our first question was whether we could record chaotic or fractal activity from the sensory cortex of rats. We applied stringent criteria in our calculation of D2 and are confident that the cortical field potentials we recorded were fractal. It is possible, however, for low-pass filtered noise to mimic fractal data so we tested for this possibility in our data. We created a surrogate data set by randomizing the phases of the Fourier transform of the original data and then taking the inverse FFT to create a new data set with the same FFT power spectrum and autocorrelation function (Theiler, 1994). We then calculated D2 for each surrogate data set using identical procedures and criteria as for the original data. If the data is not fractal but is instead low-pass filtered noise, randomizing the phase of the time series should not matter because there is no correlation between the phases of noise and the D2 estimates for both the original and the surrogate data should be nearly the same. If, however, the time series is fractal, randomizing the phase should disrupt the fractal correlations in the data, and the D2 estimates for both the original and the surrogate data should be significantly different. When we tested our data with surrogate data, we found significant differences in the D2 estimates. This provides a strong argument that the signals we recorded from the sensory cortex of rats are fractal.

As for our second question, we found evidence that we could detect changes in the underlying state of the neural system by measuring changes in the fractal properties of the cortical electrical field potential. One explanation for the change in the D2 estimate between the anesthetized and the awake states is that the anesthesia blocked the reciprocal corticocortical projections to the primary sensory areas and this block is reflected by D2. Granted, many other factors were not controlled for in this experiment, such as the effect of barbiturate anesthesia on local inhibitory circuits, which could also explain the reduction in D2 under anesthesia. However, when we consider these data in conjunction with our modeling data we see evidence that the reduction in D2 may be at least partly due to changes in the efficacy of the reciprocal connections between cortical areas.

A limitation of this particular experiment is that the field potential is a measure of the summed activity of large populations of neurons and is not sensitive to small changes in activity, particularly spike patterns. We recorded data during several types of active behavior, such as active exploration, grooming, eating, and quite rest, but we found no significant differences in D2 between these states of activity. It is likely that reciprocal corticocortical activity changes during these activities, but the D2 measure is not sensitive enough to detect any such changes. We are now planning an experiment that will record single unit activity in rat sensory cortex before and during direct pharmacological activation of the fibers in secondary sensory cortex which project back to the primary sensory cortex. By directly measuring the responses of individual neurons we will be able to directly relate our findings to our computational models. Recording individual neurons will also allow us to use more sensitive measures of the spike dynamics, such as the Fano-factor.

4. SUMMARY

Our current study used computational models of simple oscillatory neural networks and in vivo experiments in an effort to understand the function of reciprocal corticocortical connections. By carefully designing our models to be biologically realistic we were able to draw comparisons between our models and the physiological neural system. From our modeling studies, we observed that a fundamental property of reciprocally connected oscillatory neural networks is a propensity to produce fractal spike trains. Because the spike trains were fractal, we were able to quantify some of their fractal properties and relate those properties to changes in the models parameters, most notably the strength of the reciprocal connection between the neural elements. We also found evidence of fractal activity in vivo, and the fractal properties of this activity could also be related to a major parameter of the real nervous system, under anesthesia and during the awake state. We feel that this illustrates a good fusion of two approaches of understanding the nervous system.

These studies represent only the beginning of our quest to understand the function of reciprocal corticocortical connections. The conclusions we have drawn from these experiments are preliminary at best and need to be confirmed by additional experiments with more controls. Our next step is to record individual spike trains in vivo while directly manipulating the strength of the projection from the secondary sensory area to the primary sensory area. We want to see if the top-down projection can influence the response properties of primary sensory cortex neurons in response to bottom-up activation of the sensory system. The results of these studies will guide us in the selection of parameters for our computational model. The computational model will eventually be expanded to more neurons, allowing us to explore the effect of combined activity and distributed reciprocal connection patterns in a realistic model. The parameters of this larger model will be constrained by attempting to replicate the data we observed in the physiological experiment that we report here. This larger model will allow us to explore parameters that we can't measure in vivo, such as simulating possible effects of anesthesia on the response properties of the network by selectively manipulating the effect of increased inhibition and decreased efficacy of the reciprocal connection, two possible mechanisms for the effect of anesthesia on changes in D2. In this way computational modeling and electrophysiological experiments can be used in concert to help unravel some of the complex workings of the brain.

ACKNOWLEDGMENTS

Portions of this work were funded by a grant from the Whitehall foundation. We would like to thank Barry Connors and Isabelle Bulthoff for providing some of the morphological data for the construction of our compartmental neuron models. We would also like to thank Kush Paul and James Patterson for their help in the analysis of the nonlinear dynamics of the computational models.

REFERENCES

Agmon, A., & Connors, B. W. (1992). Correlation between intrinsic firing patterns and thalamocortical synaptic responses of neurons in mouse barrel cortex. *Journal of Neuroscience, 12*, 319-329.

Arnault, P., & Roger, M. (1990). Ventral temporal cortex in the rat: connections of secondary auditory areas Te2 and Te3. *Journal of Comparative Neurology, 302*, 110-123.

Babloyantz, A., & Lourenco, C. (1994). Computation with chaos: A paradigm for cortical activity. *Proceedings of the National Academy of Sciences, 91*, 9027-9031.

Bassingthwaighte, J. B., Liebovitch, L. S., & West, B. J. (1994). *Fractal Physiology*. New York: Oxford University Press.

Birbaumer, N., Flor, H., Lutzenberger, W., & Elbert, T. (1995). Chaos and order in the human brain. *Electroencephalography and Clinical Neurophysiology: Supplement, 44*, 450-459.

Bower, J. M., & Beeman, D. (1995). *The Book of GENESIS*. New York: Springer-Verlag.

Bullier, J., McCourt, M. E., & Henry, G. H. (1988). Physiological studies on the feedback connection to the striate cortex from cortical areas 18 and 19 of the cat. *Experimental Brain Research, 70*, 90-98.

Bullier, J., & Nowak, L. G. (1995). Parallel versus serial processing: new vistas on the distributed organization of the visual system. *Current Opinion in Neurobiology, 5*, 497-503.

Bush, P. C., & Sejnowski, T. J. (1993). Reduced compartmental models of neocortical pyramidal cells. *Journal of Neuroscience Methods, 46*, 159-166.

Canavier, C. C., Baxter, D. A., Clark, J. W., & Byrne, J. H. (1993). Nonlinear dynamics in a model neuron provide a novel mechanism for transient synaptic inputs to produce long-term alterations of postsynaptic activity. *Journal of Neurophysiology, 69*, 2252-2257.

Carvell, G. E., & Simons, D. J. (1987). Thalamic and corticocortical connections of the second somatic sensory area of the mouse. *Journal of Comparative Neurology, 265*, 409-427.

Cauller, L. J. (1995). Layer I of primary sensory neocortex: Where top-down converges upon bottom-up. *Behavioural Brain Research, 71*, 163-170.

Cauller, L. J., & Connors, B. W. (1992). Functions of very distal synapses: Experimental and computational studies of layer I synapses on neocortical pyramidal cells. In T. McKenna, J. Davis, & S. F. Zornetzer (Eds.), *Single Neuron Computation* (pp. 199-229). San Diego: Academic Press.

Cauller, L. J., & Connors, B. W. (1994). Synaptic physiology of horizontal afferents to layer I in slices of rat SI neocortex. *Journal of Neuroscience, 14*, 751-762.

Cauller, L. J., & Kulics, A. T. (1988). A comparison of awake and sleeping states by analysis of the somatosensory-evoked potential in postcentral area 1 of rhesus monkey. *Experimental Brain Research, 72*, 584-592.

Cauller, L. J., & Kulics, A. T. (1991). The neural basis of the behaviorally relevant N1 component of the somatosensory-evoked potential in SI cortex of awake monkeys: Evidence that backward cortical projections signal conscious touch sensation. *Experimental Brain Research, 84*, 607-619.

Clancy, B. (1996). Afferent convergence in layer I of rat sensory neocortex: Neuroanatomical support for an interactive sensory-motor paradigm (Doctoral Dissertation, University of Texas at Dallas, 1996). *Dissertation Abstracts International, 57(07), 4220B.*

Coogan, T. A., & Burkhalter, A. (1990). Conserved patterns of cortico-cortical connections define areal hierarchy in rat visual cortex. *Experimental Brain Research, 80*, 49-53.

Douglas, R. J., & Martin, K. A. C. (1992). Exploring cortical microcircuits: A combined anatomical, physiological, and computational approach. In T. McKenna, J. Davis, & S. F. Zornetzer (Eds.), *Single Neuron Computation* (pp. 381-412). San Diego: Academic Press.

Fabri, M., & Burton, H. (1991). Ipsilateral cortical connections of primary somatic sensory cortex in rats. *Journal of Comparative Neurology, 311*, 405-424.

Felleman, D. J., & van Essen, D. (1991). Distributed hierarchical processing in the primate cerebral cortex. *Cerebral Cortex, 1*, 1-47.

Fleischhauer, K., & Laube, A. (1977). A pattern formed by preferential orientation of tangential fibres in layer I of the rabbit's cerebral cortex. *Anatomy and Embryology (Berlin), 151*, 233-240.

Guckenheimer, J., Gueron, S., & Harris-Warrick, R. M. (1993). Mapping the dynamics of a bursting neuron. *Philosophical Transactions of the Royal Society of London (Biology), 341*, 345-359.

Herbert, H., Aschoff, A., & Ostwald, J. (1991). Topography of projections from the auditory cortex to the inferior colliculus in the rat. *Journal of Comparative Neurology, 304*, 103-122.

Hille, B. (1984). *Ionic Channels of Excitable Membranes*. Sunderland, MA: Sinauer Associates.

Hoppensteadt, F. C. (1989). Intermittent chaos, self-organization, and learning from synchronous synaptic activity in model neuron networks. *Proceedings of the National Academy of Sciences, 86*, 2991-2995.

Hubener, M., Schwarz, C., & Bolz, J. (1990). Morphological types of projection neurons in layer 5 of cat visual cortex. *Journal of Comparative Neurology, 301*, 655-674.

Jack, J. J. B., Noble, D., & Tsien, R. W. (1975). *Electric Current Flow in Excitable Cells*. Oxford: Clarendon Press.

Jackson, M. E., & Cauller, L. J. (1994). Anesthesia-sensitive components of the SI neocortical response to forepaw stimulation in chronically implanted rats. *Society for Neuroscience Abstracts, 20*(57.10).

Jackson, M. E., & Cauller, L. J. (1997). Evaluation of simplified compartmental models of reconstructed neocortical neurons for use in large-scale simulations of biological neural networks. *Brain Research Bulletin, 44*, 7-17.

Jackson, M. E., Patterson, J., & Cauller, L. J. (1996). Dynamical analysis of spike trains in a simulation of reciprocally connected "chaoscillators": Dependence of spike train fractal dimension on strength of feedback connections. In J. M. Bower (Ed.), *Computational Neuroscience* (pp. 209-214). San Diego: Academic Press.

Jones, E. G. (1981). Anatomy of cerebral cortex: columnar input-output organization. In F. O. Schmitt, F. G. Worden, G. Adelman, & S. G. Dennis (Eds.), *The Organization of the Cerebral Cortex* (pp. 199-236). Cambridge, MA: MIT Press.

Jones, E. G., & Powell, T. P. (1968). The ipsilateral cortical connections of the somatic sensory areas in the cat. *Brain Research, 9*, 71-94.

King, C. C. (1991). Fractal and chaotic dynamics in nervous systems. *Progress in Neurobiology, 36*, 279-308.

Koch, C., & Crick, F. H. C. (1994). Some further ideas regarding the neuronal basis of awareness. In C. Koch & J. L. Davis (Eds.), *Large-scale Neuronal Theories of the Brain* (pp. 93-110). Cambridge, MA: MIT Press.

Koralek, K. A., Olavarria, J., & Killackey, H. P. (1990). Areal and laminar organization of corticocortical projections in the rat somatosensory cortex. *Journal of Comparative Neurology, 299*, 133-150.

Larkman, A., & Mason, A. (1990). Correlations between morphology and electrophysiology of pyramidal neurons in slices of rat visual cortex I: Establishment of cell classes. *Journal of Neuroscience, 10*, 1407-1414.

Lopes da Silva, F. H., Pijn, J. P., & Wadman, W. J. (1994). Dynamics of local neuronal networks: control parameters and state bifurcations in epileptogenesis. *Progress in Brain Research, 102*, 359-370.

Lowen, S. B., & Teich, M. C. (1992). Auditory-nerve action potentials form a nonrenewal point process over short as well as long time scales. *Journal of the Acoustical Society of America, 92*, 803-806.

Lowen, S. B., & Teich, M. C. (1995). Estimation and simulation of fractal stochastic point processes. *Fractals, 3*, 183-210.

Marr, D. (1982). *Vision*. New York: W. H. Freeman.

Miller, M. W., Chiaia, N. L., & Rhoades, R. W. (1990). Intracellular recording and injection study of corticospinal neurons in the rat somatosensory cortex: Effect of prenatal exposure to ethanol. *Journal of Comparative Neurology, 297*, 91-105.

Molnar, M., & Skinner, J. E. (1992). Low-dimensional chaos in event-related brain potentials. *International Journal of Neuroscience, 66*, 263-276.

Nicoll, A., & Blakemore, C. (1993). Patterns of local connectivity in the neocortex. *Neural Computation, 5*, 665-680.

Pandya, D. N., & Yeterian, E. H. (1985). Architecture and connections of cortical association areas. In A. Peters & E. G. Jones (Eds.), *Cerebral Cortex* (Vol. 4, pp. 3-61). New York: Plenum.

Paul, K., & Cauller, L. J. (1995). Using biologically realsitic models of neuronal networks to identify neuronal chaos. *Society for Neuroscience Abstracts, 21*(64.6).

Pijn, J. P., Van Neerven, J., Noest, A., & Lopes da Silva, F. H. (1991). Chaos or noise in EEG signals; dependence on state and brain site. *Electroencephalography and Clinical Neurophysiology, 79*, 371-381.

Pockberger, H. (1991). Electrophysiological and morphological properties of rat motor cortex neurons in vivo. *Brain Research, 539*, 181-190.

Pritchard, W. S., & Duke, D. W. (1995). Measuring "chaos" in the brain: a tutorial review of EEG dimension estimation. *Brain and Cognition, 27*, 353-397.

Rall, W. (1959). Branching dendritic trees and motoneuron membrane resistivity. *Experimental Neurology, 1*, 491-527.

Rall, W., Burke, R. E., Holmes, W. R., Jack, J. J. B., & Redman, S. J. (1992). Matching dendritic neuron models to experimental data. *Physiology Review, 72*, s159-s186.

Rolls, E. T. (1989). Functions of neuronal networks in the hippocampus and neocortex in memory. In J. H. Byrne & W. O. Berry (Eds.), *Neural Models of Plasticity* (pp. 240-265). San Diego: Academic Press.

Sandell, J. H., & Schiller, P. H. (1982). Effect of cooling area 18 on striate cortex cells in the squirrel monkey. *Journal of Neurophysiology, 48*, 38-48.

Schwark, H. D., Esteky, H., & Jones, E. G. (1992). Corticocortical connections of cat primary somatosensory cortex. *Experimental Brain Research, 91*, 425-434.

Shepherd, G. M., & Koch, C. (1990). Introduction to synaptic circuits. In G. M. Shepherd (Ed.), *The Synaptic Organization of the Brain* (3rd ed., pp. 3-31). New York: Oxford University Press.

Squire, L. R., & Zola-Morgan, S. (1991). The medial temporal lobe memory system. *Science, 253*, 1380-1386.

Stratford, K., Mason, A., Larkman, A. U., Major, G., & Jack, J. J. B. (1989). The modeling of pyramidal neurones in the visual cortex. In R. Durbin, C. Maill, & G. Mitchison (Eds.), *The Computing Neuron* (pp. 296-321). Reading, MA: Addison-Wesley.

Teich, M. C. (1989). Fractal character of the auditory neural spike train. *IEEE Transactions in Biomedical Engineering, 36*, 150-160.

Theiler, J. (1994). Two tools to test time series data for evidence of chaos and/or nonlinearity. *Integrative Physiology and Behavioral Science, 29*, 211-216.

Traub, R. D., Wong, R. K., Miles, R., & Michelson, H. (1991). A model of a CA3 hippocampal pyramidal neuron incorporating voltage-clamp data on intrinsic conductances. *Journal of Neurophysiology, 66*, 635-650.

Ullman, S. (1994). Sequence seeking and counterstreams: a model for bidirectional information flow in the cortex. In C. Koch & J. L. Davis (Eds.), *Large-scale Neuronal Theories of the Brain* (pp. 257-270). Cambridge,MA: MIT Press.

Zeki, S., & Shipp, S. (1988). The functional logic of cortical connections. *Nature, 335*, 311-317.

9

An Oscillatory Model of Cortical Neural Processing

David Young
Louisiana State University

ABSTRACT

Chaotic neurodynamics in the cerebral cortex is theorized as expressing degrees of uncertainty resulting from ambiguity in computational tasks. The cortex is modeled as a nonlinear system of oscillator circuits connected in a laminar structure and selectively excited or suppressed by input stimuli. Its behavior is related to modes predicted by the theory such as low level chaotic activity believed to be the default response when no stimulation is applied to isolated areas of the cortex.

1. INTRODUCTION

The most notable characteristic about brain wave activity must certainly be its oscillation. The perpetually changing neurodynamics of the brain is a complex and intriguing subject made still more interesting by several new discoveries. One discovery of relevance to this chapter is that spatial and temporal patterns of activity appear to be encoded responses to complex sensory stimuli and not merely the frequency transformation of stimulus intensity (Freeman, 1989; Menon et al., 1996; Optican & Richmond, 1987; Richmond & Optican, 1987; Richmond, Optican, Podell, & Spitzer, 1987). Another is that whole regions and remote areas of the brain will often synchronize briefly during a range of mental activity including what some believe may be related to conscious thought (Bressler, Coppola, & Nakamura, 1993; Joliot, Ribary, & Llinas, 1994; Llinas & Ribary, 1993; Tiitinen et al., 1993). An especially important discovery is that a class of neuron activity, previously dismissed as background noise, is recognized now by many to be the dynamics of a chaotic oscillator and as such plays a more significant role in how the brain processes information (Skarda & Freeman, 1987; Yao & Freeman, 1990; Young, 1997).

It is the nature of every neuron in the body that they must always oscillate, in one mode or another, just to survive. But incredibly, very little has been done, as yet, to understand the unique computational advantages of oscillations in brain wave dynamics. Historically, research in artificial neural networks has avoided, for the most part, this natural feature of the brain. For example, the goal of most traditional neural network models is to reach the static condition of a final system state; a concept entirely alien to biological *computers*. Several new views for the usefulness of oscillatory neurodynamics are now finally being formulated. But the variety of ways that oscillations are beginning to appear in modern neural network models testifies to the fact that it remains unclear what role these dynamics play naturally. Unfortunately, no real framework exists, as yet, for how to systematically approach this complex problem. Whatever form this framework will eventually take, we believe it should consider the information theoretic aspects of unstable dynamical systems.

Our model of neurocortical information processing offers a novel interpretation for the bifurcating nature of oscillatory neurodynamics. Periodic neurodynamics appear in many of the new models seeking to be more physiologically realistic (Basak, Murthy, Chaudhury, & Majunder, 1993; Crick, 1994; Joliot, Ribary, & Llinas, 1993; Pribram, 1990; Skarda & Freeman, 1987; Sutton, 1997; Sutton & Trainor, 1988). But few treat chaotic neurodynamics as a desirable feature. One that does is Freeman's model of olfaction (odor perception); (Freeman, 1987, 1989; Shimoide & Freeman, 1995). Our view of the role played by chaotic neurodynamics in cortical processing differs from Freeman's in one important way. Specifically, we assert that chaotic activity, because of its unstable nature, represents uncertainty in the outcome of tasks performed by the cerebral cortex. What we mean by *chaotic instability* refers to the tendency of a dynamical system to depart from simple periodic motion. And *a task performed by the cerebral cortex* means simply any useful behavior.

2. CORTICAL BEHAVIOR MODELING

A number of limitations in the computational capability of traditional artificial neural networks have come to light (Freeman, 1988; Kak, 1996), that are not shared by their biological counterparts. Fortunately, there are many aspects of the brain's structural organization and its unique oscillatory dynamics that can be examined more closely for clues to how modern neural network models will overcome these limitations (Garey, Dreher, & Robinson, 1991; LeVay, Wiesel, & Hubel, 1981; Schmitt, Worden, Adelman, & Dennis, 1981). Chaotic neurodynamics have particular appeal because of properties of chaotic systems that promise to be useful in computational tasks (Moon, 1987; Pecora, 1990). The author's view that neurodynamics are best governed by information theoretic decisions made incrementally as the system state evolves (Young, 1989, 1994), has lead to the interpretation of cortical neural processing that we present in this chapter. Our theory of cortical neural processing brings together, in a novel way, issues relevant to the realistic modeling of brain function to formulate a useful view of the structure and behavior of the cerebral cortex. We consider only general structure and behavior features that we believe are commonly repeated throughout the cortex because regions of the cortex vary significantly, in certain ways, and attempts to model these now would be premature.

Our approach is to investigate oscillatory dynamics in cellular automata made in the form of a two-dimensional array of processing elements interacting according to a regular connection structure. The model is meant to represent the laminar structure of the cerebral cortex. Each neuron is modeled as a second order differential equation of the form

$$\frac{d^2}{dt^2}y_{u,v} + \frac{d}{dt}y_{u,v} + y_{u,v} = \sum_R h(Y) + I_{u,v}(t)$$

where **Y** is an array of elements $y_{u,v}$, $0 < u < n$, $0 < v < n$, and n is the size of the array; R is the *receptive field* of the element $y_{u,v}$ defined by some radius of points surrounding the point at coordinates (u, v); H is a lateral interaction function; and $I(t)$ is an input function.

The goal is to develop a model that adequately represents the behavior of the cerebral cortex. To do this we begin with a description that characterizes cortical behavior and acknowledges the usefulness of chaotic neurodynamics.

2.1. Characterization of Behavior

The activity described by our theory of cortical neural processing is bimodal in regard to the kinds of oscillations that neurons are said to exhibit. Neurons or groups of neurons working together in a local cortical circuit must be capable of both kinds of behavior described by our theory. They must have a base condition (without stimulation) of a low intensity waveform that is highly chaotic. Then as input is applied, a strong periodic, or at least quasi-periodic, signal quickly appears. Such rapid transitions are known as bifurcations. Note that the term *input* is used here in a general sense. It may refer to stimulation due to sensory receptors, such as the visual, auditory, and olfactory systems, or it may simply mean a signal that originates elsewhere in the cortex.

The mechanism of pericolumnar inhibition, as proposed by Mountcastle (1978), establishes dynamic regions within the laminar cortical structure. By dynamic regions, what is meant is that these regions form due to the immediate input signal and is not the result of learned or innate structure. This raises the issue of whether input, causing the dynamic isolation of a region, in turn causes its activity to bifurcate; or is it that input causes a bifurcation that later creates isolation. A third possibility, of course, is that both are directly produced by received input. We shall refer to a region of relative stability that is isolated from its chaotic surroundings as an *activity bubble.*

2.2. The Computational Role of Chaos

An interpretation for chaotic oscillatory behavior in physiologically realistic systems is to be found in the literature and is the source of the material in this subsection (Freeman, 1987, 1989, 1994). A vase-shaped diagram was developed by Skarda and Freeman (1987) as a representation of the state space bifurcation characteristic of his model of the olfactory process. It illustrates the action of odor perception during the normal respiratory behavior of rabbits (Freeman, 1987). A spectrum of distinct behavioral modes begins at the lowest possible level, a condition while only under *deep anesthesia*. Then comes *sleep* and *waking rest*, where the amplitude is low but considerably more complex than before. Later are *exhalation* and *inhalation*, the two states of *motivation*. Finally, the most excited state of all is *seizure*. The ability to model seizures is very important in its own right, independent of what cognitive modeling insight it may bring, because it takes medical researchers that much closer to understanding and perhaps controlling the debilitating disease of epilepsy.

An important feature to bring out of the bifurcation diagram is the number of limit cycles present at the inhalation level. This differs from the waking rest level in which only one central limit cycle can be found. The limit cycles, or spatially patterned attractors, classify respective stimulus odors to which animals are trained to respond.

From this description there come four suggested functions performed by chaotic activity in biological neural systems.

1. It provides rapid and unbiased access to all the collection of latent attractors. Any attractor may be selected, without warning, by environmental factors. The process "turns off" the low-dimensional *noise* at the moment of bifurcation to a patterned attractor, and is "turned on" again on reverse bifurcation as the patterned attractor vanishes.

2. The chaotic attractor provides for global and continuous spatio-temporally unstructured neural activity. This is vital for the survival of neurons, in periods of low demand, which parish without proper conditioning to prevent atrophy of the tissue.

3. A special pattern provides response to the contextual component of the environment. In this way any new odor stimulus, not already a member of the latent attractors, interferes with the contextual response leading to failure of convergence to any of the learned patterned attractors. The resulting chaotic activity also differs from the contextual response, signaling that what has been encountered is an unidentified stimulus. The power of this process is that classification of unknown odor stimuli can occur as rapidly as the classification of any known odor, without requiring an exhaustive search through an ensemble of classified patterns.

4. A function that deals with learning. Chaos allows the system to escape from its established repertoire of responses in order to add a new response to a novel stimulus under reinforcement. The process is analogous to the Hebbian learning rule. Chaotic activity evoked by a novel odor provides unstructured activity that can drive the formation of a new nerve cell assembly by strengthening synapses between neurons of highly correlated activity.

3. SIMULATED LAMINAR STRUCTURE

We now develop a model that is less complex than that just described. The purpose is initially to simulate the base condition of our proposed cortical processor without requiring a discouraging amount of computing overhead. Then we examine responses to a number of different stimuli. Only lateral interaction is taken into account by our simplified model. Our model is not intended to duplicate the olfactory behavior expressed in Freeman's model. But it is meant to capture some of the bifurcating nature that is so prevalent throughout the entire cerebral cortex.

We begin by setting up an n-by-n array of processing elements (neurons). The output of each is numerically calculated from a second order differential equation. The key to the equation is a coupling between neurons that reflects the lateral interaction of the cortex as seen in the right hand side of the expression:

$$\frac{d^2 y_{u,v}}{dt^2} + A\frac{dy_{u,v}}{dt} + By_{u,v} = k_1 \sum_R H(y_{u+i,v+j}) + k_2 I_{u,v}(t)$$

where ($y_{u,v}$: $u = 1, \ldots, n$; $v = 1, \ldots, n$) are the neurons of the array and R is the receptive field surrounding neuron (u, v) such that for some radius r, the *receptive field R* defines the set of points $(u+i, v+j)$ by their Euclidean distance to the point (u, v) as:

$$R = \left\{(u+i, v+j) : (u+i+n)^2_{\text{mod}_n} + (v+j+n)^2_{\text{mod}_n} \leq r^2\right\}.$$

The radius r and the function H are considered to be uniform throughout the array. Also, to eliminate edge effects, neurons near the outer limits of the array wrap around to points on the opposite edge using the modular operator mod_n. A and B are constants found experimentally that represent the natural frequency and damping coefficients, respectively. The constant gains k_1 and k_2 are also determined experimentally. The function $I_{u,v}(t)$ is an input signal applied to the neuron at coordinate (u, v), which is zero everywhere when measuring the base condition. The fourth order Runge-Kutta method of integration is used to evaluate this system of simultaneous equations. The advantage of having only one differential equation per coordinate (u, v) is to reduce the complexity of our model.

3.1. Lateral Interaction Function

Most neurons in the cerebral cortex interact with neighboring neurons through a nonlinear spatial function. The range of this interaction may extend as far as several centimeters in some cases but the majority of the influence covers a much smaller area. Specific neuron types determine the characteristics of the interaction function and most follow the same general form which may be approximated as a single gain function common to every neuron in a two dimensional array of neurons. The form of the interaction function used in our simplified model is seen in Fig. 9.1.

It is generated by taking the Kaiser function (the Bessel function of the first kind divided by the Modified Bessel function of the first kind, J_0/I_0) and scaling it along lateral dimensions. Units in the figure are in microns. Only the area covered by radius

r (microns) is used in the implementation of the function. This is accomplished with the two dimensional gain matrix depicted in Fig. 9.2.

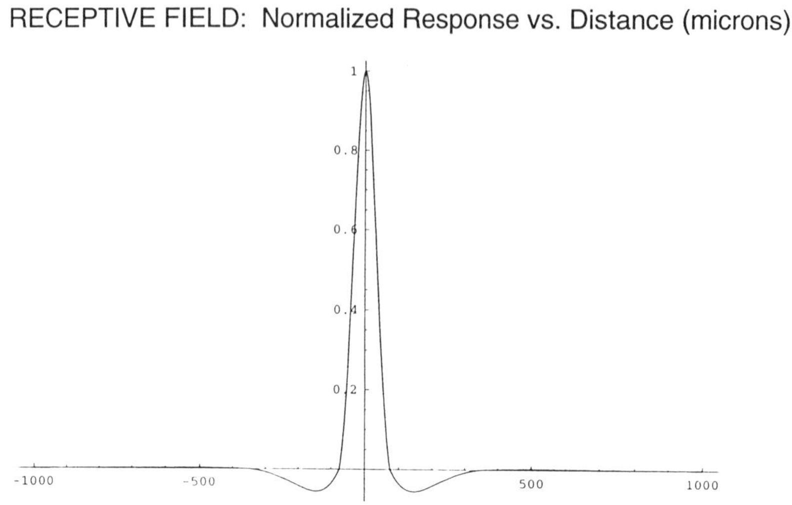

Fig. 9.1. Lateral interaction function.

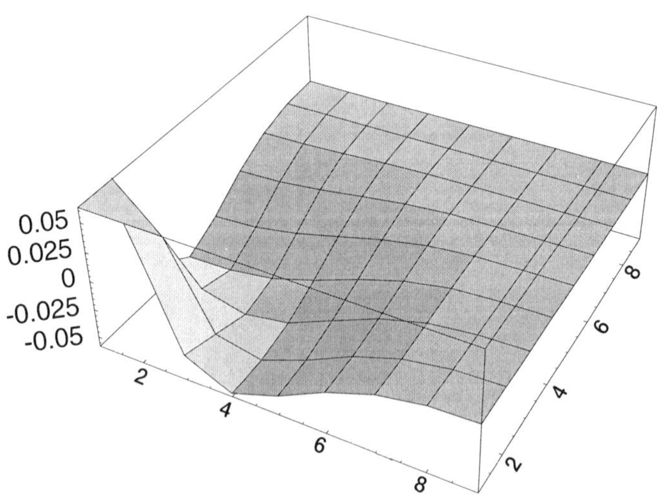

Fig. 9.2. Gain matrix (upper right quadrant).

The point (0,0) of this matrix represents the coordinates of the neuron using this gain to compute its output. To hasten the simulation of this structure, our model implements this matrix as a look-up table which avoided unnecessary calculation.

It can be seen from this figure that spatial resolution below that shown would have difficulty in representing the central peak of the interaction function while keeping the relative scale in the lateral dimension of its various features. It was for these reasons that the array is chosen to be 8-by- 8, where $n = 8$. At this scale, however, edge effects become considerable. To avoid this and yet keep the number of neurons in the model few, the modular operator is used in defining the receptive field. Only the upper right quadrant of this gain matrix, as depicted in Fig. 9.2, is stored as a look-up table. The neuron at coordinate (0,0) of this figure is evaluated with all four quadrants of the gain matrix due to the modular operator.

3.2. Simulation of Chaotic Base Condition

To observe the base response of our model, a simulation was run without applying an input stimulus. We constructed an 8-by-8 array and initialized each neuron according to a pseudorandom number generator to create the start state (y and dy/dt at $t = 0$). Parameters were set at $A = 0$, $B = 50$, $k_1 = 40$, and $k_2 = 0$. The system was integrated for 4,000 steps of size $dt = 0.01$.

To characterize this behavior and to get an idea if it is, in fact, nonperiodic, we plot the phase diagram of any two neuron responses; one against the other. Figure 9.3 is just such a phase diagram, showing the base response of $y_{3,5}$ against that of $y_{4,1}$. The

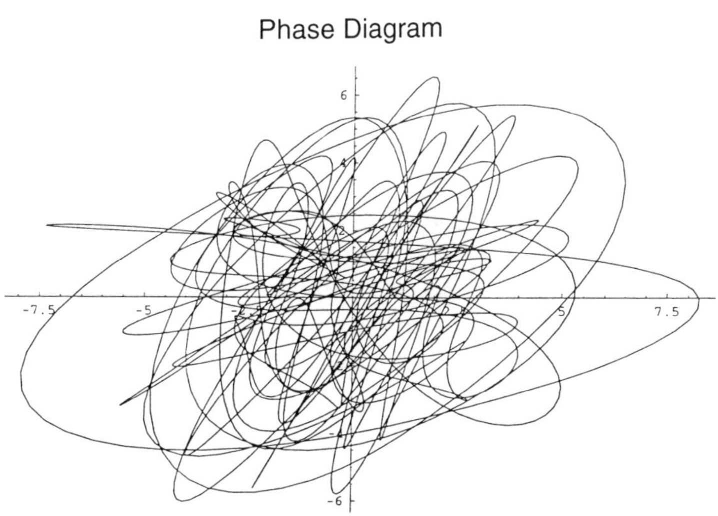

Fig. 9.3. Base response ($y_{4,1}$ vs. $y_{3,5}$); $t = 0.40$.

plot appears to be very disorderly and certainly nonrepeating over the interval of the simulation. Similar plots are obtained with other choices of neuron matrix elements.

To help determine if any long-term stabilization is occurring, another graph (Fig. 9.4) is shown for only the first 2,000 data points of the previous graph. When compared, these two graphs show that the path traced out on the phase diagram continues to have both low and high amplitude orbits, showing no indication of settling. A more conclusive determination of chaotic behavior can be had through other more computationally intensive analysis techniques such as calculation of the Lyapunov exponents of the system. In this case, over 64^2 simultaneous equations must be solved. We have not attempted such a computation at this time.

3.3. Response to Stimuli

When a sinusoidal input is applied to one or more sites within our simulated cortical array, an area of stronger response appears in the immediate vicinity of the applied input. This is similar to the stability bubbles predicted by our theory. What is more, the response appears to be much more stable than the surrounding activity. A series of experiments were done. Sinusoidal waveforms of the same frequency and phase were first applied to three pairs of locations in the array. Distances of one (adjacent locations), three and five separated the pairs of applied inputs. Also, frequency and phase shifts between the two inputs were considered. In one example, input is applied to two adjacent locations. The same frequency of $\pi/25$ is applied to both and the phase angle between the inputs is zero.

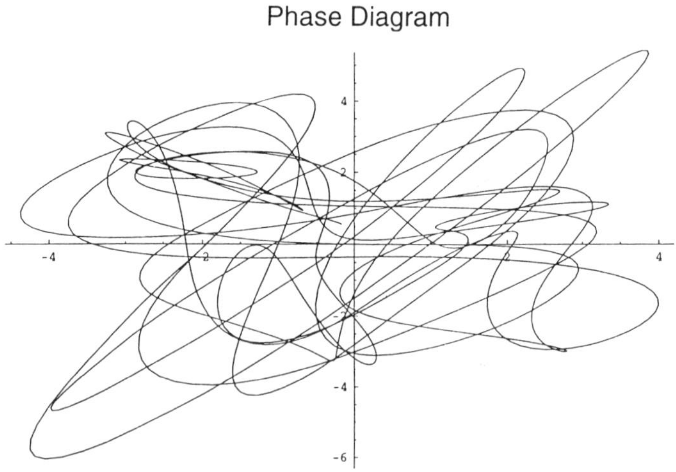

Fig. 9.4. Base response ($y_{4,1}$ vs. $y_{3,5}$); $t = 0.20$.

The left side of Fig. 9.5 depicts the time series response of each simulated neuron in an 8-by-8 array. Fourier transforms were calculated for each using fast Fourier transforms, and are shown to the right of the time series response. The base condition is certainly quasi-periodic. This is seen in the high number of spikes in their Fourier response. However, the Fourier response of the neurons to which input is applied is not as complex. Significant high-frequency response is almost nonexistent. Neurons nearby the locations where input is applied are also affected, due to the lateral interaction function.

Two frequencies are applied at a distance of 3 locations in another set of experiments. The frequency of one input is changed, $\pi/22$, in one case. The other input frequency remains at $\pi/25$. In another case, the frequencies are the same, but there is a phase angle of $\pi/4$ between them. The phase is increased to $\pi/2$ for the final case.

4. CONCLUSION

The behavior of the cerebral cortex was characterized as an interplay of chaotic and stable neurodynamics. Issues relating to the way in which chaotic neurodynamics is employed by the brain were discussed. A simulation of the lateral interaction function was shown to produce the chaotic base condition predicted by our theory. The application of periodic oscillation to our model created bubbles of stable activity. However, these bubbles were not totally isolated from the surrounding cellular array. The low-intensity interaction, experienced by neurons lying beyond the boundaries of stability bubbles, is viewed as a kind of preconscious processing.

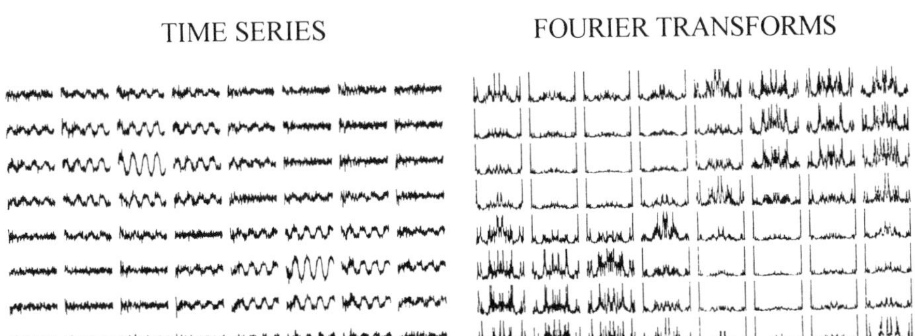

Fig. 9.5. $\omega_1 = \omega_2 = \pi/25$, $\phi = \pi$, distance = 3.

REFERENCES

Basak, J., Murthy, C. A., Chaudhury, S., & Majumder, D. D. (1993). A connectionist model for category perception: Theory and implementation. *IEEE Transactions on Neural Networks*, *4*, 257-269.

Bressler, S. L., Coppola, R., & Nakamura, R. (1993). Episodic multiregional cortical coherence at multiple frequencies during visual task performance. *Nature*, *366*, 153-156,

Crick, F. (1994). *The Astonishing Hypothesis: The Scientific Search for the Soul.* New York: Charles Scribner's Sons/Macmillan.

Freeman, W. J. (1987). Simulation of chaotic EEG patterns with a dynamic model of the olfactory system. *Biological Cybernetics*, *56*, 139-150.

Freeman, W. J. (1988). Why neural networks don't yet fly: Inquiry into the neurodynamics of biological intelligence. *Second Annual International Conference on Neural Networks, San Diego, CA.* Piscataway, NJ: IEEE..

Freeman, W. J. (1989). Perceptual Processing Using Oscillatory Chaotic Dynamics. *Advanced Topics in Neuroelectric Signal Analysis, IEEE Engineering in Medicine and Biology Society* 11th Annual International Conference, 1989.

Freeman W. J. (1994). Chaotic dynamics in neural pattern recognition. In V. Cherkassky, J. H. Friedman, & H. Wechsler H (Eds.), *From Statistics to Neural Networks. Theory and Pattern Recognition Applications* (pp. 376-394). Berlin: Springer-Verlag.

Freeman, W. J., & Vianna Di Prisco, G. (1986). Relation of olfactory EEG to behavior: Time series analysis. *Behavioral Neuroscience*, *100*, 753-763.

Garey, L. J., Dreher, B., & Robinson, S. (1991). The organization of the visual thalamus. In J. Cronly-Dillon (Ed.), *Vision and Visual Dysfunction* (Vol. 3, pp. 176-234). Boca Raton, FL: CRC.

Joliot, M., Ribary, U., & Llinas, R. (1994). Human oscillatory brain activity near 40 Hz coexists with cognitive temporal binding. *Proceedings of the National Academy of Sciences*, *91*, 11748-11751.

Kak, S. C. (1996). Speed of computation and simulation. *Foundations of Physics*, *26*, 1375-1386.

LeVay, S., Wiesel, T. N., & Hubel, D. H. (1981). The postnatal development of ocular-dominance columns in the monkey. In F. O. Schmitt, F. G. Worden, G. Adelman, S. G. Dennis, F. E. Bloom, W. M. Cowen, G. M. Edelman, & A. M. Graybiel (Eds.), *The Organization of the Cerebral Cortex* (pp. 29-45). Cambridge, MA: MIT Press.

Llinas, R. R., & Ribary, U. (1993). Coherent 40-Hz oscillation characterizes dream state in humans. *Proceedings of the National Academy of Sciences*, 90, 2078-2081.

Menon, V., Freeman, W. J., Cutillo, B. A., Desmond, J. E., Ward, M. F., Bressler, S. L., Laxer, K. D., Barbaro, N., & Gevins, A. S. (1996). Spatio-temporal correlations in human gamma band electrocortiograms. *Electroencephalography and Clinical Neurophysiology*, *98*, 89-102.

Moon, F. C. (1987). *Chaotic Vibrations: An Introduction for Applied Scientists and Engineers.* New York: Wiley.

Mountcastle, V. (1978). *The Mindful Brain.* Cambridge, MA: MIT Press.

Optican, L. M., & Richmond, B. J. (1987). Temporal encoding of two dimensional patterns by single units in primate inferior temporal cortex. III. Information theoretic analysis. *Journal of Neurophysiology*, *57*, 162-178.

Pecora, L. M., & Carroll, T. L. (1990). Synchronization in chaotic systems. *Physical Review Letters*, *64*, 821-824.

Pribram, K. H. (1990). Brain, mind, and consciousness: The science of neuropsychology. In A. Bocaz (Ed.), *Proceedings: First Symposium on Cognition, Language and Culture:*

Cross-disciplinary Dialog in Cognitive Sciences (pp. 9-38). Santiago, Chile: Universidad de Chile.

Richmond, B. J., & Optican, L. M. (1987). Temporal encoding of two dimensional patterns by single units in primate inferior temporal cortex. II. Quantification of response waveform. *Journal of Neurophysiology*, *57*, 147-161.

Richmond, B. J., Optican, L. M., Podell, M., & Spitzer, H. (1987). Temporal encoding of two dimensional patterns by single units in primate inferior temporal cortex. I. Response characteristics. *Journal of Neurophysiology*, *57*, 132-146.

Schmitt, F. O., Worden, F. G., Adelman, G., & Dennis, M. (Eds). (1981). *The Organization of the Cerebral Cortex*. Cambridge, MA: MIT Press.

Shannon, C. E., & Weaver, W. (1949). *The Mathematical Theory of Communication*. Urbana, IL: IlliniPress.

Shimoide, K., & Freeman, W. J. (1995). Dynamic neural network derived from the olfactory system with examples of applications. *IEICE Transactions on Fundamentals of Electronics, Communications and Computer Sciences*, vol. E78-A, no. 7.

Skarda, C. A., &. Freeman, W. J. (1987). How brains make chaos in order to make sense of the world. *Behavioral and Brain Sciences*, *10*, 161-195.

Sutton, J. P. (1997). Network hierarchies in neural organization, development and pathology. In W. Brandts, C. J. Lumsden, & L. E. H. Trainor (Eds.), *Physical Theory in Biology* (pp. 319-363). River Edge, NJ: World Scientific.

Sutton, J. P., & Trainor, L. E. H. (1988). Hierarchical model of memory and memory loss. *Journal of Physics A: Mathematical and General*, *21*, 4443-4454.

Tiitinen, H., Sinkkonen, J., Reinikainen, K., Alho, K., Lavikainen, J., & Näätänen, R. (1993). Selective attention enhances the auditory 40-Hz transient response in humans. *Nature*, *364*, 59-60.

Yao, Y., & Freeman, W. J. (1990). Model of biological pattern recognition with spatially chaotic dynamics. *Neural Networks*, *3*, 153-170.

Young, D. T. (1989). *Feature based retrieval for neural networks*. Unpublished master's thesis, Louisiana State University.

Young, D. T. (1994). The regulation of information as a collective property. *Proceedings of the Joint Conference on Information Sciences* (pp. 115-118). Durham, NC: Duke University.

Young, D. T. (1997). *A theory of cortical neural processing*. Unpublished doctoral dissertation, Louisiana State University.

10

Response Synchrony, APG Theory, and Motor Control

Geoffrey L. Yuen
Tennessee State University

ABSTRACT

The plausibility of using response synchronization as a mechanism for binding in the motor system is examined. The theoretical and experimental arguments for using response synchrony to solve the binding problem in movement control are first reviewed. Both types of arguments fail to present a convincing case because, response synchrony does not correlate well with routine muscle activation, does not account for the existence of command-neuron burst discharges (in motor cortex and magnocellular red nucleus), and can only be associated with tasks that involve continuous feedback control or with difficult and attention-demanding situations. An alternative theory known as the Adjustable Pattern Generator Theory (APG Theory; Houk, 1987) is presented as a candidate which would account for movement command generation and is consistent with available experimental evidence. IT is possible that motor cortical response synchrony is a complementary mode of operation to that described by the APG Theory, as the associated cortical synchrony and command burst discharge seem to occur under different circumstances. The key differences between these mechanisms are also highlighted.

1. INTRODUCTION

The arguments and experimental support for using a temporal code to "bind various visual features together have been described in detail elsewhere (Engel, König, Kreiter, Schillen, & Singer, 1992; Singer, 1994). Briefly, a time-based code appears to be able to cope with the two critical problems that any scheme to integrate visual information must overcome. First, active cells distributively representing different parts of the same visual object must be identified as belonging together ("binding" problem). Second, a mechanism is needed to avoid interference between coexisting distributed activation patterns ("superposition" problem; Gray, 1994). Although it is generally believed that the familiar arguments of "combinatorial explosion" and "superposition catastrophe" will apply also to the motor cortex, thus suggesting that a time-based code might also be needed for the motor system, experimental results from the latter have been more difficult to interpret and generalize. Thus, it would be appropriate to first review and evaluate the theoretical arguments for using a temporal code to represent movement commands.

2. THEORETICAL ARGUMENTS FOR USING A TIME CODE IN MOTOR COMMAND REPRESENTATION

2.1. Combinatorial Explosion

It is well-known that the visual system processes various features of an object (e.g., orientation, color, motion) in separate and parallel pathways, thus necessitating the "binding of these various attributes together to form a coherent percept of an object (DeYoe & Van Essen, 1988; Engel et al., 1992). The unfavorable scaling of the number of detector cells needed for a large number of objects gives rise, however, to the problem of "combinatorial explosion." This is due to the following deduction: If an object has m attributes to be detected and each attribute can take on p different values, one would need to have p^m detector neurons to identify the object. By using temporal synchrony on a fine time scale of milliseconds, one can effectively accommodate a large number of objects to be detected, because the number of usable "time bins" would be virtually infinite.

Contrary to the prevalence of neurons that are extremely feature-specific in the visual system, clear parcellations of function similar to the well-known distinct visual attributes have not been demonstrated satisfactorily in movement-related neurons. For example, although equal numbers of motor cortical neurons were found covarying with active force, displacement, and behavioral set during a holding task, a slight change in response conditions could change the parameter that correlated best with a particular neuron (Fetz, 1992). This implies that a single functional role may not be assigned to these cortical neurons (i.e., they are multifunctional). On the other hand, the number of "features" or parameters that should be integrated for a certain movement (e.g., velocity, direction, duration) does not seem to be very large. Thus theoretically, at least, the threat of combinatorial explosion is diminished in movement control.

2.2. Experimental Evidence for "Cardinal Neurons"

In the "binding by convergence" model of visual object detection, "cardinal cells" at latter processing layers or "ultimate convergent sites" are expected which should exhibit more complex constellations of features than at the earlier stages (Singer, 1994). Such a model of visual object binding appears now to be implausible because single neurons with multimodal or compound sensitivity and convergent cortical sites cannot be demonstrated unequivocally for a variety of objects. Instead, functional attributes seem to be distributively encoded in a population manner (König, Engel, Roelfsema, & Singer, 1995).

Although population coarse coding is also evident in the motor system (Georgopoulos, 1990; Mussa-Ivaldi et al., 1990; Sparks et al., 1990), neurons that assume the role of issuing commands on the cortical and subcortical levels can certainly not be ruled out. For example, "command neurons" whose firing is strongly correlated with movements and parameters of movement are well-known in the motor cortex as well as other movement-related subcortical areas such as the magnocellular red nucleus and lateral reticular nuclei (Houk, 1987; see below). Thus if one accepts these "command neurons" as the functional analog of the ethereal "grandmother cells" in the visual system, then there would seem to be a clear difference between the way the sensory and motor system are organized. On the other hand, it is legitimate to claim that command neurons similar to those found in simple nervous systems that code for specific motor patterns and behavioral sequences have not been identified in the mammalian motor cortex and other related areas (Singer, 1994).

2.3. Superposition Catastrophe

Another hypothesis of how "binding" may be achieved in vision is based on the Hebbian concept of coactivated cell assemblies, in which neurons are recruited to fire together as an active, spatiotemporally contiguous network due to correlated-firing and synaptic modification. Thus multiple attributes of an object are bound together into a coherent whole because of simultaneous activity in neurons coding for the associated attributes. This, however, prohibits the differentiation of multiple objects within a visual scene if the objects share some common attributes ("superposition catastrophe"). Does the motor system face a similar superposition catastrophe? For a number of reasons, it is unlikely that a superposition catastrophe would be expected in the motor control system. As discussed earlier, neurons in the motor system do not need to be as highly specialized with respect to their functional characteristics as visual neurons. Furthermore, topological connectivity between premotor neurons, motor neurons, and the controlled muscle suggests that there is little chance for confusion with respect to which effectors would be activated.

It is clear from the foregoing considerations that the theoretical arguments for the use of a temporal code via synchrony are less convincing when applied to the motor system as a whole. We therefore turn next to an examination of the experimental evidence for response synchronization in the sensorimotor cortex, followed by a description of an alternative theory for motor control which also depends heavily on temporal-information and dynamic-recurrent processing in oscillatory neurons.

3. EXPERIMENTAL STUDIES ON RESPONSE SYNCHRONY IN THE MOTOR CORTEX

The question of response synchronization has been experimentally investigated for the movement-related cortices. High-frequency oscillations have been observed in the frontal cortex where they occurred in relation to preparatory phases of motion (Donoghue & Sanes, 1991; Fetz, Chen & Murthy, 1994; Gaal, Sanes, & Donoghue, 1992; Murthy & Fetz, 1992), and in prefrontal cortex where they were associated with particular behavioral sequences (Aertsen et al., 1991). In general, the findings are similar to the visual cortex except in three major aspects: first, response synchronization does not seem to be correlated directly with movements or movement-related parameters (Fetz et al., 1994; Murthy & Fetz, 1992) second, synchronization is detected typically without indication of periodic oscillations in the autocorrelation function (labeled "nonoscillatory synchrony"); finally, response synchronization in the motor cortex is unique in that it is based not only on excitatory horizontal connections (as in visual cortex) but also on intrinsic pacemaker neurons (Fetz et al., 1994; Llinas, Grace, & Yarom, 1991). These differences between the two systems are not surprising given the considerations in the last section. Further details follow with respect to these differences, as well as their implications for "binding" in the motor system.

3.1. Correlation with Movement

The most common mode of firing in awake behaving monkeys is modulated firing during movements (Fetz et al., 1994). Generally, neurons in this category have firing that correlates well with either aspects of parameters of specific movements, and generally are found within topographically organized areas. In contrast, response synchronization in the gamma frequency range of 20-40 Hz is observed only transiently over wide cortical territories, including pre- and postcentral cortex in both hemispheres. Furthermore, these oscillatory episodes (average duration 4 cycles or about 150 ms) occur most often during free exploratory limb movements, fine-finger movements (retrieving raisins from a Kluver board) or from unseen locations, but seldom during repetitive movements and they are not reliably correlated to bursts of agonist muscle activity (Donoghue & Sanes, 1991; Murthy & Fetz, 1992). Synchronization between units in the frontal cortex has also been reported to occur in continuity with certain behavioral sequences in a complex delayed matching to sample task although similarly, the synchrony episodes do not correlate with movement parameters (Aertsen et al., 1991).

3.2. Nonoscillatory Synchrony

Motor cortical response synchrony is also distinguished by the lack of secondary peaks in the autocorrelation function, whereas units analyzed during synchrony episodes in the local field potential exhibit clear periodicity. However, the failure of the autocorrelation function to indicated periodicity does not rule out the presence of nonlinear oscillations, or oscillations that are not purely periodic or time-stationary (Singer, 1994). Thus this unique phenomenon is more a statement of the nonlinear properties of the neurons participating in the synchronous response being different from those observed in the visual cortex or elsewhere, in which the autocorrelation function shows both a primary peak (indicating synchrony) and secondary peaks (indicating periodic firing). It is also clear that recurrent inhibition and slow calcium-dependent potassium conductance that mediates the postburst afterhyperpolarization can give rise to bursting cycles that are not reliably detected as periodic firing with autocorrelation methods (Singer, 1994). In fact, this probably reflects the action of the intrinsic burster neurons in motor cortical response synchrony (see Section 3.3). Finally, it is also know that individual cells do not necessarily participate in every cycle of the local field potential yet can contribute to the overall synchrony (e.g., gamma oscillations in the hippocampus; Buzsáki, Horvath, Urioste, Hetke, & Wise, 1992; Ylinen et al., 1995).

3.3. Intrinsic-Burster Mechanism

Intracellular potentials recorded during motor cortical response synchrony indicate that both depolarizing and hyperpolarizing subthreshold membrane potential changes contribute to fueling the oscillations, though the extent varies in different cells. In fact, both excitatory and inhibitory neurons appear to take part in sustaining the oscillations. Furthermore, certain cortical cells exhibit a long postburst afterhyperpolarization of approximately 30 ms, which translates to a burst firing frequency of 25-35 Hz. This is a feature not observed in most other cortical neurons investigated to date (Fetz et al., 1994) and supports the view in the last paragraph that at least part of the mechanism for motor-cortical response synchrony is unique to this system.

In summary, since oscillatory episodes entrain both task-related and task-unrelated neurons equally, and since oscillatory coherence between sites does not depend on their relation to the task, nonoscillatory synchrony in the sensorimotor cortex can only reflect a binding mechanism that is superimposed on task-related modulations (Fetz et al., 1994; Murthy & Fetz, 1992). Although response synchronization has been suggested to underlie motor binding (Singer, 1994), the exact relationship between the two is not simple and much remains to be clarified. It is quite possible that oscillations may be associated with other aspects of behavior such as arousal or attention during exploratory movements or difficult tasks (Fetz et al., 1994).

4. ADJUSTABLE PATTERN GENERATOR (APG) THEORY FOR MOTOR COMMAND GENERATION

It appears from the previous section that the solution for the motor system binding problem involves mechanisms beyond those implicated in response synchronization. In particular, motor-command-generation circuitry and the existence of the command neurons are not currently addressed by this type of model for motor control. In this section, we therefore present an alternative and more traditional account of movement command generation which takes these two essential ingredients into account. The significance of this theory of motor command generation with respect to response synchronization is discussed in the final section of this chapter.

4.1. Basic Description of APG Theory

The APG theory attempts to synthesize a picture of how motor commands are generated in the brain by integrating both neuroanatomical and neurophysiological evidence relating the cerebellum to the motor cortex and premotor nuclei such as the midbrain magnocellular red nucleus. The theory can be concisely summarized in terms of the following main ideas (more complete descriptions of this theory and detail supporting references can be found in Houk, 1987; Houk & Gibson, 1987; Houk, Keifer, & Barto, 1993; Houk, Singh, Fisher & Barto, 1990).

(1) The APG model is based on the finding that the cerebellar cortex is anatomically and functionally organized into parasagittal zone is a longitudinally oriented set of Purkinje cells that receive the same parallel fiber, climbing fiber and basket cell inputs. This set of Purkinje cells exert powerful inhibition to the recurrent loop nuclei downstream from it. This recurrent loop arises from excitatory, positive feedback interactions between nucleus interpositus, red nucleus and alter reticular nucleus. Thus the entire cerebellum with the associated premotor nuclei could be thought of as a large array of parasagittally organized adjustable pattern generator modules.

(2) The basic driving force for motor commands generation is created by this recurrent positive feedback interactions in the loops between neurons in the cerebellar nuclei, lateral reticular nucleus, and red nucleus or motor cortex. The effect of the recurrent interaction is observed as long-duration burst firing in either the red nucleus or in the motor cortex. Thus the output of a typical APG unit is delivered either from the red nucleus to the limbs via the rubrospinal tract or form the motor cortex (via cerbello-ponto-cerebral connections), which in turn activates motor neurons to carry out movements via the corticospinal tract.

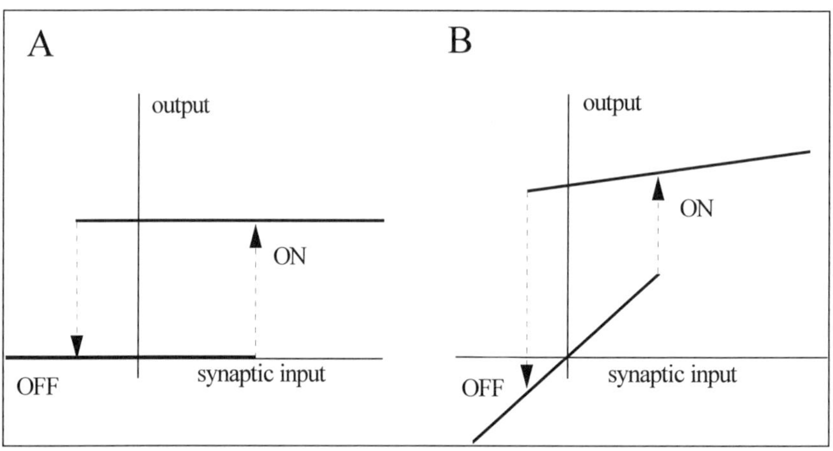

Fig. 10.1. Schematic diagram for an adjustable pattern generator. Magnocellular red nucleus (mRN) burst discharge are postulated to originate from recurrent excitatory connections from NI (nucleus interpositus) to NRTP (nucleus reticularis tegmenti pontis) to NI and from NI to mRN to LRN (lateral reticular nucleus) to NI. Inhibitory outputs from several Purkinje Cells (PKJ) is presumed to sculpt the frequency and duration of mRN burst discharges, giving rise to movement commands via the rubrospinal tract.

(3) Bursts of activity from the positive-feedback recurrent loops in (2) are sculpted by Purkinje cell inhibition to generate appropriate motor command signals (Fig. 10.1). The proper pattern of Purkinje cell activity (e.g., timing and duration) is acquired by a learning process involving the long-term depression of the parallel-fiber-to-Purkinje-cell synapse based on climbing-fiber teacher-punishment signals (Ito, 1982). The array of pattern generators must be adjustable, because the bursts of discharge in the magnocellular red nucleus have durations that covary in proportion to the duration of the movement, and the discharge rates during the burst covary according to the velocity of movement.

(4) This scheme of control can be described as quasi-feedforward because, instead of using continuous feedback from the peripheral sensors (e.g., from muscles) to modulate the force of muscular contraction and movement of the mechanical load, the system operates primarily in a predictive and feedforward mode based on discontinuous sensory trigger signals and/or internal cues (i.e., for initiation or termination of movements). The central-pattern generator properties of the proposed APG circuitry constitute the basis of feedforward predictive motor programs (see the following).

4.2. Picture of Operation

These ideas have been implemented in several computer simulations of limb movement control showing that the models can achieve endpoint control of unidirectional, planar and multiple joint/degree-of-freedom limb movements after learning (Berthier, Singh, Barto, & Houk, 1994; Dinkjaer, Wu, Barto & Houk, 1991; Houk & Barto, 1992). Movement trajectories, cosine tuning of directional sensitivity, vectorial summation of population response, and "mental" rotation of population vectors similar to that reported by Georgopoulos have also been simulated (Eisenman, Keifer, & Houk, 1992; Georgopoulos, Lurito, Petrides, Schwartz, & Massey, 1989; Georgopoulos, Schwartz, & Kettner, 1986). A typical picture of the operation of the APG controller is as follows. Prior to the arrival of a sensory or internal trigger for the starting of a motor program, the recurrent circuits described in main idea (2) are in the quiescent state. Upon arrival of any sufficiently strong trigger to any of the recurrent loop nuclei or the synchronous withdrawal of Purkinje cell inhibition, positive feedback in the all-excitatory circuit in Fig. 10.1 allows recurrent activity to build up, permitting intense and long-duration burst firing in the red nucleus. Once initiated, such a motor program is regulated only by the dynamic state, ratio, and combination of ON/OFF Purkinje cells, and it proceeds in an essentially open-loop manner until enough parallel fiber inputs turn a sufficient number of Purkinje cells back ON to quench the bursting. The appropriate patterns of Purkinje cell firing are in turn constrained by parallel-to-Purkinje synapses from training. Further details of these computer simulations describing the circuit's operations in relation to the selection, execution, and correction of motor programs for limb movements, and its relationship to movement trajectories and directional coding are available in Berthier et al. (1994) and Houk and Barto (1992).

4.3. Experimental Support

It is important to point out that the APG theory is consistent with a number of experimental findings with respect to the red nucleus, the cerebellum, and the motor cortex. Limb and movement-specific burst signals that precede movement onset by an average of 120 ms have been recorded from the magnocellular red nucleus in which the burst parameters are correlated with the movement parameters. For example, burst duration, rate, and the number of spikes in a burst are respectively correlated with movement duration, velocity, and amplitude (Gibson, Houk, & Kohlerman, 1985). Furthermore, these burst signals are not generated or continuously modulated by peripheral feedback, although the latter can influence the discharge rate during the burst (Houk & Gibson, 1987). Recurrent or reverberatory activities are also well-known for the circuitry in Fig. 10.1. For example, suppression of Purkinje cells by a GABA antagonist, long-term climbing fiber stimulation, or cooling allows recurrent activity to be initiated in the positive feedback loop nuclei (magnocellular red nucleus (mRN), nucleus reticularis tegmenti pontis (NRTP), lateral reticular nucleus (LRN) and nucleus interpositus (NT) (Allen & Tsukahara, 1974; Gibson & Houk, 1985; Tsukahara, Bando, Murakani, & Oda, 1983). A brief burst of Purkinje cell discharge also result in an initial hyperpolarization of Nucleus Interpositus (NI) cells which is then followed by a rebound depolarization that produces bursts of discharge in NI neurons.

4.4. The Role of Purkinje Cells

The model also takes into account the sensorimotor transformations that supposedly occur in cerebellar cortex. Numerous studies have documented the importance of cerebellar Purkinje cells in sensorimotor transformation and goal-directed limb movements (e.g., Gilbert & Thach, 1977; Harvey, Porter, & Rawson, 1977; Mano, Kanazawa & Yamamoto, 1986; Mano & Yamamoto, 1980). Whereas the major inputs to Purkinje cells, mossy and climbing fibers, carry sensory information (e.g., parametric and proprioceptive-corrective information for limb and joint position); (Ebner & Bloedel, 1987; Ekerot, 1984; Gellman, Gibson, & Houk, 1985), Purkinje cell discharges are much better correlated with movement parameters (e.g., movement onset, velocity of motion, or rate of force development); (Armstrong, Cogdell, & Harvey, 1973; Brooks, 1986). However, steady, intense Purkinje cell firing is observed primarily during active, self-initiated movements in contrast to passive movements (e.g., limb manipulation by experimenter). This preferential sensitivity to active movements is also evident in the interpositus nucleus of the cerebellum, a direct target of the Purkinje cells which is related to limb movements (Harvey, Porter, & Rawson, 1979; van Kan, Gibson, & Houk, 1992b). No apparent difference was noted in the mossy/parallel fiber discharges between active and passive movements (van Kan, Gibson, & Houk, 1992a), thus the same synaptic inputs are presumably transmitted to the Purkinje cells for either type of movement. Apparently, Purkinje cells become insensitive or "gated-out" to parallel fiber inputs during passive movements. This can be accounted for by postulating hysteresis in the operation of Purkinje cells so that they remain in the OFF state during passive movements and then switch to the ON state during active movements (Houk et al., 1990). On the dendritic level, the existence of intracellularly recordable plateau potentials which have long durations of 200-500 ms is also consistent with such a mode of operation. Subsequent phase plane analysis of the experimental dendritic-ion-channel data related to plateau potentials from these neurons confirmed that individual Purkinje cell dendrites can be represented, with minor simplification, as bistable elements with hysteresis (Yuen, Hochberger, & Houk, 1996); (see Fig. 10.2). In the limb control simulations mentioned above, bistable Purkinje cells seem to prevent stability problems during feedback limb control operations, which have long built-in delays. Thus, according to this computational framework, Purkinje cells can generate appropriate control signals simply by behaving as bistable elements (see also Guttman, 1991).

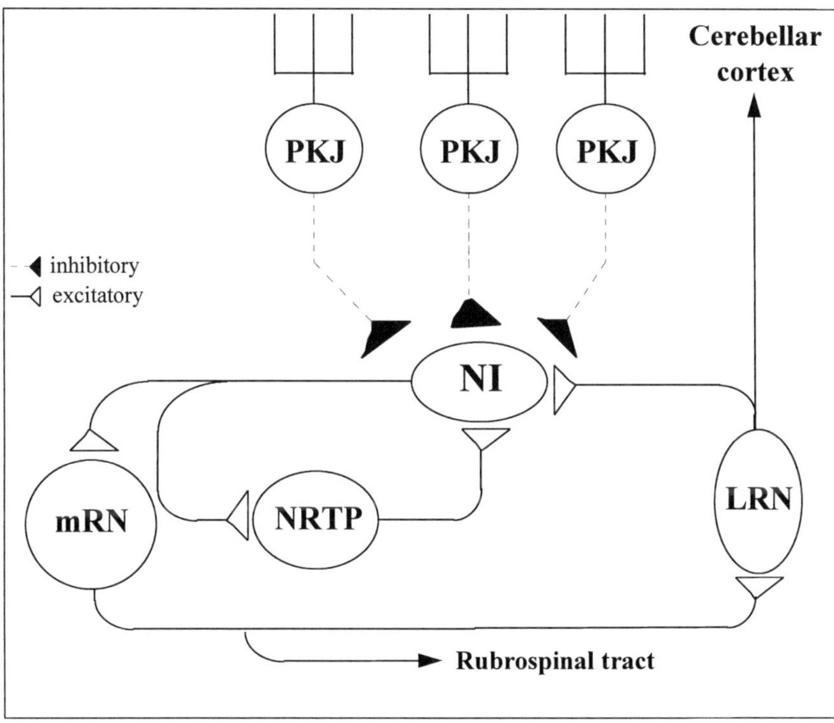

Fig. 10.2. Bistability and hysteresis in Purkinje cells. The schematic drawing illustrates the difference between (A) the Purkinje cell model as originally proposed (Houk et al., 1990) and (B) the one subsequently computed based on phase-plane and steady-state analysis of voltage clamped data of delayed rectifier potassium and high-threshold calcium channels (Yuen et al., 1996). Dashed arrows indicate system switching to the other state when given appropriate synaptic drive. The system can take on different output levels for the same input depending on the previous state. Note that nonzero resistance of OFF and ON states in (B), although bistable/hysteretic properties are essentially described as in (A).

5. RELEVANCE OF APG THEORY VERSUS RESPONSE SYNCHRONIZATION: MULTIPLE MECHANISMS FOR CONTROL?

From the preceding discussion of response synchrony and APG theory, it would appear that the two theories deal with primarily different portions of the brain: motor cortex and cerebellum/premotor areas/red nucleus. However, more recent experimental evidence suggests that the APG theory could also apply to the motor cortex as well. This extrapolation to the motor cortex is based on a number of similarities between the motor cortex and the red nucleus, which have been noted previously by a number of workers (see Miller & Houk, 1996, for references). To be specific, both the red nucleus and the motor cortex target spinal motor neurons directly, and both show prominent movement-related bursts of discharge and weaker, stimulus-locked responses to somatosensory input (Houk et al., 1993). Furthermore, recent work revealed clear tonic-firing neurons in both areas during tonic contraction of the appropriate muscles (Cheney, Fetz, & Mewes, 1991; Fromm, Evarts, Kroller, & Shinoda, 1981; Georgopoulos, Caminiti, & Kalaska, 1984; Lee & Houk, 1996). The high correlation of dynamic red nucleus firing to simultaneously recorded EMG-signal suggests that both areas could be responsible for creating muscle-coordinate-based movement command signals. Lower correlation coefficients were found for velocity and duration of the movement, suggesting that the covariation is only an auxiliary consequence of the muscle activation patterns (see main idea (4) in Section 4.1). A key difference, however, is that while the red nucleus seems to activate mostly distal and extrinsic hand extensors, the motor cortex seems to affect mostly intrinsic hand flexors (Miller & Houk, 1995). Incidently, others have reported that response averages of some sessions showed that oscillations occurred preferentially during the flexion phase (Murphy & Fetz, 1992).

Although this extension of the APG theory to the motor cortex has not been confirmed experimentally, it is conceivable that both type of mechanisms (i.e., response synchronization and cerebellar inhibitory sculpting of burst firing based on recurrent excitation) operate in the motor cortex under different circumstances. Granted that response synchronization "occurs too rarely to be essential for execution or coordination of every movement" (Fetz, 1992), so that it cannot solve the motor binding problem in general, the possibility that this mechanism is "recruited" during difficult or problem-solving situations cannot be ruled out. In fact, the results to date suggest that the two underlying mechanisms seem to occur under different behavioral circumstances. For example, whereas response synchronization in the motor cortex is most often observed during unseen or difficult reaching/retrieving tasks that require attention, red-nucleus burst firing can be observed robustly during free arm movements. It is also clear that the brain circuit subsystem involved in these two mechanisms are separate. Whereas response synchronization involves mostly cortical-cortical (and perhaps thalamic-cortical) interactions, the APG recurrent interactions involve mostly the cerebellum and either the motor cortex (through the cerebellopontocerebral connections) or the premotor nuclei (red nucleus, lateral reticular nucleus, deep cerebellar nucleus). The important differences between these two theories or mechanisms are summarized in Table 10.1.

In this chapter, we have reviewed both theoretical and experimental arguments for using response synchrony as a mechanism for binding in the motor system, described the APG theory, and made clear the crucial differences between the two theories. Both the experimental and theoretical arguments suggest that response synchrony is probably not a routine mechanism used by the brain to deliver movement commands. Instead, the evidence is currently in favor of the APG theory for this more basic role. However, the experimental conditions under which response synchrony can be observed in the sensorimotor cortex that it may nevertheless be important during movements that demand more attention or involve more strategic and sequential planning.

	Response Synchronization	**APG Recurrent Networks Theory**
Type of Movement	unseen, difficult or attention-demanding movements	unrestricted arm movements
Mode of Operation	sensory feedback	feedforward/command
Correlation to Movement	none with respect to oscillation amplitude and frequency	clear correlation with muscle activation patterns
Connectivity of Detected Sites	no clear localization	topographic regions
Time Course	transient (~150 msec/episode)	tonic (~500 msec)
Subsystems Implicated	sensorimotor cortex, association cortex, thalamus	cerebellum, cortex, premotor nuclei

Table 10.1. Comparison of Response Synchronization and APG Theory as models for motor control.

ACKNOWLEDGMENTS

The author's work is supported by the Office of Naval Research (N-00014-93-1-0636). Helpful discussions with Lee Miller, Dao-Fin Chen, and proofreading from John Kuschewski are gratefully appreciated. The author also wants to thank Center for Neural Engineering Director Dr. Mohan Malkani and Dean Decatur Rogers for their encouragement.

REFERENCES

Aertsen, A., Vaadia, E., Abeles, M., Ahissar, E., Bergmann, I., Carmon, B., Lavner, Y., Margalit, E., Nelken, I., & Rotter, S. (1991). Neural interactions in the frontal cortex of a behaving monkey: Signs of dependence on stimulus context and behavioral states. *Journal fuer Hirnforschung, 32,* 735-743.

Allen, G., & Tsukahara, N. (1974). Cerebrocerebellar communication systems. *Physiological Reviews, 54,* 957-1006.

Armstrong, D. M., Cogdell, B., & Harvey, R. J. (1973). Firing patterns of Purkinje cells in the cat cerebellum for different maintained positions of the limbs. *Brain Research, 50,* 452-456.

Berthier, N. E., Singh, S. P., Barto, A. G., & Houk, J. C. (1993). Distributed representation of limb motor programs in arrays of adjustable pattern generators. *Journal of Cognitive Science, 5,* 56-78.

Brooks, V. B. (1986). *The Neural Basis of Motor Control.* Cambridge MA: MIT Press.

Buzsáki, G., Horvath, Z., Urioste, R., Hetke, J., & Wise K. (1992). High-frequency network oscillation in the hippocampus. *Science, 256,* 1025-1027.

Cheney, P., Fetz, E., & Mewes, K. (1991). Neural mechanisms underlying corticospinal and rubrospinal control of limb movements. *Progress in Brain Research, 87,* 213-252.

DeYoe, E., & Van Essen, D. (1988). Concurrent processing streams in monkey visual cortex. *Trends in Neuroscience, 11,* 219-226.

Donoghue, J., & Sanes, J. (1991). Dynamic modulation of primate motor cortex output during movement. *Society of Neuroscience Abstracts, 17,* 407.5.

Ebner, T. J., & Bloedel, J. R. (1987). Climbing fiber afferent system: intrinsic properties and rile in cerebellar information processing. In J. S. King (Ed.), *New Concepts in Cerebellar Neurobiology* (pp. 371-386). New York: Alan Liss.

Eisenman, L., Keifer, J., & Houk, J. (1992). Positive feedback in the cerebro-cerebellar recurrent network may explain rotation of population vectors. In F. Eeckman (Ed.), *Analysis and Modelling of Neural Systems* (pp. 371-376). Boston: Kluwer.

Ekerot, C. F. (1984). Climbing fibre actions of Purkinje cells — plateau potentials and long-lasting depression of parallel fibre responses. In J. Bloedel (Ed.), *Cerebellar Functions* (pp. 268-274). Berlin: Springer-Verlag.

Engel, A., König, P., Kreiter, A., Schillen, T., & Singer, W. (1992). Temporal coding in the visual cortex: new vistas on integration in the nervous system. *Trends in Neurosciences, 15,* 218-226.

Fetz, E. (1992). Are movement parameters recognizably coded in the activity of single neurons? *Behavioral and Brain Sciences,* 15, 679-690.

Fetz, E., Chen, D., & Murthy, V. (1994). Synaptic interactions mediating coherent oscillations in primate sensorimotor cortex. *European Journal of Neuroscience, Suppl. 7,* 127-137.

Fromm, C., Evarts, E., Kroller, J., & Shonoda, Y. (1981). Activity of motor cortex and red nucleus neurons during voluntary movement. In O. Pompiano & C. A. Marsan (Eds.), *Brain Mechanisms and Perceptual Awareness* (pp. 269-294). New York: Raven Press.

Gaal, G., Sanes, J., & Donoghue, J. (1992). Motor cortex oscillatory neural activity during voluntary movement in macaca fascicularis. *Society for Neuroscience Abstracts, 18,* 355.14.

Gellman, R., Gibson, A. R., & Houk, J. (1985). Inferior olivary neurons in the awake cat: Detection of contact and passive body displacement. *Journal of Neurophysiology, 54,* 40-60.

Georgopoulos, A. (1990). Neural coding of the direction of reaching and a comparison with saccadic eye movements. *Cold Spring Harbor Symposium in Quantitative Biology, LV,* 849-859.

Georgopoulos, A., Caminiti, R., & Kalaska, J. (1984). Static spatial effects in motor cortex and area 5: Quantitative relations in a two-dimensional space. *Experimental Brain Research, 54,* 446-454.

Georgopoulos, A. Lurito, J., Petrides, M., Schwartz, A., & Massey, J. (1989). Mental rotation of the neuronal population vector. *Science, 243,* 234-236.

Georgopoulos, A., Schwartz, A., & Kettner, R. (1986). Neuronal population coding of movement direction. *Science, 233,* 1416-1419.

Ghez, C., & Kubota, K. (1977). Activity of red nucleus neurons with a skilled forelimb movement in the cat. *Brain Research, 129,* 393-398.

Gibson, A. R., Houk, J., & Kohlerman, N. (1985). Relation between red nucleus discharge and movement parameters in trained macaque monkeys. *Journal of Physiology (London), 358,* 551-570.

Gilbert, P. F. C., & Thach, W. T. (1977). Purkinje cell activity during motor learning. *Brain Research, 128,* 309-328.

Gray, C. (1994). Synchronous oscillations in neuronal systems: mechanisms and functions. *Journal of Computational Neuroscience, 1,* 11-38.

Gutman, A. M. (1991). Bistability of dendrites. *International Journal of Neural Systems, 1,* 291-304.

Harvey, R. J., Porter, R., & Rawson, J. A. (1977). The natural discharges of Purkinje cells in paravermal regions of lobules V and VI of the monkey's cerebellum. *Journal of Physiology, 271,* 515-536.

Harvey, R. J., Porter, R., & Rawson, J. A. (1979). Discharges of intracerebellar nuclear cells in monkeys. *Journal of Physiology, 297,* 559-580.

Houk, J. (1987). Model of the cerebellum as an array of adjustable pattern generators. In M. Glickstein, C. Yeo, & J. Stein (Eds.), *Cerebellum and Neural Plasticity* (pp. 249-260). New York: Plenum.

Houk, J., & Barto, A. G. (1992). Distributed sensorimotor learning. In G. E. Stelmach & J. Requin (Eds.), *Tutorials in Motor Behavior II.* Amsterdam: Elsevier.

Houk, J., & Gibson, A. R. (1987). Sensorimotor processing through the cerebellum. In J. S. King (Ed.), *New Concepts in Cerebellar Neurobiology* (pp. 387-416). New York: Alan Liss.

Houk, J., Keifer, J., & Barto, A. G. (1993). Distributed motor commands in the limb premotor network. *Trends in Neuroscience, 16,* 27-33.

Houk, J., Singh, S. P., Fisher, C., & Barto, A. G. (1990). An adaptive sensorimotor network inspired by the anatomy and physiology of the cerebellum. In T. Miller, R. S. Sutton, & P. J. Werbos (Eds.), *Neural Networks for Control* (pp. 301-348). Cambridge, MA: MIT Press.

Ito, M. (1982). Cerebellar control of the vestibulo-ocular reflex. *Annual Review of Neuroscience, 5,* 275-296.

König, P., Engel, A., Roelfsema, P., & Singer, W. (1995). How precise is neuronal synchronization? *Neural Computation, 7,* 469-485.

Llinas, R., Grace, A., & Yarom, Y. (1991). In vitro neurons in mammalian cortical layer 4 exhibit intrinsic oscillatory activity in the 10- to 50-Hz frequency range. *Proceedings of the National Academy of Sciences, 88,* 897-901.

Mano, N., Kanazawa, I., & Yamamoto, K. (1986). Complex-spike activity of cerebellar Purkinje cells related to wrist tracking movement in monkeys. *Journal of Neurophysiology, 56,* 137-158.

Mano, N., & Yamamoto, K. (1980). Simple-spike activity of cerebellar Purkinje cells related to visually guided wrist tracking in monkeys. *Journal of Neurophysiology, 43,* 713-728.

Miller, L. E., & Houk, J. (1995). Motor coordinates in primate red nucleus: Preferential relation to muscle activation versus kinematic variables. *Journal of Physiology (London), 488,* 533-548.

Miller, L. E., Sinkjaer, T., Andersen, T., Laporte, D., & Houk, J. (1991). Correlation analysis of relations between red nucleus discharge and limb muscle activity during reaching movements in space. In R. Caminiti (Ed.), *Control of Arm Movement in Space*. New York: Springer-Verlag.

Miller, L. E., Van Kan, P., Sinkjaer, T., Andersen, T., Harris, G., & Houk, J. (1993). Correlation of primate red nucleus discharge with muscle activity during free-form arm movements. *Journal of Physiology, 469,* 213-243.

Murthy, V., & Fetz, E. E. (1992). Coherent 25- to 35-Hz oscillations in the sensorimotor cortex of awake behaving monkeys. *Proceedings of the National Academy of Sciences, 89*, 2643-2647.

Mussa-Ivaldi, F., Gister, S., & Bizzi, E. (1990). Motor-space coding in the central nervous system. *Cold Spring Harbor Symposium in Quantitative Biology, LV,* 827-835.

Singer, W. (1994). Putative functions of temporal correlations in neocortical processing. In C. Koch & J. Davis (Eds.), *Large-Scale Neuronal Theories of the Brain* (pp. 201-237). Cambridge, MA: MIT Press.

Sinkjaer, T., Wu, C. H., Barto, A., & Houk, J. C. (1990). Cerebellar control of endpoint position: A simulation model. *Proceedings of the IJCNN, 2,* 705-710. Piscataway, NJ: IEEE.

Sparks, D., Lee, C., & Rohrer, W. (1990). Population coding of the direction, amplitude and velocity of saccadic eye movements by neurons in the superior colliculus. *Cold Spring Harbor Symposium in Quantitative Biology, LV,* 805-811.

Tsukahara, N., Bando, T., Murakami, F., & Oda, Y. (1983). Properties of cerebello-precerebellar reverberating circuits. *Brain Research, 274,* 249-259.

Van Kan, P. L. E., Gibson, A. R., & Houk, J. C. (1992a). Movement-related inputs to intermediate cerebellum of the monkey. *Journal of Neurophysiology, 69,* 74-94.

Van Kan, P. L. E., Gibson, A. R., & Houk, J. C. (1992b). Output organization of intermediate cerebellum of the monkey. *Journal of Neurophysiology,* 69, 57-73.

Ylinen, A., Bragin, A., Nadasdy, Z., Jando, G., Szabo, I., Sok, A., & Buzsáki, G. (1995). Sharp wave-associated high-frequency oscillation (200 Hz) in the intact hippocampus: network and intracellular mechanisms. *Journal of Neuroscience, 14*, 30-46.

Yuen, G., Hockberger, P., & Houk, J. C. (1996). Bistability in cerebellar Purkinje cell dendrites modelled with high-threshold calcium and delayed-rectifier potassium channels. *Biological Cybernetics, 73,* 375-388.

III
Oscillatory Models in Perception, Memory, and Cognition

11
Temporal Segmentation and Binding in Oscillatory Neural Systems

David Horn and Irit Opher
Tel Aviv University

ABSTRACT

Segmentation and binding are cognitive operations that underlie the process of perception. They can be understood as taking place in the temporal domain, that is, relying on features like simultaneity of neuronal firing. We demonstrate them in a system of oscillatory networks, consisting of Hebbian cell assemblies of excitatory neurons and inhibitory interneurons in which the oscillations are implemented by dynamical thresholds. We emphasize the importance of fluctuating input signals in producing binding and in enabling segmentation of a large set of common inputs. Segmentation properties can be studied by investigating the cyclic attractors of a neural system. Employing this method we show that for constant inputs full segmentation is limited to a small set of excited memories; however, fluctuating inputs can lead to approximate segmentation of a large set of memories.

1. INTRODUCTION

To introduce our subject let us start with the visual analysis of a scene as a convenient example (Malsburg & Buhmann, 1992). It is clear that a complicated picture is built out of elements that can be recognized separately. Before identification of the different elements in the scene takes place, a segmentation process is required. It separates the different elements, thus making them accessible for further processing. We define segmentation as the task of parallel retrieval of individual memorized patterns that appear together in an input. In addition to vision it should play a role in auditory signal separation such as in the cocktail party effect (Malsburg & Schneider, 1986) and odor separation in the olfactory bulb (Hopfield & Gelperin, 1989).

Once segmentation is performed, a regrouping of all elements has to take place for reconstruction of the scene. This grouping process is called binding, in reference to the relation introduced between the different elements. An example of both segmentation and binding can be found in the psychophysical paradigm of Treisman and Schmidt (1982): A subject is presented for a very short time with the pictures of a few objects, for example, a red diamond, a green circle, and a blue square. He is required to identify and recall all elements. This scene has to be segmented into all its components, both in shape and in color, and then appropriate binding (of the right colors and shapes) of the different objects has to take place. Incorrect binding leads to illusory conjunctions (e.g., red circle).

One natural mechanism for segmentation is temporal tagging, that can be easily implemented in oscillatory systems. The realization of segmentation in oscillatory networks was demonstrated by Wang, Buhmann, and Malsburg (1990) and by Horn and Usher (1991). The activities of the different memory patterns turned on by the input oscillate in a staggered fashion. In Wang et al. (1990), the elements of the networks are oscillators by themselves, composed of excitatory-inhibitory pairs of neurons. Horn and Usher have worked with neurons that possess dynamic thresholds that exhibit adaptation: These thresholds vary as a function of the activity of the neurons to which they are attached. As such, they introduce time dependence that can turn a neural network from a dissipating system that converges onto fixed points into one that moves from one center of attraction to another (Horn & Usher, 1989).

The use of dynamic thresholds leads to a variety of models that can represent cognitive functions that are more complex than content-addressable memory retrieval. It is quite obvious how this can lead to free associative transitions between memories. It may be less obvious that it allows us to model segmentation and binding. These features were obtained within an excitatory-inhibitory network described in the next section. Based on that network, we focus on how segmentation is achieved and what is needed to obtain binding. We point out the importance of noise in obtaining these goals.

To understand better the origin of these properties we turn to a symmetric model in which we investigate the segmentation mode as a particular kind of limit cycle (Horn & Opher, 1995, 1996). It becomes clear in this model why full segmentation cannot be obtained for many memories when a constant input is used. Noisy input allows us to overcome this limitation.

2. NEURAL MODELS WITH DYNAMIC THRESHOLDS

To illustrate the method of Horn and Usher (1989), consider a neural system defined by the equation of motion

$$S_i(t+1) = F\Big(\sum_j J_{ij}S_j(t) - \theta_i(t)\Big) \qquad (1)$$

where S_i is the activity of neuron *I* and J_{ij} is the weight connecting neuron *j* to *i*. *F* is a transfer function whose threshold parameter θ_i depends on the history of the neuron activity S_i at the same location:

$$\theta_i(t+1) = \frac{\theta_i(t)}{c} + bS_i(t+1) \quad . \tag{2}$$

This is an effective integration of S_i over time. θ_i saturates at the value $g = bc/(c-1)$ if S_i stays constant at 1. c is chosen to be slightly bigger than 1. If g is bigger than the input from all other neurons, it destabilizes the tendency of the system to stay in a fixed-point and leads to oscillations of the network and to movement between different patterns.

Trying to stay closer to biological models, we turn to an excitatory-inhibitory network (Horn & Usher, 1990). In this model the memory patterns are assumed to be carried by excitatory neurons only. A pattern is defined by a cell assembly of excitatory neurons that excite each other. These patterns affect one another through their joint excitation of the inhibitory neurons that, in turn, inhibit all the excitatory neurons. If the same excitatory neuron participates in two different patterns, or cell assemblies, it plays the role of a two-way pointer between these two patterns. In the absence of any such cases, that is, when all patterns are disjoint, we can derive differential equations for the patterns' activities:

$$\frac{dm^\mu}{dt} = -m^\mu + \sigma(Am^\mu - Bm^I - \theta_O^E - br^\mu + i^\mu) \tag{3}$$

$$\frac{dr^\mu}{dt} = \left(\frac{1}{c} - 1\right) r^\mu + m^\mu \tag{4}$$

$$\frac{dm^I}{dt} = -m^I = \sigma(CM - Dm^I - \theta_O^I) \tag{5}$$

$m^\mu(t)$, the activity of pattern number μ, is the fraction of the excitatory neurons in cell-assembly number μ that fire at time t. Similarly, m^I defines the fraction of all inhibitory neurons that fire. M represents the total excitatory activity, $M = \sum_\mu m^\mu$, and σ is the sigmoid function

$$\sigma(x) = (1 + e^{-x/T})^{-1}$$

where T determines the slope of the sigmoid. $\theta_O{}^E$ and $\theta_O{}^I$ are the (static) thresholds of all excitatory and inhibitory neurons correspondingly. The excitatory thresholds are assumed to have dynamic components that are represented by their average r^μ within the cell assembly μ.

In Equations (3)-(5) we have included external inputs i^μ affecting memory number μ. In other words, we operate our memory system under the influence of continuous external stimuli, and test its functioning under these conditions.

3. SEGMENTATION AND BINDING IN AN EXCITATORY-INHIBITORY NETWORK

We have described segmentation and binding in the Introduction by employing the example of psychophysical experiments (Treisman & Schmidt, 1982) in which an observer is presented with a display consisting of three colored shapes, for example, a red diamond, a blue square, and a green circle. If we suppose that shapes and colors are stored in different cortical modules (networks), we are faced with the double problem of segmentation and binding. That is, the "shape" module should recognize and segment the colors. The binding problem, then, is to provide the correct matching between the shapes and their corresponding colors. Figure 11.1 is an illustration of the problem.

The binding problem was studied (Horn, Sagi, & Usher, 1992) within a model of two coupled networks, each obeying equations of the type (3) through (5). A coupling was introduced between the inhibitory components of the two networks, in order to drive them with the same frequency, while avoiding any semantic relations between the attributes (shapes and colors) represented by the excitatory cell assemblies.

To study the segmentation we let n memories receive a common input. For suitable parameters of the system we find that memory activities aroused by the input oscillate in a staggered manner, each one peaking at different times, as displayed in the first two frames of Fig. 11.2. Thus we obtain temporal segmentation: The system identifies the mixed input by decomposing it dynamically into the different memories contained in it.

Binding is modeled by having patterns (attributes) corresponding to the same objects oscillate in phase (e.g., the activity of the pattern representing the shape "diamond" should oscillate in phase with the activity of the color "red"). To achieve

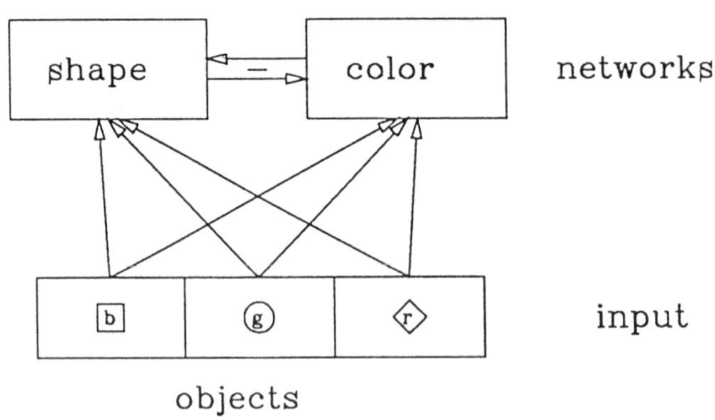

Fig. 11.1. Schematic description of a problem involving segmentation and binding.

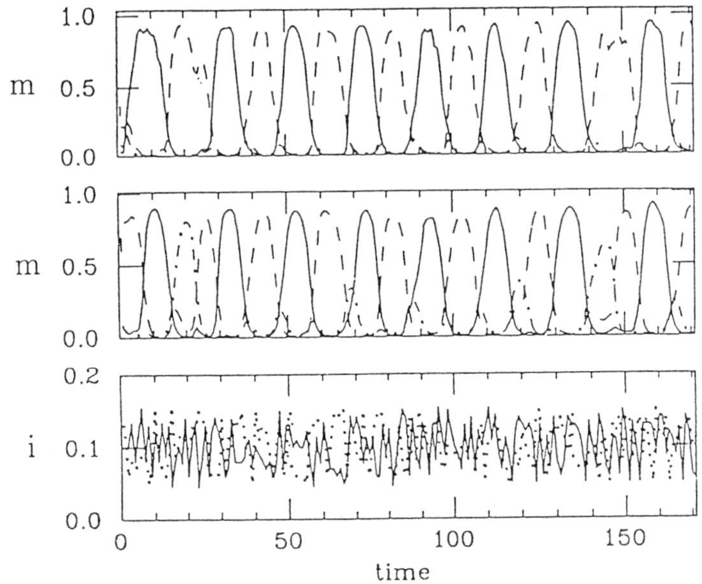

Fig. 11.2. Segmentation and binding (Horn, Sagi, & Usher, 1992). The first two frames exhibit activities of memory patterns (excitatory cell assemblies) of two coupled networks (see Fig. 11.1). The first network has five memory patterns and the second has three. The activities of the two memories excited by the input are shown by the full line and the dashed line. The dot-dashed curve represents an activated memory that does not receive an input. We observe both segmentation and binding. Segmentation means that the two different patterns in the two networks oscillate in phase. This phase locking is brought about by the common noise of the two attributes (shape and color) belonging to the same object. The inputs of the two objects are shown in the third frame.

phase locking of the attributes corresponding to the same object, one drives both by some common randomly fluctuating input. Different pairs of attributes are driven by different and uncorrelated random noises. Figure 11.2 describes results when two pairs of inputs are used. In this figure we show the two inputs in addition to the activities of the two different cell assemblies in the two networks. Note that the time scale of phase-locked oscillations is much larger than that of the autocorrelations of the fluctuating noise.

In the case of three objects, it takes more time to achieve correct binding. Moreover, the system can move out of correct binding into erroneous phase correlations. This could correspond to the phenomenon of illusory conjunctions observed in psychophysical experiments (Treisman & Schmidt, 1982).

4. SEGMENTATION VIEWED AS A LIMIT CYCLE OF A DYNAMICAL SYSTEM

To gain understanding of segmentation we have studied a system of equations that is similar in nature to (3)-(5), using methods of the type employed in dynamical systems. We consider n excitatory neurons interacting with one inhibitory neuron and receiving external inputs (Horn & Opher, 1995):

$$\frac{du^{\mu}}{dt} = -u^{\mu} + m^{\mu} - am^{I} - b^{\mu} + I^{\mu} \tag{7}$$

$$\frac{dr^{\mu}}{dt} = m^{\mu} - cr^{\mu} \tag{8}$$

$$\frac{dv}{dt} = -gv - em^{I} + f\sum_{\mu} m^{\mu} \tag{9}$$

u^{μ} denote post synaptic currents of excitatory neurons, whose average firing rates are

$$m^{\mu} = (1 + e^{-\beta u^{\mu}})^{-1} \tag{10}$$

while v and m^{I} are analogous quantities for an inhibitory neuron that induces competition between all excitatory ones. The similarity with the previous set (3)-(5) is that the variables m^{μ} (m^{I}) represent activities of excitatory (inhibitory) units normalized to the range between 0 to 1. Here each neuron plays the role of a Hebbian cell assembly in the model considered before. r^{μ} are dynamical thresholds that rise when their corresponding neurons fire. They quench the active neurons and lead to oscillatory behavior. a, ..., g, and β are fixed parameters. To study segmentation we choose $I^{\mu} = I$ as a common external input. Note that this system is now fully symmetric under the interchange of any two excitatory neurons $\mu \leftrightarrow \nu$. Figure 11.3 is a diagrammatic representation of this set of equations that displays this symmetry.

In general, this dynamical system flows into a set of dynamic attractors. Thus, for 3 excitatory elements and constant input, one finds the following types of attractors: (a) Common fixed point or common oscillatory mode. (b) Two of the elements oscillate in phase and a third out of phase. (There are three possibilities for this type of attractor corresponding to the three possibilities of choosing 2 oscillators out of 3.) (c) Staggered oscillations of all elements. (There are 2 possibilities for this attractor corresponding to the 2 possible arrangements of 3 oscillators in a ring.) The last type fits our understanding of temporal segmentation. Examples of all limit cycles are shown in Fig. 11.4, which displays different solutions of $m^{\mu}(t)$ obtained for some fixed values of parameters in the system of equations, but different initial conditions. The

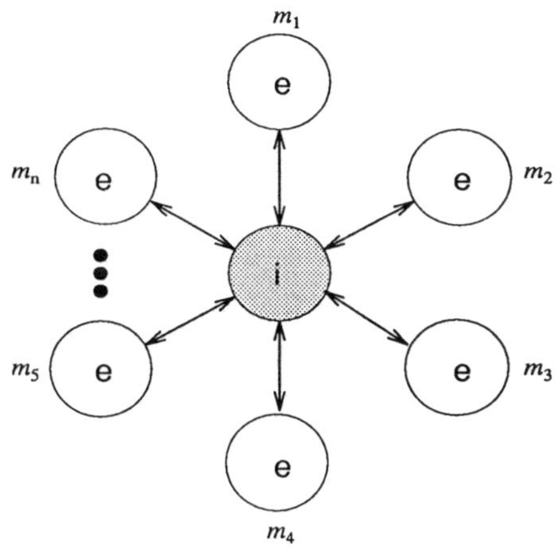

Fig. 11.3. A diagrammatic representation of the dynamical system described by Equations (7) through (10). Note that this system, that has a topological connectivity of a "star," is also symmetric under any permutation of two excitatory neurons. Its solutions break this symmetry (Horn & Opher, 1995). In particular, the segmentation solution has a "ring" structure, with different excitatory elements being activated in sequence, in spite of the fact that this structure is not imposed on the topological connectivity of the network.

segmentation mode competes here with only two other kinds of limit cycles. The choice of one or the other depends on the initial conditions of the system. It is clearly also a function of the chosen parameters.

In order to estimate the sizes of the basins of attraction of all waveforms we have chosen random initial conditions over the whole seven-dimensional space of the $n = 3$ problem, and checked onto which waveforms the system converges. Our interest is focused on the segmentation limit cycles. We found that the probability of converging onto the two waveforms of type c is 0.45 for the set of parameters specified in Fig. 11.4(c).

As n is increased, the situation becomes much more complicated. The phenomenon of full segmentation becomes less abundant and, in our simulations, stops at $n = 5$. However, partial segmentation is often obtained. This can happen in one of two ways (or a combination of both): (a) Formation of clusters of amplitudes that move in unison in a segmentation pattern. (b) Appearance of leading and non-leading amplitudes, in which the leading ones display segmentation behavior. Examples of these two types of waveforms are shown in Figs. 11.5 and 11.6.

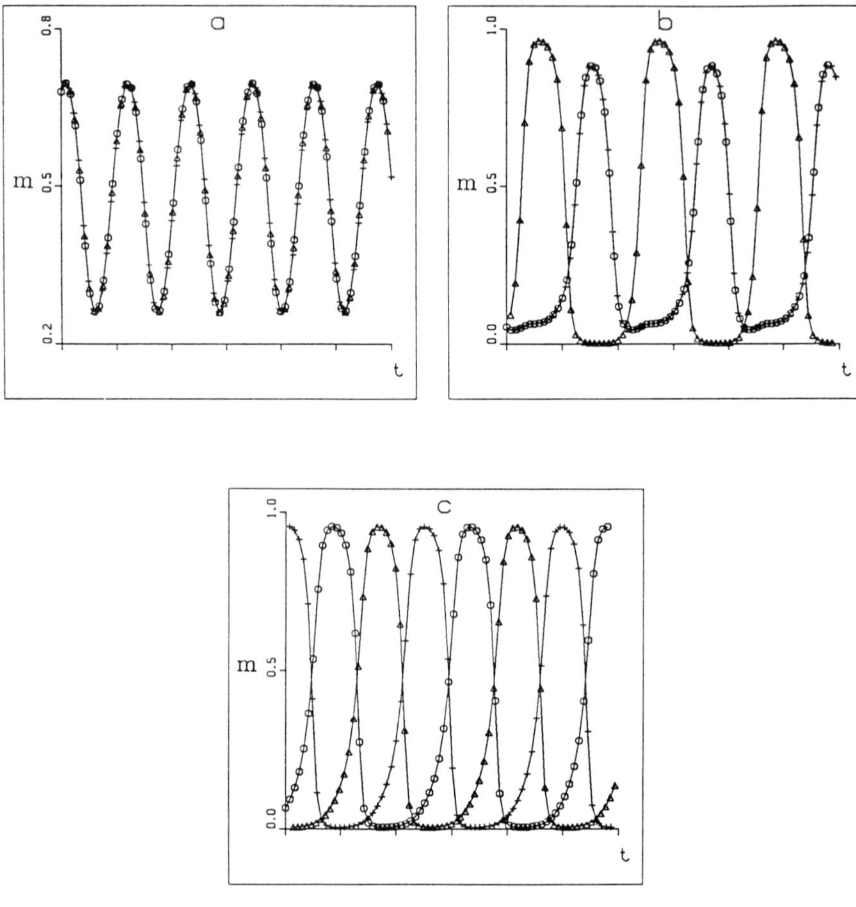

Fig. 11.4. Limit cycles of the $n = 3$ system (Horn & Opher, 1995). Parameters were the following: $a = 0.5$, $b = 0.4$, $c = 0.2$, $g = 0.1$, $e = 1.1$, $f = 0.5$, $\beta = 9$. The different m^{μ} are plotted versus time after the system has reached stability. The time scale is arbitrary but is chosen to be the same in all figures. Each m^{μ} is represented by a different symbol. The limit cycles are: (a) Fully synchronous. $I = 0.8$. (b) Partial synchronous waveform. $I = 0.4$. (c) Full segmentation. $I = 0.4$.

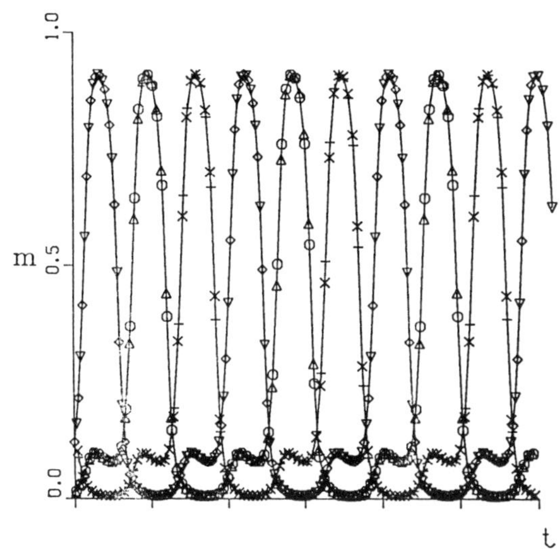

Fig. 11.5. Partial segmentation in the $n = 6$ problem through the formation of clusters of pairs that vary synchronously.

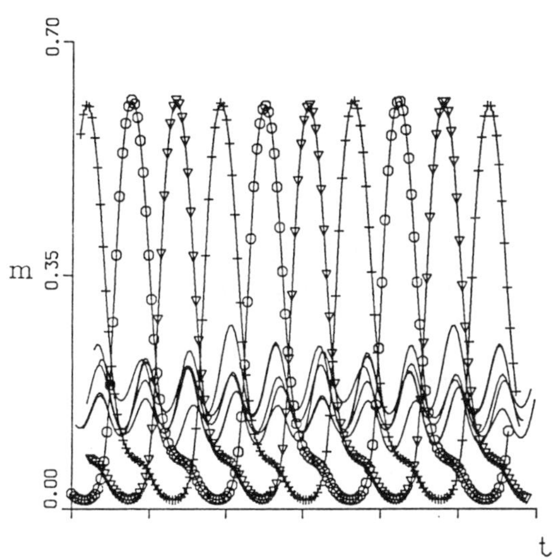

Fig. 11.6. A quasiperiodic solution of the $n = 8$ problem that displays partial segmentation. The three large amplitudes form a segmented pattern, while the low amplitudes display very different periodicities.

5. THE LIMITATION ON TEMPORAL SEGMENTATION

The fact that pure segmentation cannot be obtained in our model for $n > 5$ ties in with previous observations that temporal segmentation works only as long as n is small if the input is constant (Horn & Usher, 1991; Wang et al., 1990). This observation is valid in many variants of these models: above $n = 4$ to 6 the system loses its ability to perform temporal segmentation. It is tempting so speculate that this feature could provide an explanation for the known limits on attention and short-term memory capacity (Miller, 1956). This is the case if attention can be understood in the context of segmentation, as in the cocktail-party effect (Malsburg & Schneider, 1986), where a listener keeps his attention on several ongoing conversations. The connection with short-term memory was made by Horn and Usher (1992) who have added a potentiation term to the fatigue term of the neuron's threshold, thus allowing for continued reverberations after the stimulus is disconnected. As expected, this model of short-term memory works for only small numbers of memories that are jointly activated.

In this section we seek an explanation of the limitation within the symmetric dynamical system that we study. In the system of Equations (7) through (9), the interaction between all elements is provided by the inhibitory unit described by Equation (9). The individual excitatory unit μ, described by Equations (7) and (8), is influenced by all other units through the amplitude m^I of the inhibitory unit in Equation (9). The behavior of each m^μ in any given waveform can therefore be also viewed as the response of equations (7) and (8) to a driving term $am^I(t)$. All the waveforms that we encounter in our numerical study have an overall period τ that is roughly the same as that of the free oscillator ($a = 0$). In a segmentation mode $m^I(t)$ oscillates with a period of τ/n. This can be seen in Fig. 11.7, where we show $m^1(t)$ amd $m^I(t)$ for the $n = 5$ segmentation. m^1 has a waveform of period τ whose local peaks have widths τ/n. If we think of m^I as the driving term then the phenomenon observed here is that of subharmonic oscillation that is known to exist in nonlinear oscillating systems (Hayashi, 1964; Mandelstam & Papalexi, 1932).

A stable linear system follows the frequency of the driving term. Only nonlinear systems exhibit periodic solutions, including the subharmonic ones that are of interest to us. The nonlinear characteristics of the system determine the possible orders of the subharmonic oscillations. In particular, a subharmonic solution of order $1/k$ is likely to occur when one of the terms of the nonlinear function is of power k. Its realization depends, however, on stability conditions that must be met. Note that any such solution has ak-fold degeneracy determined by the phase that, in turn, strongly depends on the initial conditions. Full segmentation is a $1/n$-ordered subharmonic solution where each oscillator makes a different phase choice. In our case the nonlinearity is that of a sigmoid function that, in principle, contains all powers.

To test this property directly, we ran the system of equations (7) and (8) with a constant plus sinusoidal driving term h replacing m^I. In other words, we investigated solutions of the set of equations describing a single driven oscillatory, for example, $\mu =$ 1,

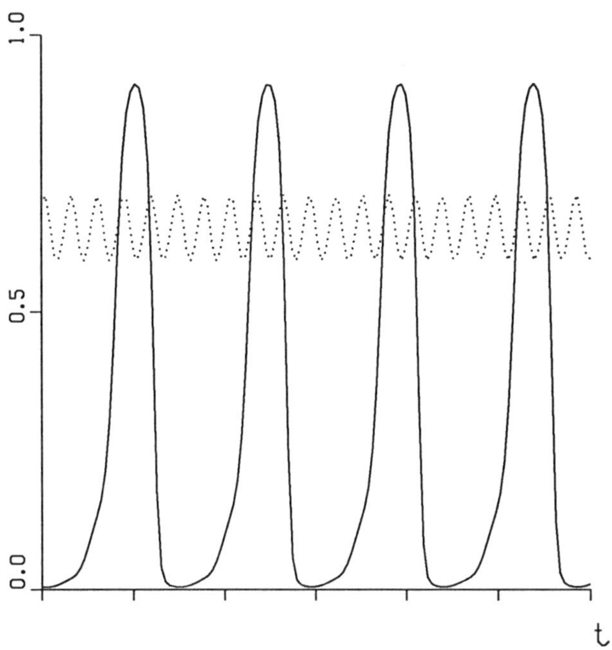

Fig. 11.7. The variation of m^1 (solid line) and the inhibitory amplitude m^I (dotted line) in the $n = 5$ fully segmented limit cycle.

$$\frac{du^1}{dt} = -u^1 + m^1 - h - br^1 + I^1 \tag{11}$$

$$\frac{dr^1}{dt} = m^1 - cr^1 \tag{12}$$

in which $h(t)$ is chosen to be similar to $am^I(t)$ of Fig. 11.7 but with a tunable frequency. We were able to generate narrow subharmonic solutions of 1/2 to 1/5. From 1/6 onwards the subharmonic solutions were no longer narrow, that is, the m^1 amplitude generated by such a driving term has width that is considerably larger than τ/m. This explains why full segmentation is limited in our system to $n \le 5$. Higher n values cannot sustain the narrow subharmonic solution needed to build segmentation.

It is interesting to find the stability of the subharmonic oscillations. We tested it (Horn & Opher, 1996) in two ways. First we ran the system with variations of the frequency ω of the pure sinusoidal driving term and measured the window $\Delta\omega/\omega$ for which subharmonic oscillations were obtained. The results show large ranges for the subharmonics 1/2 and 1/3, for which the relevant values are 0.32 and 0.11 respectively.

The other subharmonic solutions were obtained for considerable smaller frequency windows. The results for 1/4, 1/5, and 1/6 are 0.03, 0.015 and 0.013 respectively. Then we tested stability of the subharmonic solution against the mixing of a lower frequency ω-$\delta\omega$, that is the driving term of the nth subharmonic. Surprisingly the 1/2 solution turns out to be unstable, whereas higher solutions of 1/3, 1/4 and so forth have a range of stability of the order $\delta\omega/\omega \approx 0.2$. These results explain why, in partial segmentation solutions observed for high n values, three segments of leading amplitudes are dominant. The small amplitudes add a varying background to the driving term created by the large amplitudes, the ones responsible for the subharmonic solution. The fact that the 1/3 subharmonic solution has a large frequency window and is stable against admixture of several frequencies is the reason for the dominance of structures like the one displayed in Fig. 11.6.

The stability of partial segmentation into three leading components is particularly evident when we break the symmetry and use graded inputs, that is, I^μ with different values. The characteristic result, shown in Fig. 11.8, is that of three leading amplitudes (with different values reflecting the inputs) and a background of small amplitudes of the oscillators that have low inputs.

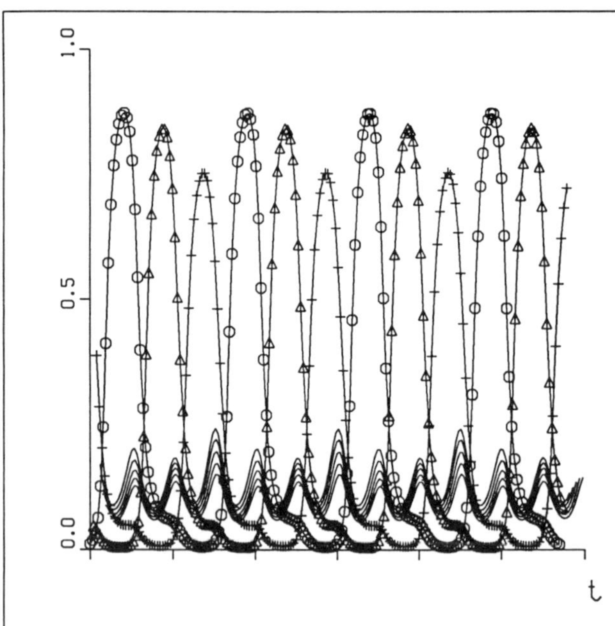

Fig. 11.8. Waveforms of an $n = 8$ system with graded inputs. I^μ were chosen as 0.6, 0.575, 0.55, 0.525, 0.5, 0.475. 0.45.0.425.

6. FACILITATION OF SEGMENTATION BY NOISY INPUTS

The effective segmentation obtained for the case of graded inputs leads us to investigate the possibility of unlimited effective segmentation for a noisy input. Looking for regularity in the oscillation patterns becomes more difficult when I^{μ} contain stochastic elements. To facilitate the study and interpretation, let us consider the correlation matrix

$$C^{\mu\nu}(\theta) = \frac{1}{T} \int_{t_1}^{t_1+T} m^{\mu}(t) m^{\nu}(t+\theta) dt \tag{13}$$

where the integral is carried out over time T larger than the characteristic period, $T > \tau$, after some transient time t_1 has elapsed, ensuring that the limit cycle has been reached. Regularity may emerge only if we allow for an integration time T that is much larger than the characteristic period. Integrating over long time scales we may hope that the fact that the system of differential equations is symmetric on average will reflect itself in some effective symmetry of the waveforms that the correlation matrix elements may reveal.

An example of $n = 3$ is shown in Fig. 11.9. Here we choose an input of $I^{\mu} = 0.4+0.1\eta^{\mu}$, where η^{μ} is a random variable that changes rapidly between 0 and 1, and obtain a regular structure that reflects full segmentation. The symmetry is obtained despite the random component in the input. Moreover, full segmentation is the only limit cycle observed. Increasing n to 4 and more, we find that the symmetry is broken. The general pattern is one of approximate segmentation, as demonstrated in Fig. 11.10. The correlation structure displays distinct peaks, as is the case in all segmentation modes, but the regularity of relative phases is broken, even to the extent that the order of different peaks can change with time.

For large n values ($n > 5$), simple noise does not induce segmentation. There exists either large overlap between different oscillators or partial segmentation in a very disordered form. In order to obtain segmentation one has to make sure that the (random) input affects not more than five oscillators at a time. We have therefore employed two random components. One assigns to each oscillator a random input, and the other selects which five oscillators will be allowed to have their input active at a given time. The two independent random sequences are chosen to have rapid variations, that is, time scales less than 0.1τ. This type of input has a random Fourier decomposition. The results are displayed in Fig. 11.11. Segmentation is quite evident: Each oscillator dominates for some time. The order of the dominant oscillators is random, yet, on the average, all oscillators are being excited. This mechanism of effective segmentation through noise activation can be used for any number of oscillators.

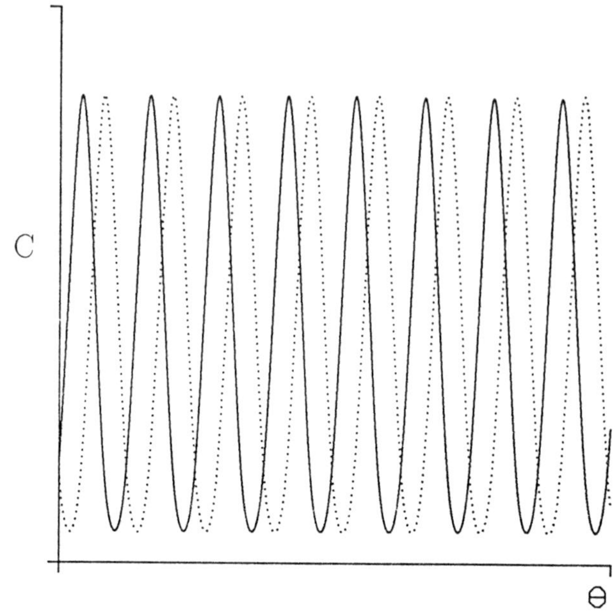

Fig. 11.9. Correlations C^{12} (solid line) and C^{13} (dotted line) versus θ for noisy input in the $n = 3$ case display almost perfect segmentation.

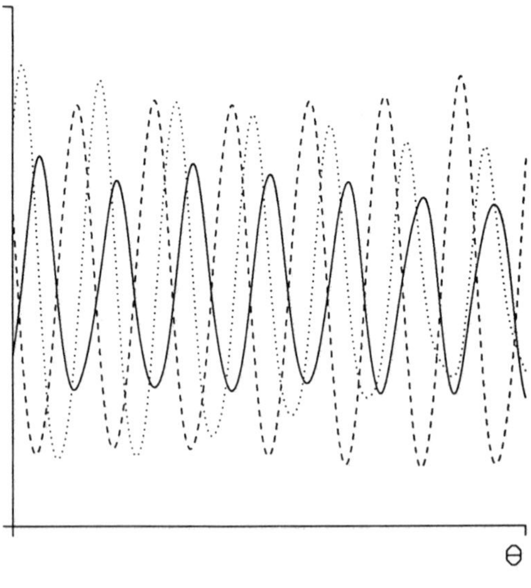

Fig. 11.10. Correlation structures for $n = 4$ of the pairs 12 (solid line), 13 (dotted line), and 14 (dashed line), show that noisy inputs lead to approximate segmentation.

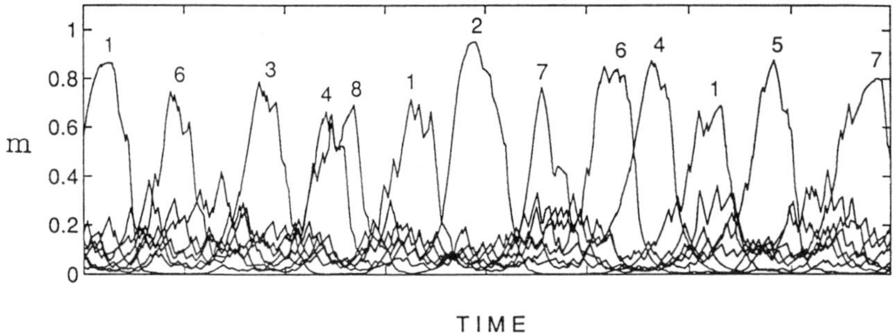

Fig. 11.11. Staggered oscillation of the $n = 8$ problem is obtained for random inputs with rapid variation affecting a few oscillators at a time. Activities of all oscillators are displayed as function of time.

7. SUMMARY: THE IMPORTANCE OF NOISE

We have seen the importance of a random component in the input for both the binding problem and the segmentation problem. For binding as formulated here, it was important to find some way to introduce information about the nonsemantic correlation between the color and shape types. This was achieved with the random noise applied to each object and reflected in the two attributes that must be bound. So far there exists no experimental foundation for such a realization of binding. Keele, Cohen, Ivry, Liotti, and Yee (1988) have shown that temporal variations on the scale of 50 ms do not facilitate binding in the visual domain. Hence they conclude that temporal variation that is relevant to binding may have to be internally generated.

We have seen that segmentation is a feature that is due to the nonlinear nature of the system. In the symmetric model described here, pure segmentation corresponds to a limit cycle whose basin of attraction disappears for $n > 5$. We have an understanding of the origin of this limitation in terms of subharmonic oscillations. We saw that it can be overcome when noisy inputs are used. The importance of noise in the segmentation problem is that it leads in a natural way to segmentation patterns rather than other limit cycles that exist in the symmetric problem. Moreover, under appropriate noisy conditions, when only a few memories are activated simultaneously, an unlimited segmentation pattern can be generated.

ACKNOWLEDGMENT

It is a pleasure to acknowledge the help of Marius Usher in the work summarized here.

REFERENCES

Hayashi, C. (1964). *Nonlinear Oscillations in Physical Systems.* Princeton, NJ: Princeton University Press.

Hopfield, J. F., & Gelperin, A. (1989). Differential conditioning to a compound stimulus and its components in the terrestrial mollusc *Limax maximus. Behavioral Neuroscience, 103,* 329-333.

Horn, D., & Opher, I. (1995). Dynamical symmetries and temporal segmentation. *Journal of Nonlinear Science, 5,* 359-372.

Horn, D., & Opher, I. (1996). Temporal segmentation in a neural dynamical system. *Neural Computation, 8,* 375-391.

Horn, D., Sagi, D., & Usher, M. (1992). Segmentation, binding and illusory conjunctions. *Neur*al *Computation, 3,* 509-524.

Horn, D., & Usher M. (1989). Neural networks with dynamical thresholds. *Physical Review A, 40,* 1036-1044.

Horn, D., & Usher, M. (1990). Excitatory-inhibitory networks with dynamical thresholds. *International Journal of Neural Systems, 1,* 249-257.

Horn, D., & Usher, M. (1991). Parallel activation of memories in an oscillatory neural network. *Neural Computation, 3,* 31-43.

Horn, D., & Usher, M. (1992). Oscillatory model of short-term memory. In J. E. Moody, S. J. Hanson, & R. P. Lippmann (Eds.), *Advances in Neural Information Processing Systems 4* (pp. 125-132). San Mateo, CA: Morgan Kaufman.

Keele, S. W., Cohen, A., Ivry, R., Liotti, M., & Yee, P. (1988). Tests of a temporal theory of attentional binding. *Journal of Experimental Psychology: Human Perception and Performance, 14,* 444-452.

Malsburg, C. von der, & Buhmann, J. (1992). Sensory segmentation with coupled neural oscillators. *Biological Cybernetics, 67,* 233-242.

Malsburg, C. von der, & Schneider, W. (1986). A neural cocktail party processor. *Biological Cybernetics, 54,* 29-40.

Mandelstam, L., & Papalexi, N. (1932). Uber resonanzerscheinungen Beifrequenteilung. *Zeitschrift fur Physik, 73,* 223-248.

Miller, G. A. (1956). The magical number seven, plus or minus two: Some limits on our capacity for processing information. *Psychological Review, 63,* 81-97.

Treisman, A. M., & Schmidt, H. (1982). Illusory conjunctions in the perception of objects. *Cognitive Psychology, 14,* 107-141.

Wang, D., Buhmann, J., & Malsburg, C. von der (1990). Pattern segmentation in associative memory. *Neural Computation, 2,* 94-106.

12

Perceptual Framing and Cortical Synchronization

Alexander Grunewald
California Institute of Technology

Stephen Grossberg
Boston University

(Adapted from Stephen Grossberg and Alexander Grunewald, "Cortical Synchronization and Perceptual Framing," *Journal of Cognitive Neuroscience, 9:1* (January, 1997), pp. 117-132. © 1997 by the Massachusetts Institute of Technology.)

ABSTRACT

How does the brain reliably represent the timing of visual information in a dynamic environment? Because the features defining an object are processed at different rates, different feature attributes belonging to the same object may not be processed simultaneously in cortex. In other words, visual information may get desynchronized. However, if a population code about the timing of visual information is used, then this problem can be avoided. To use a population code for timing it is necessary to define temporal frames that localize the neural activities in time. Perceptual framing is a process that resynchronizes object features by the synchronization of cortical activities corresponding to the same visual object, and thus it helps establishing a population code. A neural network model is presented in which desynchronized neural activities can rapidly be resynchronized. The model shows how psychophysical data can be explained through neural mechanisms. Simulations of the model quantitatively explain perceptual framing data, including psychophysical data about temporal order judgments. The properties of the model arise when fast long-range cooperation and slow short-range competition interact via nonlinear feedback with cells that obey shunting equations.

1. INTRODUCTION

Early stages of the primate visual system process the visual environment by decomposing images into local features, such as contrast, orientation, and motion. This analysis is carried out in several stages. At the retina, visual input is transduced into contrast information. This is transmitted to the lateral geniculate nucleus (LGN) and from there to the striate cortex (V1). In V1, orientation information is extracted, among other types of information. How are temporal attributes coded in the visual system? The response onset latency of retinal and geniculate neurons strongly varies from trial to trial, even when identical stimuli are being used (Sestokas & Lehmkuhle, 1986; Shapley & Victor, 1978). Moreover, the precise parameters of the stimulus strongly influence the response onset latency. For example, less luminant stimuli are processed slower than more luminant stimuli, and higher spatial frequencies are processed slower than lower spatial frequencies (Bolz, Rosner, & Wässle, 1982; Sestokas & Lehmkuhle, 1986). Because most images from a real environment contain a variety of luminances and spatial frequencies, processing of different parts of an image may happen at different rates, so that the cortical representation of the image may be desynchronized. As long as the retinal image is constant, this does not cause serious problems. However, when there is motion in the retinal image, the visual system needs to ensure that all the parts corresponding to the same retinal image are processed together, to avoid illusory conjunctions of features belonging to subsequent images that could impair recognition of objects in a scene. This problem is illustrated in Fig. 12.1. Under extreme conditions, such as the rapid presentation of visual stimuli, it can happen that illusory conjunctions do occur (Intraub, 1985). Why are illusory conjunctions not observed all the time?

Perceptual framing is the process whereby the parts of an image are resynchronized (Varela, Toro, John, & Schwartz, 1981). In the present study, a neural network model is presented that exhibits perceptual framing, so that inputs to the network are resynchronized if they are temporally offset by less than a critical delay. The present study also shows that perceptual framing can be implemented with the same type of bipole cell cooperative connections that have been postulated in a model of form perception and perceptual grouping (Grossberg & Mingolla, 1985a, 1985b) and reported in neurophysiological experiments on area V2 of the primate visual cortex (von der Heydt, Peterhans, & Baumgartner, 1984).

The perceptual framing model developed herein shows how two very different sets of data can both be understood in a unified way. First, physiological data show that neural activities synchronize across wide regions of visual cortex in cats (Eckhorn et al., 1988; Gray, König, Engel, & Singer, 1989) and monkeys (Freeman & van Dijk, 1987; Kreiter & Singer, 1992) with a period of about 15 ms. The meaning of this synchronization is unclear at present. The model offers an interpretation of this cortical synchronization within the context of perceptual framing. Second, psychophysical temporal order judgment data suggest that at about 20 ms stimulus onset asynchrony (SOA) subjects begin to obtain a reliable representation of the temporal order of two brief stimuli (Hirsch & Sherrick, 1961). The model shows how temporal order judgments can be a way to probe perceptual framing. It is possible to extend the model to account for spatiotemporal interactions, and to show robustness in the presence of competition and noise (Grossberg & Grunewald, 1995).

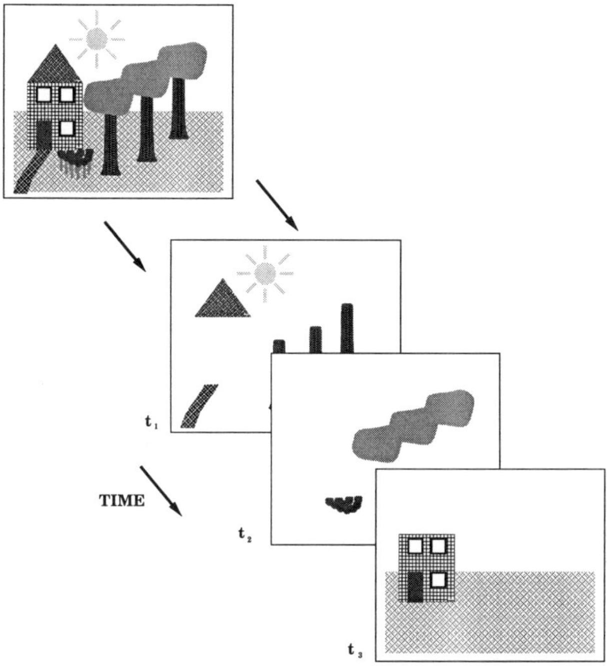

Fig. 12.1. An illustration of the temporal framing problem. Some stimulus attributes are processed faster than others. Since real world scenes contain a whole spectrum of attributes it is possible that different parts of a single image get processed at different times.

2. PERCEPTUAL FRAMING AND TEMPORAL ORDER JUDGMENTS

This section provides a brief review of neurophysiological data which shows that early stages of neural processing are temporally inaccurate, but later stages are not. A review of psychophysical data on temporal aspects of visual perception suggests that the temporal precision of visual processing is quite accurate.

2.1. Neurophysiological Data Concerning Temporal Dynamics

Latencies of neuronal responses in the retina and in the lateral geniculate nucleus (LGN) vary to a considerable extent for identical stimuli (Sestokas & Lehmkuhle, 1986;

Shapley & Victor, 1978). The standard deviation of response onset latencies in the LGN has been reported to vary between 10 and 50 ms depending on the stimulus, and the standard deviation of the response peak latency has been shown to be even bigger (Bolz et al., 1982; Sestokas & Lehmkuhle, 1986). In other words, the timing of neural events at early stages of visual processing seems quite crude. If the neuronal responses in the visual cortex were independent, and based only on independent feedforward activation from the LGN, then one would expect the geniculate variances of the response onset latencies to add, thus yielding even greater uncertainty as to the precise onset of neuronal responses. Several neurophysiological studies addressed this issue and concluded that the standard deviation of combined response onset latencies in the visual cortex is just 10 ms (Celebrini, Thorpe, Trotter, & Imbert, 1993; Maunsell & Gibson, 1992; Vogels & Orban, 1991). A careful analysis of the response onset latencies (Maunsell & Gibson, 1992) by cortical layer showed that the standard deviation is as small as 6 ms. These data suggest that, contrary to the expected increase in variability, there is a decrease. In other words, the activities in visual cortex cannot be independent, and some form of interaction reduces earlier levels of temporal uncertainty. A recent study by Nowak, Munk, Girard, and Bullier (1995) reported recordings from the primate visual cortex in areas V1 and V2 in which higher values for the standard deviation were obtained, even when they took into account the cortical layer within which a neuron is situated. At first sight, these data appear puzzling, and in direct contradiction to the primate data cited earlier. However, the differences may be accounted for by the animal preparation used. The animals in the study by Maunsell and Gibson (1992) were awake and behaving monkeys, while Nowak et al. (1995) used anesthetized monkeys. It is possible that the anesthesia had an adverse effect on the response accuracy of cells. Recordings from the retina and from the LGN show that processing speed also depends on stimulus characteristics. Very luminant stimuli are processed substantially faster than less luminant stimuli (Bolz et al., 1982; Sestokas & Lehmkuhle, 1986), and gratings with lower spatial frequency are processed faster than gratings with higher spatial frequencies (Sestokas & Lehmkuhle, 1986). This effect has been studied when only a small stimulus is in the image.

These physiological results suggest that the temporal accuracy of neurons is initially rather low, and consequently one would expect low temporal resolution at the perceptual level if individual neurons code the perceived timing of events. A population code may get around this limitation. This is further discussed in Section 2.3.

2.2. Psychophysical Data Concerning Temporal Dynamics

One partially informative way to study temporal dynamics in visual perception is to use reaction time (RT) studies. The reaction time paradigm has been used to study the dependence of reaction time on the contrast of a flash of light, and it was found that the reaction time decreases with increasing contrast (Bukhardt, Gottesman, & Keenan, 1987), even if the energy of the flash is kept constant. Similarly the reaction time depends on the wavelength of the stimulus (Ueno, Pokorny, & Smith, 1985) and the spatial frequency (Gish, Shulman, Sheehy, & Leibowitz, 1986).

Such RT studies show that changing the stimulus along a feature dimension may change the rate of processing. In a display with several stimuli characterized by differences along the same feature dimension, these results would carry over if processing of the image were independent for each stimulus. However, spatiotemporal interactions occur during image processing, including brightness illusions and effects of filling-in (Arrington, 1994). Thus RT studies of single feature processing cannot be directly used to predict the temporal dynamics of composite images or realistic scenes.

Temporal order judgment (TOJ) is another paradigm that has been used to compare the rates at which two different stimuli are processed. In this paradigm, observers are presented with two flashes of light at different locations in rapid succession, and they have to indicate which stimulus appeared first. Usually the duration of the stimuli is kept constant, but the stimulus onset asynchrony (SOA) is varied. The result of such an experiment is a psychometric curve, where the probability for correct detection is given as a function of SOA.

Two points of that psychometric function are of particular importance: the point of subjective simultaneity (PSS), and the threshold for accurate TOJ perception. The PSS is the point at which the psychometric function crosses the 50% level. If the two stimuli are identical, then the PSS will lie at 0 SOA, and it will shift if the two stimuli are processed at different rates. By convention, the point at which the psychometric function is 75% is often used as a threshold value for simultaneity. An influential study by Hirsch and Sherrick (1961) showed that the threshold lay at about 20 ms under optimal conditions. Their subjects were highly trained, and the stimuli used were bright dots with high ambient illumination.

Sternberg and Knoll (1973) developed the independent channels model of TOJs. According to this model, each stimulus is processed independently, and stimuli only interact at the site at which the temporal order is actually determined. Several decision functions at that site distinguish between different versions of the independent channels model.

Recent investigations comparing RT and TOJ data have investigated whether the two paradigms yield equivalent results. Jaskowski (1993) varied the onset rise times of visual stimuli, and compared that to a stimulus with zero rise time. The RT study showed that the rise time had only a small effect, whereas the TOJ experiments showed a clear slowing down of processing as rise time increased. Similarly, Tappe, Niepel, and Neuman (1994) found that if gratings were used as stimuli, then RT increased as a function of spatial frequency, whereas PSS stayed constant.

In summary, RT studies and TOJs do not yield the same results about relative rates of processing. It is possible that the dependence of motor reaction time on the visual stimulus may corrupt RT times too much for them to be a useful tool in the present context. For this reason, TOJ results are preferable over RT results as an explanatory target. The results from TOJs suggest that temporal perception is remarkably accurate.

Rapid serial visual presentation (RSVP) is a different paradigm that can employ realistic scenes. Observers are presented with a sequence of visual stimuli at various frame rates. Several tasks are used in conjunction with RSVP. Observers may be asked to detect a particular stimulus, they may be asked to identify which stimulus had a particular feature, which feature followed a particular cue, et cetera. The nature of the paradigm lends itself to the study of how subsequent stimuli interact when they are being rapidly processed.

Intraub (1985) employed an RSVP paradigm in which observers had to recognize which object was surrounded by a frame (see Fig. 12.2). The motivation for that study was to investigate how difficult it is to perceive a single visual stimulus as a whole. She found that subjects were quite reliable at this task until she increased the frame rate to very high levels (about 10 Hz). In that case, observers often reported that the frame appeared around an object that preceded or followed the correct object. These illusory conjunctions do not seem to depend on attentional manipulation. This experiment also indicates that only under extreme conditions do the processing of the object and the surrounding frame not occur together. Similar observations using colored digits have also been reported (McLean, Broadbent, & Broadbent, 1982). These experiments, in which observers had to identify the color of a target digit in a stream of digits, showed that observers sometimes reported the color of an earlier or later digit.

RSVP data thus indicate that illusory conjunctions occur rarely, which suggests that the perceived timing of events is quite accurate. This further corroborates the high temporal resolution that follows from studies using the TOJ paradigm.

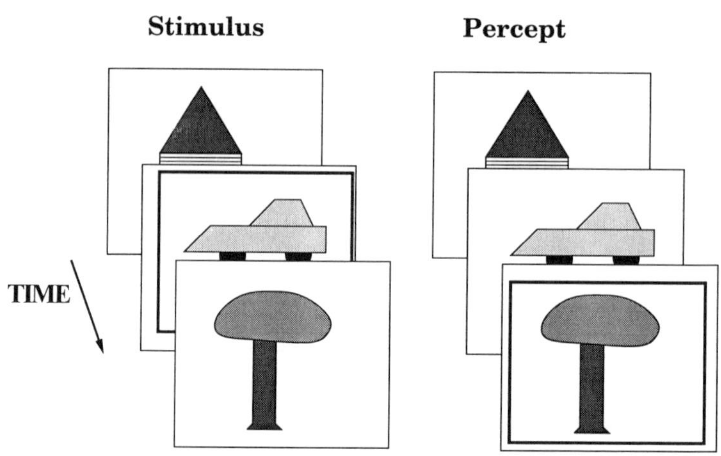

Fig. 12.2. Illusory conjunctions can occur under extreme conditions, as shown by (Intraub, 1985). In that study, observers were shown sequences of images at high presentation rates (9 Hz). One of those images was surrounded by a frame, and observers had to report which image was surrounded by a frame. Observers often reported objects before or after the correct object.

2.3. Perceptual Framing as Resynchronization

Based on the psychophysical findings in the TOJ and RSVP paradigms one has to conclude that the temporal accuracy of the visual system is remarkably high. This suggests that the accuracy of the underlying neural processes should be quite high. Alternatively, it may be that perceptual timing is coded via the timing not of individual neurons, but of an entire ensemble. However, a temporally distributed code would lead to an ambiguity as to which time a neural event belongs to. This ambiguity can be reduced if frames are defined in time. All neural information that falls within such a frame belongs to the same perceptual time.

The physiological data reviewed earlier suggest that the accuracy of neural events is quite low, and that it strongly varies with stimulus attributes. This makes it impossible to use individual neurons to code timing, and hence a distributed code has to be used. As a consequence, it appears that a process such as perceptual framing (Varela et al., 1981) is necessary to correctly identify to which time the activity of a given neuron belongs. The data suggest that perceptual framing occurs only in the presence of several stimuli within the visual field. In other words, perceptual framing is inherently a spatiotemporal phenomenon wherein spatial interactions between visual events in time somehow resynchronize them.

3. MECHANISMS FOR PERCEPTUAL FRAMING

This section discusses several candidate neural mechanisms that may subserve perceptual framing. It is shown how the cortical synchronization of activities can subserve perceptual framing.

3.1. Central Clock

One possible mechanism is a central clock that determines the processing cycles during which perceptual information could be processed (Wiener, 1961). Any stimuli that fall within a single cycle would be considered as belonging to the same image. On the other hand, two stimuli that belong to different processing cycles would be considered as belonging to different images. This mechanism predicts that the perception of simultaneity would be influenced not only by the temporal difference between two stimuli, but also by the state of the internal clock. If two stimuli fell within the same processing cycle, they should be perceived as simultaneous, otherwise they should be perceived as sequential. An experiment showing an interaction of the phase of the alpha rhythm and the perception of simultaneity has been reported (Varela et al., 1981), but the same laboratory later found evidence that spoke against this (Gho & Varela, 1989).

A central clock as outlined above implies that there is a shortest stimulus-independent length of time that can be perceived, which has been called a perceptual moment (Allport, 1968). This is in contradiction to results by Efron and Lee (1971), who showed that no such stimulus independent time interval exists. Building on the concept of perceptual moment, Allport (1968) proposed a view according to which there is a traveling moment, that starts as soon as a stimulus comes on. Thus, the clock that times perception is no longer internal, but stimulus-locked. Moreover, the precise timing parameters can be influenced by the stimulus. This view still assumes that there is some central clock, that it is stimulus-driven, and that its parameters depend on the stimulus. But is there a need for this assumption? After all, there is very little evidence for a central clock regulating visual processing. Moreover, the assumption of a central clock poses a host of problems, such as the mechanism by which the clock obtains the stimulus-dependent parameters. These problems can be avoided if the central clock is replaced by local clocks or oscillations (one clock corresponding to each local feature detector). Perceptual framing can then be achieved by synchronization of these clocks. This is the view put forward and further investigated in this chapter.

3.2. Synchronization in the Visual Cortex

Could cortical synchronization be the resynchronization of local processing alluded to earlier? Several findings point in this direction. First, cortical synchronization occurs only when a stimulus is presented (Gray & Singer, 1989). Without a stimulus, there is no need for perceptual framing. Second, neurons can synchronize with different partners depending on the stimulus, suggesting flexibility in the synchronization process. Third, synchronization occurs across several millimeters of cortical tissue within the same hemisphere (Gray et al., 1989), and across several centimeters between hemispheres (Engel, König, Kreiter, & Singer, 1991). Fourth, synchronization occurs very rapidly (Gray & Singer, 1989), suggesting that if it contributes to visual processing, it is probably related to some time-critical aspect of visual processing.

In conclusion, it appears that the cortical synchronization of neuronal activities is a viable candidate for a mechanism subserving perceptual framing. In this view the main function of cortical synchronization is not to achieve figure-ground segregation. Instead, all visual information perceived simultaneously is synchronized. Synchronization does not occur only between objects that are segmented, or bound, together, but between all features within the same visual image. Synchronization does not indicate to which object a given feature belongs, but to which perceptual frame. The next section introduces a neural network model in which this possibility is explored using computer simulations.

4. A MODEL OF PERCEPTUAL FRAMING

The model we propose is an extension of a model introduced by Grossberg and Somers (1991) to explain how cortical activity can quickly be synchronizedwithout a central rhythm generator. That model is a simplification of the Boundary Contour System (BCS) for emergent boundary segmentation of (Grossberg & Mingolla, 1985a, 1985b). Synchrony can only be established with neural activities that vary over time. The simplest time-varying dynamics are oscillations, which are employed in the present model for convenience. However, more complex dynamics, such as quasi-periodic or chaotic systems, may also be used as carrier signal for synchronization.

The goal of Grossberg and Somers (1991) was to simplify the BCS model as a much as possible to expose the core mathematical mechanism behind fast resynchronization. They thereby demonstrated how this key property could be used to explain cortical neural data on synchronization (e.g., Eckhorn et al., 1988; Freeman & van Dijk, 1987; Gray et al., 1989; Kreiter & Singer, 1992) using a perceptual theory that had already been used to suggest explanations of many other types of perceptual and neural data. The present work continues this strategy to strengthen the linking hypothesis between perceptual and neural data that both probe the synchronization process. To the present time this is the only model of which we are aware that makes the linking hypothesis. Indeed, the model demonstrates fast synchronization. Fast synchronization means that the model can resynchronize desynchronized cell activities within a few cycles of the oscillation. Grossberg and Somers (1991) demonstrated synchronization within a few cycles. Such rapid synchronization enables the model to carry out perceptual framing. In addition, the model provides an explanation of cortical neural data about synchronization, perceptual data about synchronization, and perceptual data about grouping processes other than synchronization.

The BCS contains a feedforward filter followed by a feedback grouping network. The simplified BCS contains only a variant of the feedback grouping network. It contains three types of cells (Fig. 12.3). The first two cell types are fast excitatory cells (cells that react quickly) and slow inhibitory cells (cells that react slowly) that are coupled together through reciprocal pathways (Fig. 12.3). An excitatory cell excites itself, an inhibitory interneuron, and a third type of cell, called a bipole cell, that couples excitatory cells together. An inhibitory cell inhibits only the excitatory cell from which it derives its excitation. Inputs to the excitatory cells are capable of triggering oscillations within such a network. Each excitatory cell obeys an equation which includes multiplicative, or shunting, interactions between the cell potential and its input and feedback signals (Grossberg, 1973). Each slow inhibitory cell obeys a simpler additive equation that linearly time-averages signals from the excitatory cell. This combination of fast shunting and slow addition was first used in Ellias and Grossberg (1975) to simulate oscillatory dynamics. A mathematically related type of dynamics was proposed by Morris and Lecar (1981) to explain voltage oscillations in an invertebrate preparation. Somers and Kopell (1993) have analyzed mathematically how the Ellias-Grossberg and Morris-Lecar models generate fast resynchronization (e.g., synchronization within one processing cycle), whereas sinusoidal oscillators do not.

The third cell type, called a bipole cell, couples the excitatory cells together via long-range cooperative feedback. Bipole cells have tripartite receptive fields. Two of these subfields branch in a laterally oriented direction from the bipole cell body. The third inputs directly to the cell body. The bipole cell fires if at least two of the three subfields are activated by excitatory cells. If the two oriented branches are excited, then a bipole cell can help to complete a boundary between these branches. If one branch and the cell body are activated, then a bipole cell can be activated at a line end. The present study refines that of Grossberg and Somers (1991) by using a tripartite, rather than a bipartite, bipole cell receptive field and a sigmoidal signal function in the fast-slow oscillator, rather than the threshold-linear signal function that was previously used, to quantitatively simulate psychophysical data. The tripartite bipole cell facilitates

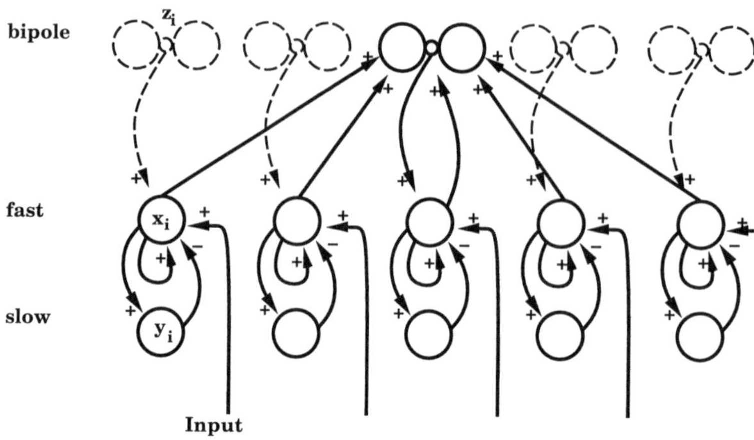

Fig. 12.3. The architecture of the fast synchronization model. A layer of fast-slow oscillators is recurrently coupled to a layer of bipole cells.

synchronization near line ends. The sigmoid function enables low levels of activity spread out over space to collectively generate sufficiently high activity in the bipole cells to trigger feedback signals. In this way, small and temporally desynchronized signals that converge on bipole cells can induce large and synchronous network responses. The model is defined mathematically later in the chapter.

5. SIMULATION OF TEMPORAL ORDER JUDGMENTS

As noted in Section 2.1, one way to test the notion of perceptual framing is to link it to temporal order judgments (TOJs) between two visual stimuli. When perceptual framing breaks down, two stimuli can be perceived as successive, whence observers can identify their temporal order. Hirsch and Sherrick (1961) found that the point at which subjects reach threshold in a TOJ task lies at about 20 ms SOA for highly trained subjects using bright stimuli with high ambient illumination. See Fig. 12.4, which also shows that the model closely approximates their data.

Figure 12.5 provides a finer description of how synchronization is related to the plot of Fig. 12.4. This simulation plots the time difference between the internal

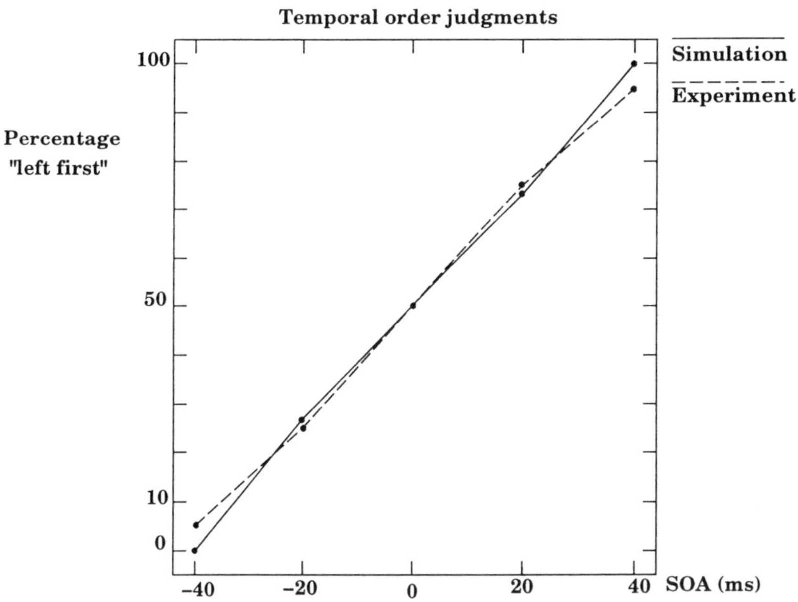

Fig. 12.4. Percentage left first of temporal order judgments as a function of SOA. Comparison between experimental results (Hirsch & Sherrick, 1961) and model simulation. SOA indicates the time by which stimulus one (e.g., the "left stimulus") leads the other stimulus in a two stimulus presentation task. The ordinate gives the percent responses that stimulus one appeared first. Solid line: results from simulation of the model. Dashed line: results from experimental study. Positive SOA means that the "left" stimulus was presented first, negative means that the "right" stimulus was presented first.

representations of two external stimuli as a function of their SOA. The solid line shows the effects of synchrony on small SOAs. For different SOAs, we found the internal time difference Δt for the corresponding neural signals in the model.

The time of maximum response corresponding to each of the two stimuli is a random variable, and the mean of the difference between the two random variables corresponding to the two stimuli is the internal time difference Δt. The probability that each of those neural signals occurs at any given time follows the normal distribution. The standard deviation of the time of the maximum response σ is the same for both, and has been reported to be 6 ms (Maunsell & Gibson, 1992; Zack, 1973). The probability that the signal corresponding to the first stimulus is perceived first can be found by taking the difference of the two random variables, which is also a normal distribution, with mean Δt and standard deviation $\sqrt{2}\sigma$. Thus the probability that the first stimulus in a two-stimuli paradigm is perceived first, and hence that the temporal order of the stimuli is perceived correctly, is given by

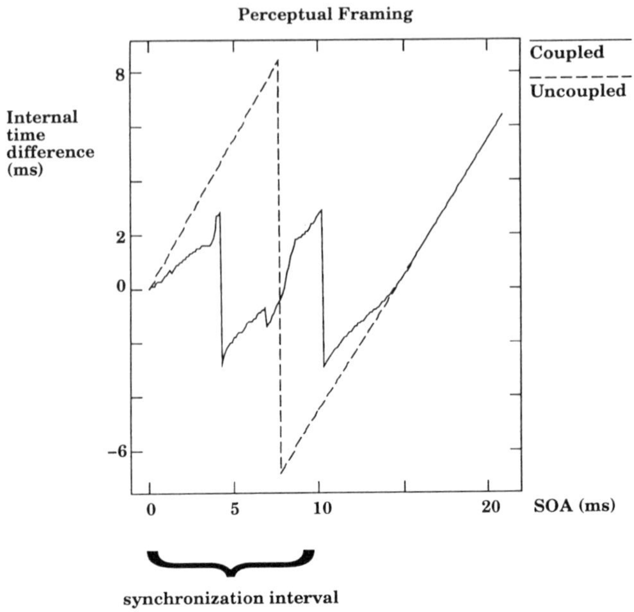

Fig. 12.5. Perceptual framing, The abscissa indicates the SOA (in simulated ms) between two stimuli, and the ordinate gives the resulting time difference (in simulated ms) between peaks of activity in the internal representations of the two stimuli. Solid line: performance in the presence of bipole coupling. Dashed line: performance in the absence of bipole coupling. The oscillatory nature of the underlying network processing is reflected in the fact that both curves cross the x-axis several times for nonzero SOAs.

$$P = \Phi\left(\frac{\Delta t}{\sqrt{2}\sigma}\right), \tag{1}$$

where Φ is the cumulative normal distribution function,

$$\Phi(x) = \frac{1}{\sqrt{2\pi}} \int_{-\infty}^{x} e^{-\frac{1}{2}s^2}\, ds. \tag{2}$$

6. MODEL EQUATIONS AND PARAMETERS

Each SOA leads to a different value for Δt, and hence a different probability P. In Fig. 12.4 the experimental results of Hirsch and Sherrick (1961) about temporal order judgments and the simulation results are compared. The simulations match the data closely.

Because bipole cells carry out oriented cooperation, the main model properties can adequately be demonstrated through one-dimensional simulations. In particular, model simulations used 64 oscillators arranged in a ring. Each oscillator consists of two nodes each, one fast and one slow. The activity of the fast node is denoted by x_i and of the corresponding slow node by y_i. The index i denotes the position of the oscillator and ranges from 1 to 64. Oscillators with indices differing by one are neighbors. Because the oscillators are arranged as a ring, units indexed by 1 and 64 are also neighbors. This structure was chosen to avoid edge effects. Care was taken to ensure that input was sufficiently far removed from the wrap-around position to avoid interactions around the whole ring. The input to x_i is denoted by I_i and it is position specific. Associated with every oscillator is a bipole cell whose activity is denoted by z_i (see Fig. 12.3). The activities x_i, y_i, z_i can also be interpreted as the mean potential of a population of cells, which is in accord with recent evidence suggesting that neurons that synchronize do not necessarily oscillate at each cycle (Eckhorn & Obermueller, 1993). The equations governing the oscillators are:

Fast Shunting Excitatory Neuron

$$\frac{dx_i}{dt} = -Ax_i + (B - x_i)(Cf_a(x_i) + f_a(z_i) + I_i) - Dx_i f_a(y_i) \quad (3)$$

Slow Additive Inhibitory Neuron

$$\frac{dy_i}{dt} = E(x_i - y_i) \quad (4)$$

where the sigmoid signal function f_a in (3) is given by

$$f_a(x) = \frac{x^{n_a}}{Q_a^{n_a} + x^{n_a}}. \quad (5)$$

Quantities A, B, C, D, E, n_a, and Q_a are parameters of the network. Equation (3) is a shunting equation that describes the influences of positive feedback $f_a(x_i)$ from the ith excitatory cell population to itself, positive feedback $f_a(z_i)$ from the ith bipole cell, input I_i, and negative feedback from the ith inhibitory interneuron; see Fig. 12.3. The terms $(B - x_i)$ and $(- Dx_i)$ are the shunting terms that automatically gain control the excitatory and inhibitory inputs, respectively. Equation (4) says that the ith inhibitory interneuron slowly time-averages input from the ith excitatory cell.

The equation governing the bipole cells is:

Bipole Neuron

$$z_i = \left[f_b(L_i) + f_b(R_i) + Ff_b(C_i) - \Gamma\right]^+ \quad (6)$$

where $[x]^+ = \max(x, 0)$ and the bipole signal function is

$$f_b(x) = \frac{x^{n_b}}{Q_b^{n_b} + x^{n_b}} \tag{7}$$

Equation (6) is expressed as an algebraic equation because it is assumed that the bipole cell responds quickly to its input signals. The terms $f_b(L_I)$ and $f_b(R_I)$ describe input signals to the ith bipole cell from its left and right receptive fields, respectively. The term $Ff_b(C_I)$ describes a direct input to the location of the cell body. Each input term in (6) has a finite maximum due to the squashing effect of the sigmoid signal f_b. The output threshold is chosen so that at least two out of three of these receptive field parts must be active before the cell could fire. In principle, parameter F could be chosen so that a single input at the location of the bipole cell could also fire it. The terms L_i, R_i, and C_i that represent these bottom-up inputs to each bipole cell are given by

$$L_i = \frac{1}{w}\sum_{j=1}^{w} f_a(x_{i-j}) \tag{8}$$

$$R_i = \frac{1}{w}\sum_{j=1}^{w} f_a(x_{i+j}) \tag{9}$$

$$C_i = f_a(x_i) \tag{10}$$

where w is the halfwidth of the kernel. Taken together, Equations (3) through (10) define a system of Ellias-Grossberg oscillators (Ellias & Grossberg, 1975) coupled together with bipole feedback.

Scaling of time was done by taking into account that the period of oscillations should be about 15 ms. This is in line with the recent finding suggesting that oscillations in the primate have a considerably higher frequency (60-90 Hz) than in the cat (30-50 Hz) (Eckhorn et al., 1993). It was found that putting a time step of 1 unit in the model equal to 1 ms yielded good results. Numerical integration was performed using a fixed step Runge-Kutta method. The integration step size used was $H = 0.1$ ms. The parameters used throughout this report are $A = 1$, $B = 1$, $C = 20$, $D = 33.3$, $\Gamma = 1$, $w = 6$. The initial conditions of the network were chosen to be $x_i = y_i = z_i = 0$ for all i, except in the simulation showing synchronization, where the initial conditions were chosen at random.

In the simulations of synchronization across the network (Fig. 12.6), 20 nodes received an input of $I_i = 0.5$. All other nodes received background input of $I_i = 0$. The initial conditions of the network where chosen to lead to random phases if an input would come on. Hence x_i was chosen at random between 0 and 0.15, y_i was chosen at random between 0.15 and 0.55, and $z_i = 0$ for all i. See Grossberg and Somers (1991) for additional simulations of the earlier model showing fast synchronization in response to two disjoint input bars and creation of an illusory contour between them.

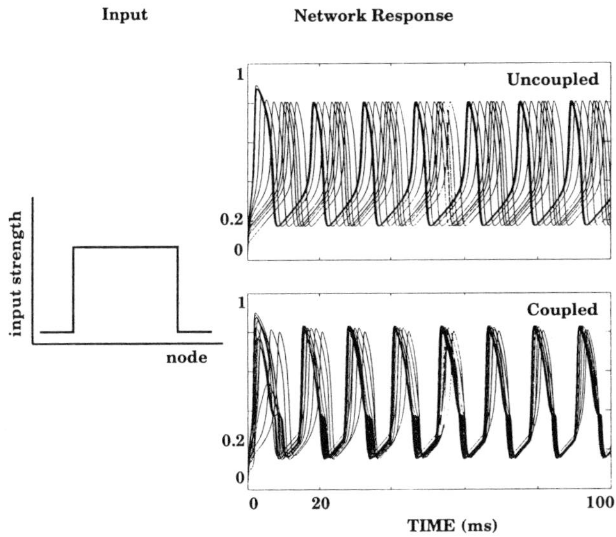

Fig. 12.6. Simulation of synchronization of the network when the input is a bar stimulus. Initial conditions were randomly distributed. The input is shown left. The resulting network activities are shown on the right. When there is no coupling via feedback, network cells remain in random phases (top). With coupling, network cells synchronize rapidly from random initial conditions (bottom).

In the simulations of perceptual framing, two nodes received an input ($I_i = 0.8$) which lasted for 250 ms. The first input ($i = 31$) came on at simulation onset, the second input ($i = 34$) came on later at the SOA. The background activity of the network was zero. In Fig. 12.5, it is shown how much time there was between the last peak of the activity corresponding to the first stimulus, and the peak closest in time of the activity corresponding to the second stimulus. This explains why some times are negative. The simulation of TOJ was based on the simulation shown in Fig. 12.5 and was obtained as described in the text. The outcome is shown in Fig. 12.4.

The network model is made up of 128 coupled differential equations. Such a large system can exhibit very complex dynamics. In the present simulations, network dynamics were affected only quantitatively, but not qualitatively, by modest changes in network parameters. In general, the network parameters (A, B, C, D, E, Γ, w) in the present study were the same as those employed in earlier studies (Ellias & Grossberg, 1975; Grossberg & Somers, 1991), mainly to maintain continuity and to allow comparison. The slow-variable rate parameter E in equation (4) was used to calibrate time in the network. It was chosen to yield realistic oscillation frequencies. Parameter F in equation (6) allows boundaries to cooperatively complete and synchronize at the ends of input bars. The parameters and in (5) define the signal function; they were chosen to approximate the signal function used previously (Grossberg & Somers, 1991).

The bipole signal function in equation (6) is defined by parameters and, to achieve a balance between allowing feedback signals to occur when the inputs to the network was small, yet not saturating the oscillators due to excess feedback when large inputs occurred.

7. OTHER MODELS OF CORTICAL SYNCHRONIZATION

What sorts of mechanisms could, in principle, achieve cortical synchronization? Bottom-up convergence of signals in visual cortex does not suffice as a mechanism for synchronization, if only because cortical cells have a fast rate of integration (Mason, Nicoll, & Stratford, 1991). Yet the responses of cortical cells within the first 5 ms after response onset is a 95% accurate predictor of the entire response strength (Celebrini et al., 1993; Oram & Perrett, 1992). It has also been shown that synchronization cannot be mediated by a clocking mechanism such as the cortical alpha rhythm (Gho & Varela, 1989), because triggering stimuli in a TOJ task to the alpha rhythm did not affect performance.

Here we model how synchronization of distributed cortical activities by recurrent cooperative-competitive interactions can temporally realign out-of-phase image parts. The results model data showing that cortical activities synchronize in the cat and in the monkey when a stimulus is present in the visual field (Eckhorn et al., 1988; Gray & Singer, 1989), even when the receptive fields of the units recorded do not overlap. Specifically, when the receptive fields of the cells from which recordings were made did not overlap, then synchronization nonetheless occurred when a bar that extended across both receptive fields was swept through the image. Weak synchronization also occurred when the bar was occluded in the middle (i.e., the area that lies between the receptive fields). No synchronization occurred if two separate bars were swept through both receptive fields simultaneously in opposite directions. Similar results were also found in the awake monkey (Kreiter & Singer, 1992). Synchronization has been shown to occur across wide cortical distances (Gray et al., 1989), and even across hemispheres (Engel et al., 1991). Initially it was postulated that synchronization occurs between oscillating cell sites (Gray & Singer, 1989), a claim that has been controversial (Ghose & Freeman, 1992; Young, Tanaka, & Yamane, 1992).

These experiments have inspired a large number of models of cortical synchronization (Baldi & Meir, 1990; Eckhorn, Reitboeck, Arndt, & Dicke, 1989; König & Schillen, 1991). The present model differs from these alternative models in several important respects. First and foremost, the present model is part of a larger neural theory of visual perception that already has been used to explain and predict many psychophysical and neural data; see for example Francis, Grossberg, and Mingolla (1994). Here we show that a variant of the same boundary segmentation process can also explain data about perceptual framing. Other models of cortical synchronization have not yet been used to parametrically simulate perceptual data. Without such a behavioral linking hypothesis, such models cannot be said to explain the binding problem of visual object perception.

Second, the present model achieves fast synchronization of desynchronized and distributed data. As noted before, Grossberg and Somers (1991) first demonstrated this property with computer simulations, and Somers and Kopell (1993) have proved it mathematically. Fast synchronization is needed to frame together desynchronized object parts before they can be incorrectly bound with incorrect parts of other objects, as Intraub (1985) has shown can occur among image parts from different images in very rapidly presented image sequences, as in Fig. 12.2. The present work builds on the results of Grossberg and Somers (1991). Various other synchronization models have not demonstrated fast synchronization, or do not represent neuron dynamics, but instead use formal equations for phase synchronization (Baldi & Meir, 1990; Lumer & Huberman, 1992; Niebur, Schuster, Kammen, & Koch, 1991). Terman and Wang (1995) described an oscillator that shares some mathematical properties with the Ellias-Grossberg oscillator. Their model uses local cooperation and global competition, rather than our long-range cooperation and short-range competition, to rapidly synchronize locally connected image figures and to desynchronize spatially disjoint figures. This mathematical study does not attempt to explain any perceptual data or to explain how neurons with spatially separated receptive fields can synchronize. One reason for these gaps in other models may be that they do not view the synchronization task as one of perceptual framing, or of fast resynchronization of temporarily desynchronized object parts. Rather, they attribute all binding properties to the very existence of a synchronous oscillation between object parts. In many such models, the phase of the oscillation is taken to encode all the features that belong within a single object. Some models also require that attention be focused on an object or object part before it can oscillate synchronously (Crick & Koch, 1990). It is hard to understand, however, how an object's phase can remain constant as its image size and position on the retina change radically, while the same is happening to other objects, due to changes in their distances and angles with respect to an observer. It is also well known that segmentation of unfamiliar objects can occur preattentively before attention is engaged.

In the present account, the ability to resynchronize asynchronous object parts, not the existence of oscillations per se, becomes the focus of interest. Here, key properties of framing are attributed to cooperative interactions of long-range bipole cells. Although we simulate this model in a parameter range where oscillations occur, segmentation can also occur using the present type of model in parameter ranges where oscillations do not occur (Grossberg & Mingolla, 1985a, 1985b). In the present model, oscillations provide an extra degree of freedom that calibrates how asynchronous object parts can become and still be rapidly resynchronized, or framed, together. It is important to reiterate at this point that all features and objects corresponding to the same image synchronize, and that the phase is not used as a code to segment the visual image.

Using bipole cells, textured objects can be bound together (Grossberg & Mingolla, 1985b). In a textured scene, objects are often defined by spatially disjoint textural elements. Moreover, the textural elements belonging to different objects may be as close together as the elements belonging to the same objects. In order to separate such objects from one another, a mechanism is needed that can bridge the featureless spaces between texture elements, and can use properties such as texture orientation, size, depth, and alignment across space to distinguish which textures belong to which objects. The

Boundary Contour System of which bipole cells form a part has been shown capable of grouping under these conditions. It is hard to see how a mechanisms using unoriented nearest-neighbor cooperation and global competition, as in Terman and Wang (1995), can accomplish this. All simulations of their model use simple connected figures that are widely separated from one another.

Finally, one influential binding model, that of Malsburg (1981), suggests that binding requires a type of ultrafast synaptic plasticity that has not yet been experimentally observed; see also Terman and Wang (1995). The present model synchronizes without the benefit of fast plasticity. On the other hand, its synchronous, or resonant, neural states have been proposed to initiate synaptic learning on a slower time scale (Carpenter & Grossberg, 1993; Grossberg, 1976) that is consistent with known properties of long-term potentiation or LTP (Bliss & Collingridge, 1993). Perceptual framing may thus be utilized not only for perception, but also for learning about the visual environment. Indeed it is known that perceptual learning can occur within hours, with effects lasting for a long time (Karni & Sagi, 1993).

Data about temporal order judgments are quantitatively simulated using a neural model of cortical grouping via cooperative-competitive interactions. This process leads to fast synchronization of cortical activities that defines a perceptual frame in which features belonging to the same object are temporally realigned. This model shows how a distributed code can be used to carry information about the timing of visual events, even when the underlying neural machinery does not have good temporal accuracy.

The first BCS computer simulations of boundary segmentation used V2 model bipole cells to simulate the long-range interactions that help to form illusory contours (Grossberg & Mingolla, 1985a, 1985b). More recently, similar cooperative interactions, albeit on a smaller spatial scale, have been reported in cortical area V1 (Gilbert, 1993; Gilbert & Wiesel, 1990). Grosof, Shapley, and Hawken (1993) have reported, moreover, that illusory contour completion can be supported over a shorter spatial range by V1 cells. Ross, Grossberg, and Mingolla (1995) have described a refinement of the BCS that explains all these data sets. In this model, shorter-range bipole interactions in V1 and longer-range bipole interactions V2 coexist within cooperative-competitive feedback networks at each cortical level. As in the earlier BCS model, the model V2 bipole cells help to achieve long-range boundary completion. The model V1 bipole interactions are mediated by complex cells and are hypothesized to help stabilize the development of orientational and disparity tuning properties in V1 while suppressing network noise. The bipole cells of the present model could, in principle, act at either or both of the V1 or V2 levels, since our results explore key mathematical properties of this mechanism wherever it may be found in the brain.

ACKNOWLEDGMENTS

The authors wish to thank Eric Schwartz for helpful discussions and Diana Meyers and Robin Locke for their valuable assistance in the preparation of the manuscript. AG was supported in part by the Air Force Office of Scientific Research (AFOSR F49620-92-J-0334 and AFOSR F49620-92-J-0225), the Advanced Research Projects Agency (ONR N00014-92-J-4015), and the Office of Naval Research (ONR N00014-91-J-4100).

SG was supported in part by the the Advanced Research Projects Agency (ONR N00014-92-J-4015) and the Office of Naval Research (ONR N00014-92-J-1309, ONR N00014-95-1-0409, and ONR N00014-95-1-0657).

REFERENCES

Allport, D. A. (1968). Phenomenal simultaneity and the perceptual moment hypothesis. *British Journal of Psychology*, *59*, 395-406.

Arrington, K. F. (1994). The temporal dynamics of brightness filling-in. *Vision Research*, *34*, 3371-3387.

Baldi, P., & Meir, R. (1990). Computing with arrays of coupled oscillators: An application to preattentive texture discrimination. *Neural Computation*, *2*, 458-471.

Bliss, T. V. P., & Collingridge, G. L. (1993). A synaptic model of memory: Llong-term potentiation in the hippocampus. *Nature*, *361*, 31-39.

Bolz, J., Rosner, G., & Wässle, H. (1982). Response latency of brisk-sustained (X) and brisk-transient (Y) cells in the cat retina. *Journal of Physiology(London)*, *328*, 171-190.

Bukhardt, D. A., Gottesman, J., & Keenan, R. M. (1987). Sensory latency and reaction time: dependence on contrast polarity and early linearity in human vision. *Journal of the Optical Society of America A*, *4*, 530-539.

Carpenter, G., & Grossberg, S. (1993). Normal and amnesic learning, recognition and memory by a neural model of cortico-hippocampal interactions. *Trends in Neurosciences*, *16*, 131-137.

Celebrini, S., Thorpe, S., Trotter, Y., & Imbert, M. (1993). Dynamics of orientation coding in area V1 of the awake primate. *Visual Neuroscience*, *10*, 811-825.

Crick, F., & Koch, C. (1990). Towards a neurobiological theory of consciousness. *Seminars in the Neurosciences*, *2*, 263-275.

Eckhorn, R., Bauer, R., Jordan, W., Brosch, M., Kruse, W., Munk, M., & Reitboeck, H. J. (1988). Coherent oscillations: A mechanism of feature linking in the visual cortex? *Biological Cybernetics*, *60*, 121-130.

Eckhorn, R., Frien, A., Bauer, R., Woelbern, T., & Kehr, H. (1993). High frequency (60-90 Hz) oscillations in primary visual cortex of awake monkey. *NeuroReport*, *4*, 243-246.

Eckhorn, R., & Obermueller, A. (1993). Single neurons are differently involved in stimulus-specific oscillations in cat visual cortex. *Experimental Brain Research*, *95*, 177-182.

Eckhorn, R., Reitboeck, H. J., Arndt, M., & Dicke, P. (1989). A neural network for feature linking via synchronous activity. In R. M. J. Cotterill (Ed.), *Models of Brain Function* (pp. 255-272). New York: Cambridge University Press.

Efron, R., & Lee, D. N. (1971). The visual persistence of a moving stroboscopically illuminated object. *American Journal of Psychology*, *84*, 365-375.

Ellias, S. A., & Grossberg, S. (1975). Pattern formation, contrast control, and oscillations in the short term memory of shunting on-center off-surround networks. *Biological Cybernetics*, *20*, 69-98.

Engel, A. K., König, P., Kreiter, A. K., & Singer, W. (1991). Interhemispheric synchronization of oscillatory neuronal responses in cat visual cortex. *Science*, *252*, 1177-1179.

Francis, G., Grossberg, S., & Mingolla, E. (1994). Cortical dynamics of feature binding and reset: Control of visual persistence. *Vision Research*, *34*, 1089-1104.

Freeman, W. J., & van Dijk, B. W. (1987). Spatial patterns of visual cortical fast EEG during conditioned reflex in a rhesus monkey. *Brain Research*, *422*, 267-276.

Gho, M., & Varela, F. J. (1989). A quantitative assessment of the dependency of the visual temporal frame upon the cortical rhythm. *Journal of Physiology (Paris)*, *83*, 95-101.

Ghose, G. M., & Freeman, R. D. (1992). Oscillatory discharge in the visual system: Does it have a functional role? *Journalof Neurophysiology*, *68*, 1558-1574.

Gilbert, C. D. (1993). Circuitry, architecture, and functional dynamics of visual cortex. *Cerebral Cortex, 3*, 373-386.

Gilbert, C. D., & Wiesel, T. N. (1990). The influence of contextual stimuli on the orientation selectivity of cells in primary visual cortex of the cat. *Vision Research, 30*, 1689-1701.

Gish, K., Shulman, G. L., Sheehy, J. B., & Leibowitz, H. W. (1986). Reaction times to different spatial frequencies as a function of detectability. *Vision Research, 26*, 745-747.

Gray, C. M., König, P., Engel, A. K., & Singer, W. (1989). Oscillatory responses in cat visual cortex exhibit inter-columnar synchronization which reflects global stimulus properties. *Nature, 338*, 334-337.

Gray, C. M., & Singer, W. (1989). Stimulus-specific neuronal oscillations in orientation columns of cat visual cortex. *Proceedings of the National Academy of Sciences, 86*, 1698-1702.

Grosof, D. H., Shapley, R. M., & Hawken, M. J. (1993). Macaque V1 neurons can signal "illusory" contours. *Nature, 365*, 550-552.

Grossberg, S. (1973). Contour enhancement, short term memory, and constancies in reverberating neural networks. *Studies in Applied Mathematics, 52*, 213-257.

Grossberg, S. (1976). Adaptive pattern classification and universal recoding, II: Feedback, expectation, olfaction, illusions. *Biological Cybernetics, 23*, 187-202.

Grossberg, S., & Grunewald, A. (1995). *Cortical synchronization and perceptual framing* (Tech. Rep. CAS/CNS TR-94-025). Boston University.

Grossberg, S., & Mingolla, E. (1985a). Neural dynamics of form perception: Boundary completion, illusory figures, and neon color spreading. *Psychological Review, 92*, 173-211.

Grossberg, S., & Mingolla, E. (1985b). Neural dynamics of perceptual grouping: Textures, boundaries, and emergent segmentations. *Perception & Psychophysics, 38*, 141-171.

Grossberg, S., & Somers, D. (1991). Synchronized oscillations during cooperative feature linking in a cortical model of visual perception. *Neural Networks, 4*, 453-466.

Hirsch, I. J., & Sherrick, C. E. (1961). Perceived order in different sense modalities. *Journal of Experimental Psychology, 62*, 423-432.

Intraub, H. (1985). Visual dissociation: An illusory conjunction of pictures and forms. *Journal of Experimental Psychology: Human Perception and Performance, 11*, 431-442.

Jaskowski, P. (1993). Temporal-order judgment and reaction time to stimuli of different rise times. *Perception, 22*, 963-970.

Karni, A., & Sagi, D. (1993). The time course of learning a visual skill. *Nature, 365*, 250-252.

König, P., & Schillen, T. B. (1991). Stimulus-dependent assembly formation of oscillatory responses: I. Synchronization. *Neural Computation, 3*, 155-166.

Kreiter, A. K., & Singer, W. (1992). Oscillatory neuronal responses in the visual cortex of the awake macaque monkey. *European Journal of Neuroscience, 4*, 369-375.

Lumer, E. D., & Huberman, B. A. (1992). Binding hierarchies: A basis for dynamic perceptual grouping. *Neural Computation, 4*, 341-355.

Malsburg, C. von der (1981). *The correlation theory of brain function* (Tech. Rep. 81-2). Max-Planck-Institut, Göttingen.

Mason, A., Nicoll, A., & Stratford, K. (1991). Synaptic transmission between individual pyramidal neurons of the rat visual cortex in vitro. *Journal of Neuroscience, 11*, 72-84.

Maunsell, J., & Gibson, J. R. (1992). Visual response latencies in striate cortex of the macaque monkey. *Journal of Neurophysiology, 68*, 1332-1343.

McLean, J. P., Broadbent, D. E., & Broadbent, M. H. P. (1982). Combining attributes in rapid serial visual presentation tasks. *Quarterly Journal of Experimental Psychology, 35A*, 171-186.

Morris, C., & Lecar, H. (1981). Voltage oscillations in the barnacle giant muscle fiber. *Journal of Biophysics, 35*, 193-213.

Niebur, E., Schuster, H., Kammen, D., & Koch, C. (1991). Oscillator-phase coupling for different two-dimensional network connectivities. *Physical Review A, 44*, 6895-6904.

Nowak, L. G., Munk, M. H. J., Girard, P., & Bullier, J. (1995). Visual latencies in areas V1 and V2 of the macaque monkey. *Visual Neuroscience, 12*, 371-384.

Oram, M. W., & Perrett, D. I. (1992). Time course of neural responses discriminating different views of the face and head. *Journal of Neurophysiology, 68*, 70-84.

Ross, W., Grossberg, S., & Mingolla, E. (1995). A cortical architecture for real and illusory contour processing in areas V1 and V2. *Investigative Ophthalmology and Visual Science, 36*, 2187.

Sestokas, A. K., & Lehmkuhle, S. (1986). Visual response latency of X- and Y-cells in the dorsal lateral geniculate nucleus of the cat. *Vision Research, 26*, 1041-1054.

Shapley, R. M., & Victor, J. D. (1978). The effect of contrast on the transfer properties of cat retinal ganglion cells. *Journal of Physiology(London), 285*, 275-298.

Somers, D. C., & Kopell, N. (1993). Rapid synchronization through fast threshold modulation. *Biological Cybernetics, 68*, 393-407.

Sternberg, S., & Knoll, R. L. (1973). The perception of temporal order: Fundamental issues and a general model. In S. Kornblum (Ed.), *Attention and Performance* IV (pp. 629-685). New York: Academic Press.

Tappe, T., Niepel, M., & Neuman, O. (1994). A dissociation between reaction time to sinusoidal gratings and temporal order judgment. *Perception, 23*, 335-347.

Terman, D., & Wang, D. (1995). Global competition and local cooperation in a network of neural oscillators. *Physica D, 81*, 148-176.

Ueno, T., Pokorny, J., & Smith, V. C. (1985). Reaction times to chromatic stimuli. *Vision Research, 25*, 1623-1627.

Varela, F. J., Toro, A., John, E. R., & Schwartz, E. L. (1981). Perceptual framing and cortical alpha rhythm. *Neuropsychologia, 19*, 675-686.

Vogels, R., & Orban, G. A. (1991). Quantitative study of striate single unit responses in monkeys performing an orientation discrimination task. *Experimental Brain Research, 84*, 1-11.

von der Heydt, R., Peterhans, E., & Baumgartner, G. (1984). Illusory contours and cortical neuron responses. *Science, 224*, 1260-1262.

Wiener, N. (1961). *Cybernetics: or Control and Communication in the Animal and the Machine* (2nd ed.). Cambridge, MA: MIT Press.

Young, M. P., Tanaka, K., & Yamane, S. (1992). On oscillating neuronal responses in the visual cortex of the monkey. *Journal of Neurophysiology, 67*, 1464-1474.

Zack, J. L. (1973). Estimation of the variability of the latency of responses to brief flashes. *Vision Research, 13*, 829-835.

13

Attention, Depth Gestalts, and Spatially Extended Chaos in the Perception of Ambiguous Figures

David DeMaris
University of Texas at Austin

ABSTRACT

Ambiguous percepts have often been explained by simple satiation or fatiguing of neural circuitry coding the percept. More recently, theories based on nonlinear dynamics have appeared. The Necker cube literature indicates that satiation is unlikely in early stages of the visual system, that the formation of depth gestalts is a local process, and that there are correlations between attention, eye movement fixation times, switching time distributions, and residency times in the reversible states. It is proposed that spatially mediated bifurcation parameter fluctuations in spatially extended, coupled nonlinear cell assemblies embody depth gestalts as oscillation cluster gradients. The gradients may be organized by intrinsic spatial flows mediated by forms that imply a perspective. Initial simulations exploring these conjectures are reported, along with a brief review of relevant visual psychophysics and an introduction to the coupled map lattice methods for modeling nonlinear neural networks.

1. INTRODUCTION

Gestalt psychology catalogued many fundamental phenomena in vision and posited a qualitative field-oriented model of perception, but to date no mathematical formulation explaining the rich psychophysics of gestalt formation has emerged. Since the Gestalt era, analytic or computational models in biological and machine vision have predominantly treated early stages of the visual system as linear filter channels or other specialized feature detectors, leading up to computational modules that group and recognize objects (Treisman et al., 1990). Ambiguous or multistable percepts in depth perception (the Necker cube) and figure-ground reversals (the Rubin vase/faces image) are anomalies that have prompted theorists to consider nonlinear models, in contrast to other visual phenomena more easily explained by linear systems theory. Models for multistability have ranged from straightforward circuits with some component which fatigued (Attneave, 1971) to more sophisticated analyses based on catastrophe theory applied to psychophysical data (Ta'eed, Ta'eed, & Wright, 1988). Recently a nonlinear model with attention parameters reset by coupling to order parameters, which might be considered a more richly elaborated fatigue mechanism, has been proposed (Ditzinger & Haken, 1986; Haken, 1988). Analytical techniques from nonlinear dynamics for dimension estimation have recently been used to analyze time series of perceptual reversals, suggesting that low dimensional deterministic chaos could play a role in both depth interpretation and in the magnitude of sequential saccadic eye movements (Richards, Wilson, & Sommer, 1994). None of these studies has addressed the full range of psychophysical data, especially variations of scale and reversal time series; nor have they tried to integrate multistable phenomena into a broader theory of what the components of the visual system are trying to do when it gets stuck in a multistable percept. I argue that existing theories relating gestalt formation and feature binding (Gillam, 1980) should now be married with insights from *spatially extended* nonlinear dynamics to present a comprehensive view uniting gestalt formation (as evidenced in grouping, figure-ground and construction of a depth map), attention (as evidenced in spontaneous eye movements), and binding. The depth gestalt is defined to be a spatial mapping from two-dimensional retinal input to a three-dimensional segmentation of the visual field (Marr, 1982) or simply a gradient in two-dimensional space biasing the perceived distance to an object or region of space.

The understanding of the inherent dynamical complexity of coupled chaotic oscillators that might underlie perceptual phenomena has emerged in recent years based on observations from abstract network dynamics studies (Kaneko, 1989) and as explicit models of perceptual and cognitive systems (Gregson, 1988; Skarda & Freeman, 1989). In addition to the interest in chaotic oscillations, observations of synchronized gamma band oscillations have generated considerable attention in recent years and have been identified as possible signatures of attentional processes and feature binding (Eckhorn, 1992; Grossberg & Somers, 1991).

The interaction of gestalt formation with attention is well documented in the case of reversible depth perception with the Necker cube. It is argued here that it may be helpful to consider depth perception and attention as a unified field constructed from the interaction of visual forms and gradients in a spatially distribution of oscillation clusters. This formulation may provide insight into the complex interaction of switching and residency times with attention (as evidenced by eye fixation), depth gestalt, and spatial scale dependencies in multistable phenomena. The recently developed dynamics of coupled nonlinear oscillating systems may provide a sufficiently rich foundation to model such systems.

This chapter first introduces the range of psychophysical data associated with luminance and spatial scale on reversible depth percepts. Next, the interactions between attention, as indicated by eye fixation points, and the perception of the Necker cube and the Mueller-Lyer size distortion illusion are considered. Some historical (precomputational) theory relating the underlying processes of perspective decoding, spatial illusions, and the role of eye movements in memory formation is noted. In the third section, the terminology and mathematical basis of coupled map lattices are outlined, including the extensions to anisotropic bifurcation fields mediated by the entrainment of oscillations in neighboring assemblies. Simulations of the evolution of the lattice dynamics with Necker cube patterns as initial conditions are presented, followed by a comparison to other nonlinear models of ambiguous percepts.

The ideas advanced here are in early stages of investigation and can only be considered as steps toward a framework employing spatially extended nonlinear dynamics to the computational perception of forms and to modeling brain dynamics. It was demonstrated in related work (DeMaris, 1995) that the evolution of spatial patterns used as initial conditions in a chaotic coupled map lattice is useful in characterizing the pattern without conventional feature detection. Initial oscillatory patterns, interacting in weakly chaotic regimes, evolve to produce a unique state distribution that characterizes similarity of patterns via a Euclidean distance metric without explicit feature analysis or representation. The overall plan of this research is to extend this computation of oscillations derived from local geometric features to a final representation utilizing feature linking via intermittency. The attentional and depth gestalt work introduced here serves to highlight regions of interest in a visual form and to modify shape determined oscillations to bind their location in space. The architecture resembles conventional modular approaches, but attention is conceived (in one of its forms) as a self-organized fluctuation between chaotic and periodic oscillations. When in spatially focused periodic oscillation modes, this attention module plays roles in both the formation of depth gestalts and the process of binding oscillations into a composite perception.

2. DEPTH PERCEPTION AND MULTISTABLE PERCEPTS

The *satiation* or *fatiguing* theory of multistable percepts (Attneave, 1970) is probably the most commonly cited in visual psychology texts today. This essentially states that the neural signal carrier of the percept becomes depleted, saturated, or otherwise enters a refractory period allowing the alternative percept to emerge. Prior to examining more complex dynamics, the fundamental evidence against this simple explanation should be cited. The effect of luminance variation over three orders of magnitude on reversal rate, including scotopic (night vision) conditions in which cones were completely inactive, has been studied by Riani and colleagues (Riani, Oliva, Selis, Ciurlo, & Pietro, 1984). Prior studies over smaller magnitude ranges had shown contradictory results, with some studies claiming no effect, others reporting effects up to a 100% increase in reversal rate. The Riani et al. study, carefully designed to operate in the stable or plateau reversal regime (Brown, 1955), showed no effect on reversal rate. This was considered as strong evidence against a fatiguing effect in early levels of the visual system, up to area V1. Although simple satiation in brain regions encoding higher level percepts cannot be ruled out, it is clear that spatial form rather than intensity is the determining factor.

2.1. Eye Fixations in Viewing the Necker Cube

In an attempt to resolve a long standing dispute on whether eye movements were an *effect* or *cause* of reversals, Ellis and Stark (1978) undertook a study of the location and duration of fixations during reversals. Subject fixations were allowed to range freely over a fairly large (12-degree) cube while recording fixation points, duration, and reversal times. They demonstrated that fixations are attracted along diagonals in the cube, had longer duration during reversal events (600-800 ms in contrast to 350-700 ms for other fixations), and that fixations near (but not on) a central vertex forced its interpretation as part of the near face; they summarize scanning behavior as "back and forth between temporally changing externally appearing corners." Qualitatively described in their study are motion effects related to fixation and stability. Moving the cube, which interferes with fixation, can prevent reversals. The presence of a moving distractor bar in a large cube (visual angle 20 degrees) also prevents reversals from occurring.

Experiments indicating a strong causal relationship of fixation point on reversal dynamics have been reported (Kawabata, Ymagami, & Noaki, 1978). In one, subjects were instructed to fixate on one of the two central vertices that could be interpreted as the front face of a cube, and their fixation point was measured. The fixated vertex was perceived as part of the front face for roughly 70% of the time, and the reverse perception was held for 30%. When other vertices were fixated, the residence times in each percept were nearly equal. In a second study, subjects fixated on a target in a blank field prior to the cube being flashed for 200 ms in various positions; subjects then reported the perceived orientation. In this case, when the target point is near one of the possible front vertices it clearly induces the perception of that vertex in the near field, with probability of the alternative percept falling off with distance.

2.2. Effect of Visual Angle Subtended by a Necker Cube

Size effects on reversal rate means and distributions have been studied with careful control to measure the plateau reversal rate by Borsellino et al. (1982). Cubes with sizes subtending a wide range of angles in the visual field were presented to subjects. They found a rapid decrease in the reversal rate for 0 to 5 degrees, with a plateau between 5 and 30 degrees. Intriguingly two distributions of response are found for angles over 30 degrees: some subjects exhibited a strong trend of decreasing rate, others a much weaker trend. Their model posited three component processes combining to produce the response: a constant term independent of angle, a retinal term, and a cortical term "interpreted as due to the spreading of excitation with the characteristic of a filling in pattern," with the perturbation that provokes spreading assumed to arise from different scanning strategies which come into play at larger angles. This conception is influential in the model described in the next section, in which scanning and the spreading excitation process are considered to be intimately linked, but the temporal differences are determined by characteristic times of wave interactions.

Cognitive explanations, in which a globally consistent perceptual framework enforces a top-down schema for perspective, vied with fatigue theories prior to demonstrations involving multiple cubes which showed that multiple conflicting perceptions could exist in the same visual field (Long & Toppino 1981). If schema operate on the neural substrate, they must at least be relatively localized and do not imply any consistent interpretation of identical stimuli over a broad field. Since that work, evidence has accumulated for local processes; von Grunau and coworkers (von Grunau, Wiggin, & Reed, 1984) estimate the effective spatial extent of the process at about 3 degrees of visual field, based on a series of experiments aimed at influencing the time during which the same or opposite orientations were perceived for two Necker cubes by a process of adaptation to a nonambiguous perspective. While they concluded that local processes dominated, they interpreted their results as supportive of satiation theories.

2.3. Attention, Spatial Illusions, and Eye Movements

Attention and monocular depth perception processes have been invoked in attempts to explain illusory effects. Gillam (1980) accounts for such size distortion illusions as the Ponzo and Poggendorff illusions and foreshortening effects as part of a natural process of perspective decoding. She argued that the figures are perceived as *illusory* because of the removal of contextual details that reinforce a three-dimensional interpretation, and provides a figure illustrating the imbedding of several illusions in a three-dimensional scene where they appear well integrated. Such a form-based depth-gestalt system could play an important role in conditions where conditions are inadequate to establish depth through texture gradients (such as navigating through branches devoid of foliage).

In reviewing explanations of the origins of illusions, Gillam mentions *activity theories* which posit that illusions arise as a pretext for a behavioral response; in particular the *efferent readiness* theory (Festinger et al., 1967). Festinger and colleagues contend that the process by which the visual system prepares to initiate a saccade is the source of illusions. These are presumed to be strictly preparatory steps, not actual movements; that eye movements themselves play no determining role in most illusions is considered well established. They also argued that some attentional foci are constructed by the visual system but may not actually initiate saccades; this should be contrasted with the earlier review of Necker cube reversal, where saccades and fixations are shown to correlate with reversals. Finally they noted that when subjects attempt to fixate on ends of Mueller-Lyer figures, they fixate within the arrowheads rather than at the intersection points. They suggested that this has the result of lengthening the inward pointing arrows and shortening the outward pointing arrows. Coren and Porac (1983) demonstrated that saccades to the fixation targets at the center of a Mueller-Lyer figure systematically overshoot the actual target for the lengthened percept of an arrow pair. A related study used a modified figure with color or line type variations in a figure so that either the left or right half of the figure is perceived as longer if subjects were instructed to attend to the appropriate stimulus; saccades in this case, with the same visual stimulus present, were still subject to the overshoot effect corresponding to the attention mediated percept. The importance of this finding with respect to ambiguous perception is simply to indicate again that features distant from the saccade target cooperate to distort both spatial perception and an attentional process.

Noton and Stark (1971) measured scan paths for subjects forced to look at pictures in the near visual field such that eye movements were required to view the whole picture, and developed a theory of object coding and recognition based on serial coding and matching. If a fixed visitation order of features were required, scan paths should be repeatable for individual subjects viewing the same image; they found this to be generally the case, though there was some variation. They observed that when shifts of attention occur for objects subtending smaller angles in the visual field, no eye movements are required; they suggested that a common attentional mechanism underlies both saccade and nonsaccade attention processes. The variability in scan paths and the fact that in some recognition events no scan paths were observed were considered as problematic for the theory, but such variability would naturally accompany a process founded on deterministic chaos.

Gillam's perspective decoding framework and Festinger's observations regarding the apparent fixation-inducing action of diagonal junctions and rotated Mueller-Lyer-like forms in the Necker cube point toward an architecture in which an emerging spatial interpretations and eye movements are mutually determining. In the model (Fig. 13.2) developed in Sections 3 and 4, it is proposed that flows in the coherence (transient periodicity) and fluctuating *gradients in the relative population* of particular oscillation frequencies (clusters) emerge in the response of cell assemblies through lateral interactions governed by the extracted edges of a visual form. In this scenario, genetically determined structure and perceptual-motor actions during development combine to establish the network topology and parameter ranges. In turn, these allow the brain networks to respond rapidly to such a stimulus by forming an attentional focus to guide visual behavior, such as scanning for junctions with vertical lines where stereo judgments can resolve ambiguous depth, or preparing for motor behavioral response to nearby objects in a particular region of the visual field. The emergence of periodically oscillating "foreground" regions triggered by such scene features in a larger field of chaotic and thus incoherent "background" domains could serve to direct foveal attention and to tune visual-motor parameter gradients. Because the system is essentially fluctuating and nonstationary, periodic and chaotic descriptions apply only in a fuzzy sense — a particular region in a modular layer spending more time in the periodic oscillations regime, or with a greater proportion of assemblies in a cluster that is oscillating periodically, would be supporting a foreground interpretation.

2.4. Oscillations, Attention, Feature Binding, and Saliency

Koch and Crick (1994) discussed a possible role for synchronized gamma band oscillations (40-80 Hz) such as those measured in cat visual cortex. They postulate that these oscillations are the mechanism for binding different temporal coded features into a unified percept. A detailed model is not specified, only that modulation of selected perceptual encodings would result in modification of the temporal microstructure of the signal in some way. The source of the attentional signal is postulated to come from an extra-cortical saliency map that identifies regions containing features of interest for binding by temporal coding. The question of how salient features are extracted from the visual field for a young organism with no ready made cognitive framework is not addressed, however.

Expanding on Freeman's chaotic oscillations paradigm (Freeman, 1986; Freeman & van Dijk, 1987), Baird (1991) suggested that oscillations such as 40 Hz (gamma) might serve as a clock for averaging of local field potentials between cell assemblies during perceptual encoding. Some investigators propose models in which 40 Hz is a natural resonance time in small networks or in a recurrent corticothalamic loop (Llinas & Ribary, 1994; Mannion & Taylor, 1992). If the native oscillation period of cell assemblies operating in the periodic phase regime were near 40 Hz, one could envision that the oscillations are modulated based on phase coherence between spatial regions when adjacent assemblies receive bursts of activity. This may allow interassembly lateral coupling (corresponding to an entrainment process) at a clocked interval; between this interval, coherent gamma-band oscillations inside each assembly might be a special state reached only under certain conditions, when the lateral interactions, assembly dynamics and perturbation by early areas (V1) cooperate to produce transient coherence in selected spatial locations in a retinotopically mapped area. Thus the control of binding, as suggested by Koch and Crick, may still come into play; but the saliency map and source of oscillatory control may emerge, in the absence of conscious search, by the lateral interactions and recurrent feedback in an early visual area dedicated to that task. Oscillations inducing spatial bifurcations appear to be the cortically determined *cause*, rather than an effect, of the foreground interpretation, and could trigger activation or parameter changes in a layer or area dedicated to binding the oscillatory encodings of the surrounding larger regions. A possible dynamics of feature linking and binding via intermittent dynamics in nonequilibrium networks is described by Tsuda (1991). In a chaotic link binding theory, the periodic synchronized oscillations might trigger parameter changes in a binding module (lattice) to move the dynamics to an intermittency regime, linking oscillations of adjacent regions with rich spectral clusterings into a unified oscillation pattern. After a memory has been constructed from such a bound representation, it could be fed back into the early visual layers as a search *bias signal.*

The next section presents the dynamics of a family of nonlinear oscillating networks used to explore the influence of Necker cube size on the statistical evolution of oscillations.

3. NONLINEAR DYNAMICS AND NEURAL MODELING

Neural networks in which the global state vector evolves to a static condition might be termed convergent or equilibrium, in the sense that during recognition of learned categories they remain in the same convergent phase regime due to stationary parameters in the network dynamics. The Hopfield network with symmetric connections and multilayer back propagation networks are examples of equilibrium networks in this sense, with the weights stabilized by training to a stationary state. To jump out of the equilibrium state encoding a recognized memory, in order to process continuing sensory input, such networks must be reset. Typically some supervisory process is proposed. In contrast, biological networks exhibit continual nonstationary dynamical activity, with intrinsic resetting or cyclic behavior of dynamical control parameters governed by perception, attention, mood, and intrinsic cycles such as breathing (Elbert et al., 1994). Even when dynamical control parameters are stationary, much of the work on such dynamic pattern networks explores the chaotic and intermittent dynamical regimes to explain cognitive and perceptual phenomena.

Some basic concepts needed to understand the dynamical models are now introduced. For more detailed presentations of nonlinear dynamics emphasizing their application as a basis for cognition and learning the reader is referred to Mainzer (1994), Abraham (1991), and Gregson (1988). Also, MacGregor (1993) describes a theory of neuronal encoding with oscillation modes that has some features in common with the modeling style in this chapter.

3.1. One-Dimensional Nonlinear Maps

A *map* is an iterated difference equation

$$S_{t+1} = f(S_t)$$

where S is a real-valued state, f is some function mapping S within a subset of the real number domain R, and t is a discrete time step. Iteration implies that the result of applying the function at time t is fed back into the computation at time t+1. Nonlinear maps use some nonlinear function f, resulting in diverse asymptotic behaviors after transients of a duration that depends on the initial condition and parameters of the equation.

An *attractor* of a map is the asymptotic state or state sequence after many iterations. The *basin* of an attractor is the set of all states that converge to the same attractor after some number of iterations. This basin structure can be considered as an intrinsic categorization by partitioning the input states into categories corresponding to the attractors.

A dynamical system with attractors can be used as a model for perceptual and memory processes. Training a supervised neural network consists of shaping the dynamics of a network so that the attractor basins map input states into the categories (attractors) desired. Although learning and memory capacity in attractor networks is a major area of research, here the emphasis is on pattern formation and spatial computations that modify the dynamics prior to learning episodes.

The logistic map is a well-studied map used as a network node (cell, neuron unit, site) in the models described below (see Figs. 13.1 and 13.2).

The equation for the logistic map is

$$S_{t+1} = 1 - bS_t^2$$

subject to the constraints $-1 < S < 1, 0 < b < 2$; where b is a bifurcation parameter; changing the parameter forces a structured transition between phases following the sequence {fixed point: limit cycles: intermittency: chaos}. Typically the transition points between phase regimes are visualized by bifurcation trees for systems with one bifurcation parameter, and by phase space plots for spatially extended systems with multiple parameters.

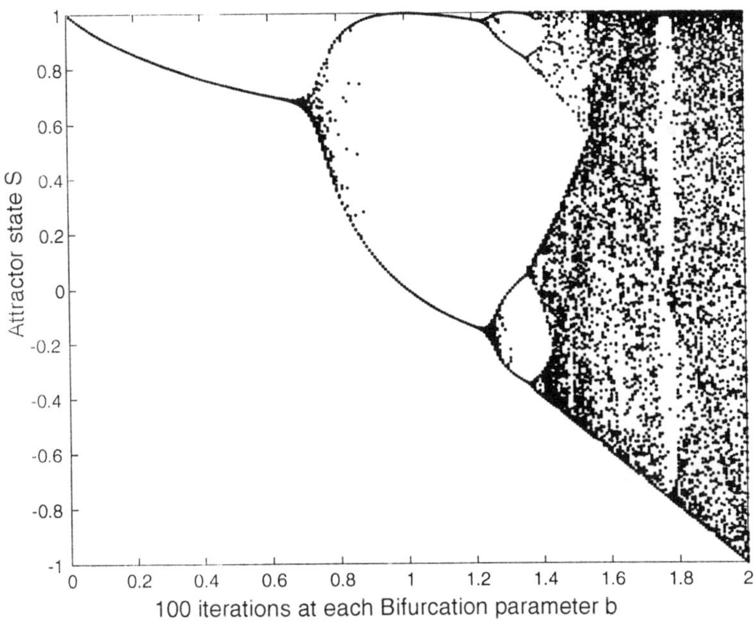

Fig. 13.1. Bifurcation tree showing asymptotic states of attractors as the parameter b is increased. Random initial points are chosen and the system is run for 100 time steps at each b value to produce this plot. Where multiple state S points exist for the given b, a periodic, intermittent or chaotic attractor exists; the actual state values are cycling as shown in the time series. In the periodic regimes, such as where $b = 1$, the cell assembly in a biological network would be in some burst mode, oscillating between low and high average frequencies.

Depending on the bifurcation control parameter b, the attractor state sequence may be a single state (fixed point), periodic oscillation between a few states (limit cycle), unstable sequences of periodic oscillations linked by pseudorandom sequences (intermittency), or a pseudorandom visitation of the state space points but within a bounded area (strange attractor, chaotic attractor). Each of the attractor types can be considered as a *phase* or *phase regime* (bifurcation range, interpreted as excit-atory-inhibitory ratios of local networks), analogous to thermodynamic phase in classical physical systems. These phase regimes are bounded by critical values of the control parameters. When a control parameter is modulated to cross a point where attractors appear or disappear the crossing event is known as *bifurcation*. Bifurcations between qualitatively different regions of phase space, such as crossing the transition from limit cycles to chaotic behavior, are termed *phase transitions*.

3.2. Spatially Extended Systems: Spatiotemporal Chaos

Although the map introduced in Fig. 13.1 illustrates a dynamical system containing a single state variable, the definitions can be extended to networks of coupled real-valued nodes, known as *coupled map lattices (*CML*)*. The *network* attractor is then a vector or array of the states of all nodes. In such networks, a bifurcation behavior at the level of the entire network is evident, emerging from the interaction of each site, neighboring sites, and the initial conditions or coupled external forcing values. This network-level bifurcation may be tuned by controlling the phase regime of the individual nodes, the number of connections between nodes (neighborhood size), the ratio of excitatory to inhibitory connections, or the coupling strength between nodes.

Various network topologies have been explored for spatiotemporal chaotic systems. Network nodes may be *locally coupled* to adjacent nodes, *diffusively coupled* to a small region of the lattice, *globally coupled* to every node in the lattice, coupled to a random set of neighbors, or some blending of these conditions. The globally coupled map topology (GCM) has been extensively studied (Kaneko, 1990) and is the architecture proposed here to encode depth (Fig. 13.2).

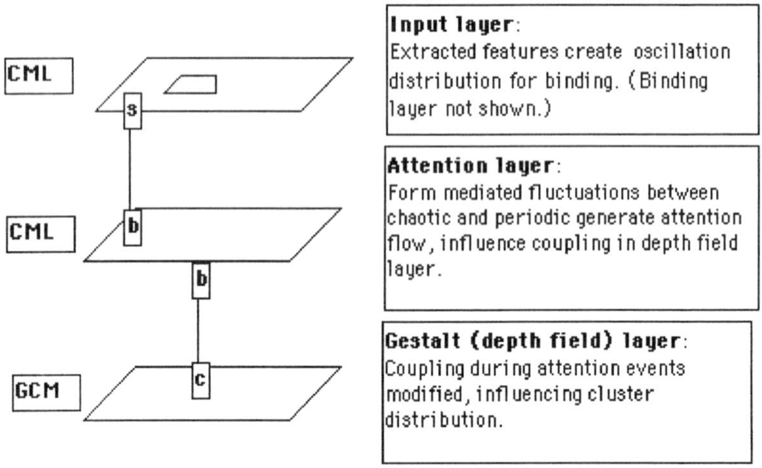

Fig. 13.2. Three layer coupled map architecture for simulating interactive formation of attention foci and depth gestalt formation. The first layer represents the shape processing reaction diffusion layer described in equations (1-3). The second layer represents the emerging attention foci when the fluctuations of equation (3) fall below a threshold indicating periodic oscillations. This layer drives both layer 1 and controls the coupling parameter in layer 3 (equation (6)). A third layer and set of equations is used to encode the actual depth mapping or depth gestalt, by the spatial distributions of clusters (particular oscillation modes) when the entire lattice is oscillating near the edge of its coherent regime, supporting only a few oscillation modes.

In addition to the tuning of the entire lattice to a particular type of oscillation phase regime, the dynamical evolution with certain initial conditions and parameter ranges may result in spatial bifurcations or pattern formation, where certain spatial regions are effectively segmented into sets of interacting sites, separated by domain boundaries that inhibit interaction between neighbors. Pure numerical studies of such pattern formation and applications to such diverse subjects as fluid dynamics and ecological population dynamics have been performed, where the distribution and stability of such regions and patterns are the chief quantities of interest. It is this (relatively unexplored) level of network pattern formation that is of most interest in modeling perceptual dynamics of spatial forms, with their sensitivity to the details of orientation and spatial scale.

Each variable (site or unit) in a field (the lattice) represents a quantity associated with an aggregate of microscopic units. This kind of representation, common in statistical mechanics or fluid dynamics, is known as a *macrostate* variable. Temperature or instantaneous velocity of a fluid, for example, might be macrostate variables in a CML fluid dynamics study. In this chapter the macrostate variable S is associated with the ensemble activation (average spike train frequency of a connected ensemble). Modeling of network details with spiking activation functions and membrane transfers via numerical solutions of ordinary differential equations has been employed by Kowalski, Albert, Rhoades, and Gross (1992) and Chapeau-Blondeau and Chauvet (1992) to demonstrate oscillating, chaotic, and sometimes synchronized chaotic behavior. Such oscillations in small networks have been subsumed in the macrostate variables in the coupled map models and simulations described here, in order to devote computational resources to the higher level spatial pattern formation mechanisms. Siegel (1990), using a nonlinear signal analysis technique of delay embedding on spike train sequences, noted similarities between their phase space plots and those obtained by analyzing single sites of a CML system.

When a physical system is simulated with a coupled map model, a sequence of processes is decomposed into simple parallel dynamics at each lattice point, with each process carried out successively. In the present model, this means that at each iteration, a diffusion step is performed modeling lateral entrainment of cell assemblies, then a reaction step representing local evolution within each assembly. The bifurcation parameter for the logistic map at each site is also a variable parameter in this system and is updated at a slower rate based on the local neighborhood evolution.

The entire diffusion step can be expressed as:

$$S_d(x,y) = (1-c)S_t(x,y) + \frac{c}{4}\left[S_t(x,y+1) + S_t(x,y-1) + S_t(x+1,y) + S_t(x-1,y)\right] \tag{1}$$

where S_d is the intermediate diffusion array, t is the current time step, x, y are the spatial indices of the pixel array S at the center of the diffusion neighborhood, S is the state variable at each pixel of the array, and c is the coupling constant restricted to the range (0.0 to 1.0). The factor $(1-c)$ scales the state at each node prior to summing the neighbor states, to insure that the states remain within numerically stable bounds. In practice the step is implemented by a diffusion and scaling step followed by the application of the map.

The second computational unit applied in each time step is the logistic map:

$$S_{t+1}(x,y) = 1 - bt(x,y)\{Sd(x,y)\}^2 \tag{2}$$

where S, t, x, and y are as above and where b is the bifurcation parameter, restricted to the range $(0.0 < b < 2.0)$. S is restricted to the range $(-1.0 < S < 1.0)$.

In Kaneko's studies the lattice dynamics are characterized in the space of bifurcation and coupling, with each held constant in a particular simulation run. In contrast, in the model here b is itself variable at each lattice site, leading to $b(x, y)$, computed from the local evolution of the map according to the following equation:

$$\begin{aligned} b_{t+1} = b_t * (1-c)\frac{c}{4}[1 + \{S_t(x,y+1) + S_t(x,y-1) \\ + S_t(x+1,y) + S_t(x-1,y)\}] * S_t(2-bt) \end{aligned} \tag{3}$$

where b, c, S, x, and y are as previously defined. The second factor is simply the neighborhood average S previously computed for this iteration, now used in a multiplicative fashion to influence the bifurcation state in the next cycle, with the addition of 1 causing this to be an excitatory factor, balanced by the inhibitory factor $(2-b)$. The combination of the two terms results in *spatially mediated fluctuations* around an unstable periodic mean value. From a programming and visualization standpoint, the S and b evolution equations are implemented as two separate two-dimensional lattices. These are represented as modular layers in the system architecture in Fig. 13.2.

The equations governing the globally coupled map (GCM) depth encoding layer and interactions with the second (bifurcation fluctuation attention layer) are given below.

$$g_m(x,y) = 1 - b_g\{g_t(x,y)\}^2 \tag{4}$$

where g_m is an intermediate product, representing the nonlinear map evolution prior to mean-field coupling. much like the S_d term in Equation (1). The term b_g is a separate bifurcation parameter active at all sites, and may be considered a kind of arousal state of the network. It is currently set at 1.54, near the transition to chaos for the map

$$gc_t(x,y) = .1 + .27 * \{1 \text{ iff } b(x,y) < b_{thresh},\ 0 \text{ otherwise}\} \tag{5}$$

gc_t is the global coupling term which is allowed to vary over space, under the control of the b layer.

A partial mean field (mean of the active, most coherent sites) is computed:

$$gmean_t = \left\{ \sum_{i=1}^{N} (g_{sub\text{-}thresh}(x,y)) \right\} / N \qquad (6)$$

where N is the number of sites in the b lattice which are below the threshold as defined in Equation (5). The sites in g whose x,y coordinates in the b lattice are below the threshold are the only ones used in computing the mean, hence those sites tend to pull others into their basin of attraction.

Finally the next state g is computed by:

$$g_{t+1}(x,y) = (1 - gc_t(x,y)) * g_m(x,y) + gc_t(x,y) * gmean_t \qquad (7)$$

4. SIMULATION RESULTS

Simulations are underway in the author's MATLAB based multilayer coupled map lattice system to test the approach outlined here. Although the results are still rather inconclusive, it is hoped that the reader will understand the general style of investigation, which is relatively novel. No systematic attempt to reproduce and understand the full range of Necker cube psychophysics surveyed above has been made, but an initial attempt was undertaken at fusing the investigation of attentional fluctuations coupled to a layer embodying the depth perceptual gestalt. With this model, the influence of size has a parameter has been examined. Two cubes of different sizes are evolved in the lattice with an initial gradient established to simulate a depth organization bias such that the bottom of the visual field is nearer. The reaction diffusion layer is updated at every time step, while the bifurcation parameters are updated every four steps, following suggestions by Baird (1991) that the framing rate of parameter changes should be slower than the diffusion (entrainment) interactions. If gamma band (40-80 Hz) frequencies correspond to the fundamental lattice iteration time step, constraining the b and gc parameter lattices to be updated every four steps corresponds to changes in the alpha (10 Hz) frequency band of the EEG.

Figure 13.3 shows the effect of allowing the b parameter to fluctuate deterministically (henceforth referred to as *autobifurcation*) on the dynamics of a single logistic map, equivalent to one site in the lattice. Figures 13.4 and 13.5 monitor the evolution of the bifurcation field in a small region around the corners of a large and small Necker cube centered in a b-parameter field with a slight gradient around the transition to chaos. The cube pattern is represented by initial states corresponding to strongly and weakly activated patterns, assumed to have been extracted by conventional early vision edge detection mechanisms. Another reasonable strategy, not explored yet, would be to periodically drive the lattice with the pattern of interest.

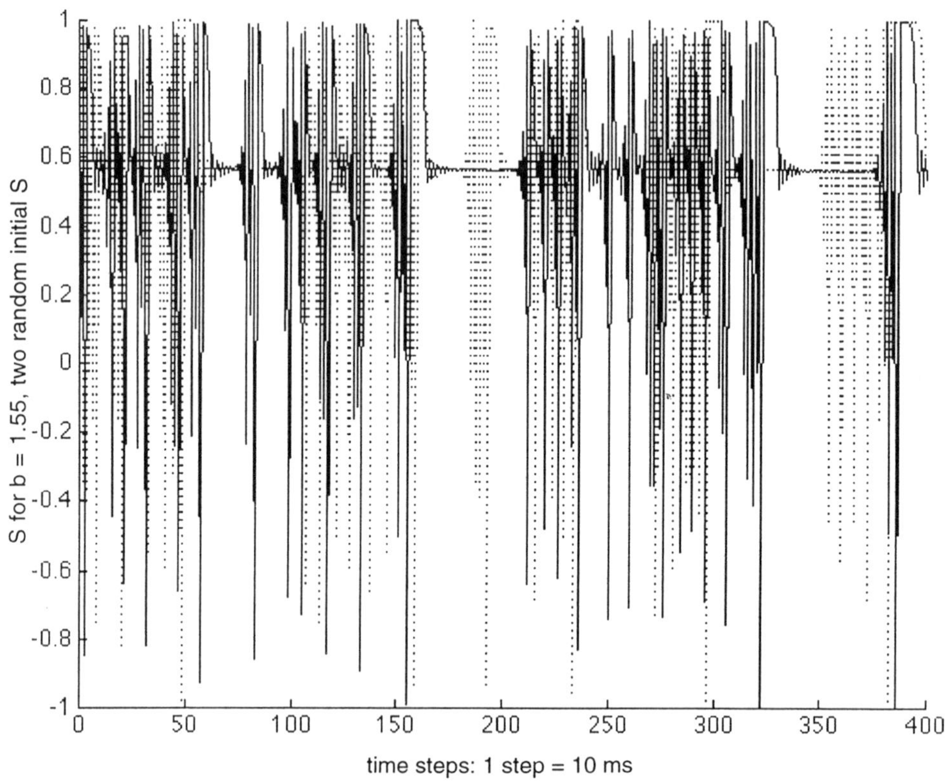

Fig. 13.3. Autobifurcation cycles induced in a single, uncoupled logistic map by evolving the b parameter at each time step according to $b = b * (a{+}1) * (2{-}b)$. Initial b is 1.55. This figure show two random initial conditions evolving in the autobifurcating mode, revealing the sensitivity to initial conditions.

Figure 13.6 shows the way in which the distribution of the time between fluctuation minima events in the second layer are correlated with the size of the initial cube pattern. The trend of the data seems to be sharper peak and tighter distribution for the smaller cube. Because these minima — claimed to be correlated with attention and fixations when oscillating in the periodic regime — drive the dynamics of the third depth layer, it is expected that similar correlations in cluster switching time distributions may be found. The minima events are the precursors that may force a switch in the spatial distribution of oscillation clusters in the third layer, if conditions are suitable.

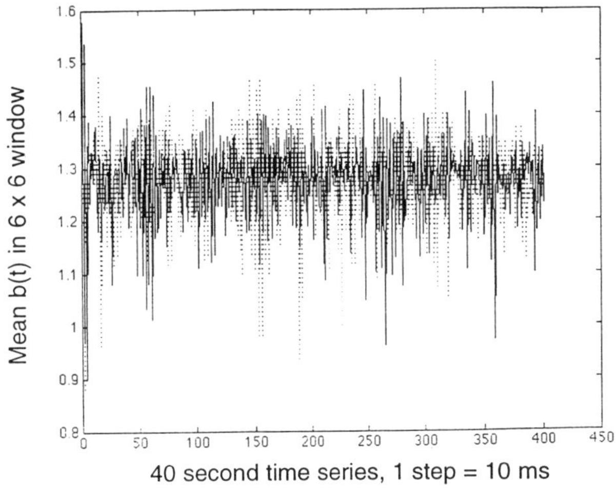

Fig. 13.4. Big cube mean b value of 6 x 6 window around both "possible front" corners, under autobifurcation cycle with initial $b = 1.6$, gradient 1.55 top to bottom of image, $c = 0.3$, for 400 time steps. Minima of b should correspond to greater temporal coherence in S. Deep minima or temporally clustered minima may correspond to figure reversal and presaccadic attention focus formation. Lower left corner is solid, upper right corner dotted.

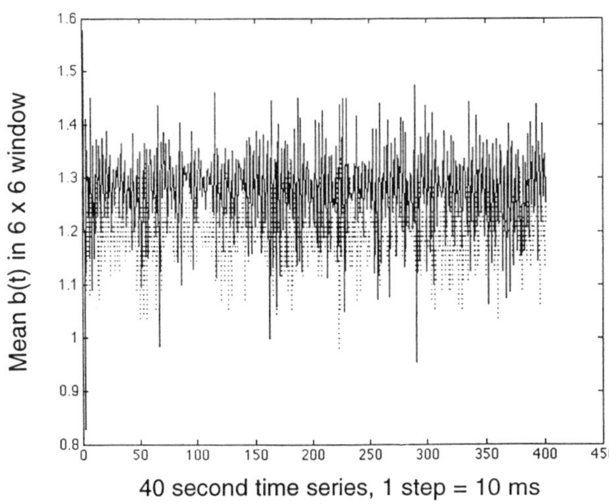

Fig. 13.5. Small cube mean b value of 6 x 6 window around both "possible front" corners, under autobifurcation cycle with initial $b = 1.6$, gradient 1.55 top to bottom of image, $c = 0.3$. 400 time steps are shown. Minima of b should correspond to greater local coherence in S. Lower left corner is solid, upper right is dotted line.

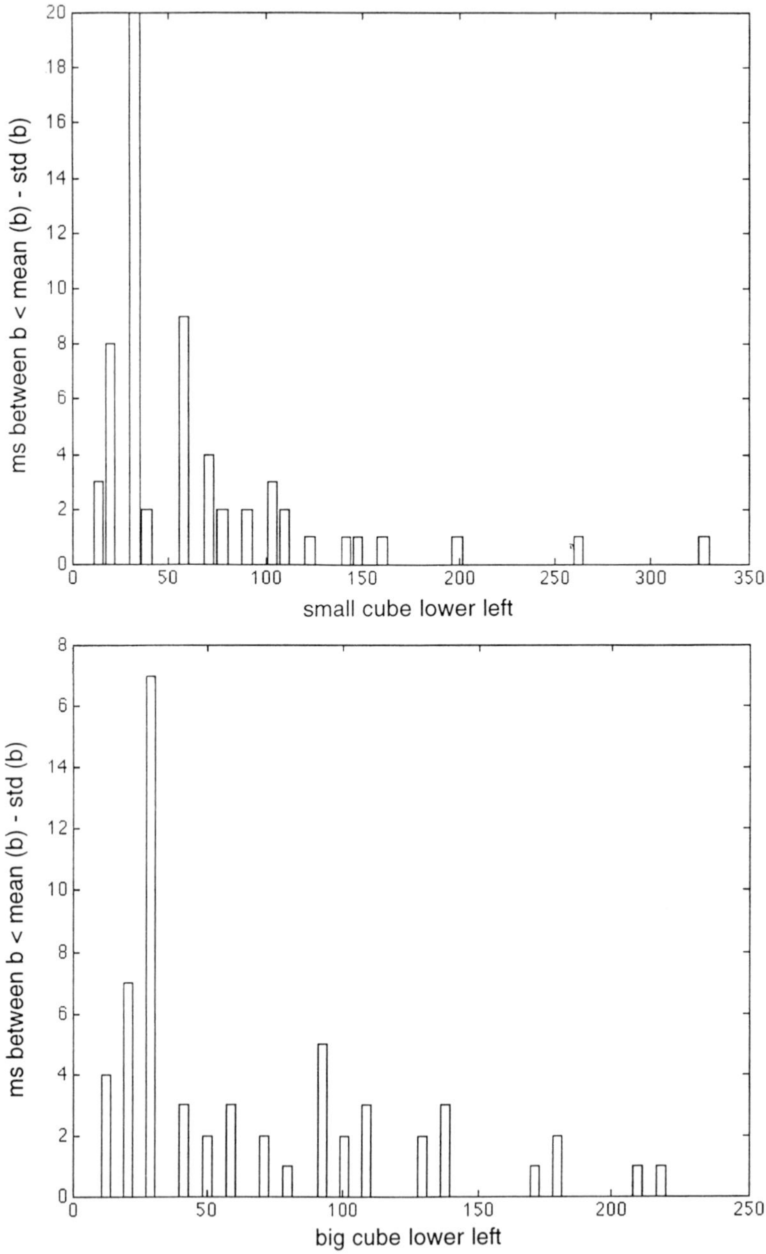

Fig. 13.6. Distribution of time differences between minima events where mean *b* in lower left 6 x 6 window < threshold = (mean(*b*)-- standard deviation(*b*)). This is one possible interpretation of switching events (or their precursors, also depending on spatial clustering). Note that the distribution is tighter for the small cube and flatter for the large, in agreement with the findings in Borsellino et al. (1982).

Figure 13.7 shows the evolution of the mean state values in the horizontal rows in the lattice where the two interior corners were monitored in the large cube. It can be seen that the signals drift in and out of synchronization; the time series suggests that when the signals are synchronized, the same clusters (oscillation modes) predominate and the space occupied by one corner has been pulled into the attractor basin of the other. Further statistics gathering is required to evaluate the relationship of the spatial and temporal evolution of the depth layer to the parameters of the Necker cube.

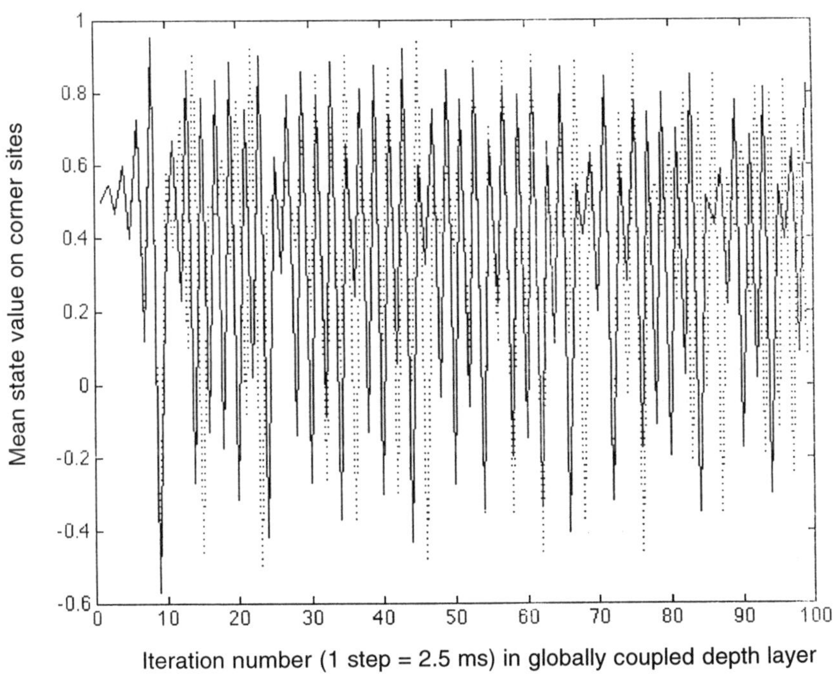

Fig. 13.7. Evolution of the row mean values of the state of the GCM depth gestalt layer in the rows corresponding to the ambiguous corners on the large cube. It can be seen that the signals drift in and out of synchronization; the time series suggests that when the signals are synchronized, the same clusters (oscillation modes) predominate and the space occupied by one corner has been pulled into the attractor basin of the other.

5. DISCUSSION

The time series depicted in Figs. 13.4 and 13.5 of the evolving patterns on the reversible corners of a Necker cube as the lattice initial condition suggests alternative interpretations. One scenario is that the deep minima in *b* correspond to reversal events, or at least to impulses that initiate the switch through still more complex dynamics. It is also evident that there are episodes where relatively periodic motion is sustained over a relatively long time period (indicated by several adjacent minima), which could correspond to switching events while individual deep minima, perhaps clustered in space, correspond to formation of attention focus and fixation targets.

The spatial evolution of patterns has also been monitored during simulation runs. The visualization in that case plots lattice coordinates in which the *b* parameter is below some threshold, (currently one standard deviation below the mean value). Visually, there appears to be significant fluctuation in the spatial density of these *b*-minima, lending some support to a hypothesis that sustained spatial clustering of relatively coherent oscillations corresponds to a fixation event, and that certain regions around a form may emerge as focal points which attract fixations.

The approach here is similar in some respects to that advanced in the Ditzinger and Haken (1986) model for figure-ground reversal, but attempts to introduce a spatial dimension and focusing of chaos toward periodicity to account for the effects of cube size on the oscillations and apparent links between depth organization and eye fixations. In their model, relationships between attention parameters and an order parameter are defined such that there is a saturation nonlinearity of an attention parameter when an order parameter (corresponding to a particular percept of figure) increases, forcing a "reset" in the attention state variable. This in turn triggers a dynamical reorganization and emergence of the alternate attractor in the order parameter.

Haken noted that a time constant in the equation, linking order parameters and attention, controls the reversal times between percepts. The simulation of a single map in the fluctuating bifurcation parameter scenario advanced in this paper suggests that reversal times may be governed by the initial spatial state, rather than governed by a network time constant. The extension here in which the bifurcation state is continually updated by the local oscillations toward a quasi-stable fluctuation around the transition to chaos might better account for the association of transition time and fluctuations with the spatial scale of the cube. In addition, the association of attention to higher coupling in the present model helps to account for Kawabata et al. (1978) findings on the biasing of the initial percept of the cube of an attended corner to the front. This is particularly so if one assumes that the spatial encoding uses more coherent signals to represent nearer locations in space. This seems a good assumption, as it would allow for a kind of priming of search and attention toward nearby space when a spatial memory was fed back into the system.

Kaneko (1990) suggested that globally coupled maps may provide a good model for switching between ambiguous figure-ground percepts. The phenomenon of *cluster switching* is offered as a mechanism. Input on a single site can induce reorganization of the entire cluster. A cluster in this context refers to lattice sites synchronized in the same attractor. In contrast, the present study explores the combination of oscillations in a locally coupled map selectively changing the (coupling) bifurcation parameter in specific regions of a globally coupled map, to establish *cluster gradient*s corresponding to a depth gestalt.

The diverse and sometimes contradictory phenomena seen in multistable perception and spatial illusions, compounded with the number of degrees of freedom afforded by the CML modeling strategy, constitute a challenging modeling problem. The resultant mass of data allows for varied interpretations, and of course there is no language-using subject to query about whether the cube flipped; one must rely on visualization of the spatiotemporal behavior to gain insight into dynamics that would correspond to depth gestalt formation. The prospect of a relatively simple model with deterministic changes in perception coupled to actions like eye movements is attractive, both for the understanding of vision and perhaps as a foundation for understanding the dynamics underlying higher cognitive phenomena. Linguists in the early part of the century noted links between body-centered spatial perception, self-object categorical distinctions, and specific phoneme assignments within language groups (Cassirer, 1955). An understanding of the way spatial context modifies the dynamics of attention and form could be an important link in bridging perception to the roots of categorical thought, which may lead directly to the biological substrate for grammars. Extending this line of research on the origins of language in intuition and expression, Langer (1982) proposed that ambiguous visual perceptions (and whatever dynamics underlie them) are a crucial phenomena at the root of self-consciousness. Ambiguous perceptions may underlie the ability to choose to see something in one or another way and to know that a *self* exists to make the choice.

REFERENCES

Abraham, F. D. (1991). *A Visual Introduction to Dynamical Systems Theory for Psychology.* Santa Cruz: Aerial Press.

Attneave, F. (1971). Multistability in perception. *Scientific American, 225*, 62-71.

Baird, B. (1990). Bifurcation and category learning in network models of oscillating cortex. *Physica D, 42*, 365-384.

Borsellino, A., Carlini, F., Riani, M., Tuccio, M. T., De Marco, A., Penengo, P., & Trabucco, A. (1982). Effects of visual angle on perspective reversal for ambiguous patterns. *Perception, 11*, 263-273.

Brown, K. T. (1955). Rate of apparent change in a dynamic ambiguous figures a function of observation time. *American Journal of Psychology, 68*, 358-371.

Cassirer, E. (1955). *The Philosophy of Symbolic Form.* New Haven: Yale University Press.

Chapeau-Blondeau, F., & Chauvet, G. (1992). Stable, oscillatory and chaotic regimes in the dynamics of small neural networks with delay. *Neural Networks, 5*, 735-743.

Chua, L. O., & Yang, L. (1988). Cellular neural networks: Theory. *IEEE Transactions on Circuits and Systems, 35*, 1257.

Coren, S., & Porac, C. (1983). The creation and reversal of the Mueller-Lyer illusion through attentional manipulation. *Perception, 12*, 49-54.

DeMaris, D. (1995). Computing shape similarity with chaotic reaction diffusion spectra. In *Proceedings of 1995 World Congress on Neural Networks* (Vol. 1, pp. 270-273). Mahwah, NJ: Lawrence Erlbaum Associates.

Ditzinger, T., & Haken, H. (1986). Oscillations in the perception of ambiguous figures. *Biological Cybernetics, 61*, 279-287.

Eckhorn, R., Schanze, T., Brosch, M., Salem, W., & Bauer, R. (1992). Stimulus specific synchronizations in cat visual cortex: Multiple electrode and correlation studies from several cortical areas. In E. Basar & T. H. Bullock (Eds.), *Induced Rhythms in the Brain*. Boston: Birkhauser.

Elbert, T., Ray, W. J., Wowalik, Z. J., Skinner, J. E., Graf, K. E., & Birbaumer, N. (1994). Chaos and physiology: Deterministic chaos in excitable cell assemblies. *Physiological Reviews, 74*, 1-40.

Ellis, S. R., & Stark, L. (1978). Eye movements during the viewing of Necker cubes. *Perception, 7,* 575-581.

Festinger, L., Burnham, C.A., Ono, H., & Bamber, D. (1967). Efference and the conscious experience of perception. *Journal of Experimental Psychology Monograph 74* (4 Pt. 2).

Freeman, W. J. (1986). Simulation of chaotic EEG patterns with a dynamic model of the olfactory system. *Biological Cybernetics, 56*, 458-459.

Freeman, W. J., & van Dijk, B. W. (1987). Spatial patterns of visual cortical fast EEG during reflex in a rhesus monkey. *Brain Research, 422*, 267-276.

Gillam, B. (1980). Geometrical illusions. *Scientific American, 242*, 102-111.

Gregson, R. A. M. (1988). *Nonlinear Psychophysical Dynamics*. Hillsdale, NJ: Lawrence Erlbaum Associates.

Grossberg, S., & Somers, D. (1991). Synchronized oscillations during cooperative feature linking in a cortical model of visual perception. *Neural Networks, 4*, 453-460.

Haken, H. (1988). Synergetics in pattern recognition and associative action. In *Neural and Synergetic Computers* (pp. 2-16). Berlin: Springer-Verlag.

Kaneko, K. (1986, 1993). *Collapse of Tori and Genesis of Chaos in Dissipative Systems* (Enlarged ed.). Singapore: World Scientific.

Kaneko, K. (1989). Spatiotemporal chaos in one and two dimensional coupled map lattices. *Physica D, 37*, 1-41.

Kaneko, K. (1990). Clustering, coding, switching, hierarchical ordering and control in network of chaotic elements. *Physica D, 41*, 137-142.

Kaneko, K. (1993). Overview of coupled map lattices. *Chaos, 2* (3), 279-282.

Kawabata, N., Ymagami, K., & Noaki, M.(1978). Visual fixation points and depth perception. *Vision Research, 18*, 853-854.

Koch, C., & Crick, F. (1994). Some further ideas regarding the neuronal basis of awareness. In C. Koch & J. L. Davis (Eds.), *Large-Scale Neuronal Theories of the Brain*. Cambridge MA: MIT Press.

Kowalski, J. M., Albert, G. L., Rhoades, B. K., & Gross, G. W. (1992). Neuronal networks with spontaneous, correlated bursting activity: Theory and simulations. *Neural Networks, 5*, 805-822.

Langer, S. (1982). *Mind: An Essay on Human Feeling* (Vol. III). Baltimore: Johns Hopkins University Press

Llinas, R. R., & Ribary, U. (1994). Perception as an oneiric-like state modulated by the senses. In C. Koch & J. L. Davis (Eds.), *Large-Scale Neuronal Theories of the Brain*. Cambridge, MA: MIT Press.

Long, G. M., & Toppino, T. C. (1981). Multiple representations of the same reversible figure: Implications for cognitive decisional interpretations. *Perception, 10*, 231-234.

MacGregor, R. J. (1993). *Theoretical Mechanics of Biological Neural Networks*. San Diego: Academic Press.

Mainzer, K. (1994). *Thinking in Complexity: The Complex Dynamics of Matter, Mind, and Mankind*. New York: Springer-Verlag.

Mannion, C. L. T., & Taylor, J. G. (1992). Information processing by oscillating neurons. In J. G. Taylor & C. L. T. Mannion (Eds.), *Coupled Oscillating Neurons*. London: Springer-Verlag.

Marr, D. (1982). *Vision: A Computational Investigation into the Human Representation and Processing of Visual Information*. San Francisco: Freeman.

Noton, D., & Stark, L. (1971). Eye movements and visual perception. *Scientific American, 224*, 34-43

Peréz, J. C. (1988). *De Nouvelle Voies Vers L'intelligence Arificielle: Pluri-disciplinarite, Auto-organization, Reseau Neuronaux*. Paris: Masson.

Peréz, J. C., & Massotte, P. (1987). Chaos fractal attractor. Personal communication.

Riani, M., Oliva, M.A., Selis, G., Ciurlo, G., & Pietro, R. (1984). Effect of luminance on perceptual alteration of ambiguous patterns. *Perceptual and Motor Skills, 58*, 267-274.

Richards, W., Wilson, H. R., & Sommer, M. A. (1994). Chaos in percepts? *Biological Cybernetics, 70*, 345-349.

Siegel, R. M. (1990). Non-linear dynamical system theory and primary visual cortex processing. *Physica D, 42*, 385-395.

Skarda, C., & Freeman, W. J. (1987). How brains make chaos in order to make sense of the world. *Behavioral and Brain Sciences, 10*, 161-195.

Ta'eed, L., Ta'eed, O., & Wright, J. E. (1988). Determinants involved in the perception of the Necker cube: An application of catastrophe theory. *Behavioral Science, 33*, 97-115.

Treisman, A., Cavanagh, P., Fischer, B., Ramachandran, V.S., von der Heydt , R. (1990). Form perception and attention: striate cortex and beyond. In L. Spillman & J. S. Werner (Eds.), *Visual Perception: The Neurophysiological Foundations*. San Diego: Academic Press.

Tsuda, I. (1992). Dynamic link of memory: Chaotic memory map in nonequilibrium neural networks. *Neural Networks, 5*, 313-326.

von Grunau, M. W., Wiggin, S., & Reed, M. (1984). The local character of perspective organization. *Perception and Psychophysics, 35*, 319-324.

Yao, Y., & Freeman, W. J. (1990). Model of biological pattern recognition with spatially chaotic dynamics. *Neural Networks, 3*, 153-170.

14

Oscillatory Neural Networks: Modeling Binding and Attention by Synchronization of Neural Activity

Galina Borisyuk
Institute of Mathematical Problems of Biology, Russian Academy of Sciences

Roman Borisyuk
Institute of Mathematical Problems of Biology, Russian Academy of Sciences, and University of Plymouth

Yakov Kazanovich
Institute of Mathematical Problems of Biology, Russian Academy of Sciences

Gary Strong
National Science Foundation

ABSTRACT

This chapter presents some mathematical models in support of the hypothesis that there is a general principle of information processing at the levels of both preattention and attention. It is claimed that, at both levels, information processing is based on the coherent (synchronous) activity of neurons, neural populations, and brain structures. The level difference is presumed to relate to how synchronization is realized. At the level of preattention, synchronization results from the self-organization of cortical activity, whereas at the level of attention, synchronous activity is controlled by special brain structures that act as a central executive. Two types of oscillatory neural networks are developed to model preattention and attention phenomena. In preattention modeling we concentrate on the binding problem. To solve this problem, a two-layer network of neural oscillators is developed which is able to generate two-frequency envelope oscillations, where the amplitude of high-frequency oscillations is modulated by a lower frequency. This network synchronizes regions of oscillatory activity at high and low frequencies according to the type of stimulation. Such synchronization gives feature binding for both simple and complex stimuli. Networks of phase oscillators with a central element are used to describe a different dynamical behavior that is associated with attention focus formation and switching. For input to the attention system represented by two stimuli, we give a complete description of conditions when a specific attention focus can be formed. The results are interpreted and discussed in terms of attention modeling. This includes the interpretation of psychological experiments on visual selective attention, the problem of attention focus formation, and the possibility of spontaneous attention switching.

1. INTRODUCTION

This work is based on a hypothesis that is now supported by many brain researchers that assumes two relatively independent levels of information processing in the brain. A *low level* (associated with preattentive processing) is responsible for extracting features from input stimuli and for providing simple combinations of features. At this level, the brain structures operate in parallel without preselection of input components. A *high level* (associated with attention) is responsible for forming complex representations of reality. At this level, the information fragments supplied by sensory modalities, memory, and motor components are bound into meaningful patterns that are recognized and memorized. A characteristic feature of this level is its serial form of processing. At any moment, attention is focused on a portion of information that is analyzed more carefully and in greater detail than the other information that is available. The attention focus then moves from one object to another with a preference for new, strong, and important stimuli.

Later, we present some mathematical models in support of the idea that there is a general principle of information processing common to both the low and high levels. It is claimed that processing can be based on the coherent (synchronous) activity of neurons, neural populations, and brain structures at both the preattention and attention levels (see, e.g., Basar & Bullock, 1992). The presumed difference between the levels lies mostly in how synchronization is realized. We believe that, at the low level, it results from self-organization of cortical activity whereas, at the high level, synchronous activity is controlled by a special cortical brain structure that acts as a central executive.

The features of an object differ in their origin. They can be related to geometrical or spectral characteristics of an image or even belong to different (e.g., visual or auditory) modalities. Such features are processed in separate parts of the cortex (Damasio, 1989; Zeki & Shipp, 1988). Therefore one should explain how features are later bound into a complex representation of an object. This is called the *binding problem*. A possible solution to this problem is the hypothesis of Malsburg (1981): Labeling the features of an object is implemented through coherent activity of neural populations that code these features.

The labeling hypothesis was indirectly confirmed by experiments where stimulation induced synchronous oscillations in stimulus-specific cortical regions (Eckhorn et al., 1988; Gray, König, Engel, & Singer, 1989; Gray & Singer, 1989). Gray et al. (1989) reported that a simple visual stimulus represented by a moving light bar induces coherent periodic firing of adjacent neurons in the first visual cortical area (area 17). In the case of a complex stimulus formed by two simultaneously moving bars, synchronization depends on similarity of orientation, continuity, and coherency of motion. If a receptive field that is shared by several neurons with differing orientation preferences is simultaneously crossed by two differently oriented bars, these neurons form two groups. Within each of the groups, neural activity is synchronous, but there is no synchrony between the groups. Activities of neurons whose receptive fields do not overlap do not synchronize unless the stimuli passing these fields are identically oriented and move in the same direction (Gray et al., 1989).

Experiments with simple stimuli are usually explained by the existence of phase-locking between locally coupled neurons. In the case of a complex stimulus, however, synchronization of nonadjacent neural populations could be achieved by direct nonlocal connections between these populations. Unfortunately, such arguments fail if binding includes features represented by populations that have a small or empty set of direct interconnections. To overcome this difficulty, Damasio (1989) presumed that feature binding occurs as a result of coherent neural activity in multiple regions of the neocortex that are linked through activation of common convergence zones. Such zones, which are located in the higher levels of the neocortex, communicate through feedforward and feedback pathways to earlier zones of the primary cortex, where features of the stimulus are represented.

The idea of Damasio looks very attractive but its application may meet the following difficulty. It is known (Gray et al., 1989) that a moving light bar with a large enough gap in the middle elicits two patches of oscillatory activity in the primary visual cortex (area 17). The oscillations are synchronous in each patch but there is no evidence of synchronization (in the sense of a constant phase difference) between the patches. Consider an imaginary experiment in which an object is represented by a light rectangular contour moving along the plane. Suppose that one side of this contour has a gap and that the direction of movement is orthogonal to this side. From the *local* point of view, the bar with a gap should elicit the same type of activity independently of being included or not in a connected contour. Therefore, logically speaking, extrapolating the results of real experiments (Gray et al., 1989), one should not expect synchronous activity of neural populations representing two parts of the bar. On the other hand, according to Damasio, synchronization should take place because these areas represent the features of a rigid object.

To solve this contradiction, we suggest taking into account multifrequency (in particular, two-frequency) oscillations of neural activity (Borisyuk et al., 1992, 1994); (note that the EEG spectrum is usually represented by several oscillations distributed in a wide frequency range). In the case of a complex stimulus, feature binding can be obtained by synchronization at a lower frequency independently of nonsynchronous high-frequency oscillations. To implement this idea, we use feedback signals between convergent zones not for synchronization of the entire frequency band but only to obtain synchronous modulations at a lower frequency. When complex nonhomogeneous stimuli are used, the cortex does not exhibit obligatory synchronization of all responses in all reacting subregions. If two bars are the elements of one object (e.g., the sides of a square), synchronization between convergent zones representing these bars may occur at a low frequency. On the other hand, synchronization of high-frequency oscillations in the cortical regions activated by moving bars will not take place. Thus, which areas are involved in synchronous oscillations at different frequencies will depend not only on the stimulus local characteristics but also on the "context."

Serial processing of information at the high level has been attributed by some researchers to participation of a central executive. According to Cowan (1988), the focus of attention is represented by a subset of short-term memory storage that is controlled by a central executive. Kryukov (1991) proposed that the selection of features that form an attention focus can be realized through synchronization. The synchronous ensemble should include a central oscillator plus those populations of cortical neurons that are activated by these features. This results in the synchronous activity of populations themselves. According to Kryukov, such a network for attention modeling can be designed as a system of peripheral oscillators (PO) coupled with a central oscillator (CO) by feedforward and feedback connections. It is presumed that the septo-hippocampal region plays the role of the CO, while the POs are represented by cortical columns. The use of a central executive is in agreement with Damasio's hypothesis that the hippocampus is the vertex of a convergent zone pyramid. A similar idea is advocated by Miller (1991) who formulated a theory of representation of information in the brain based on cortico-hippocampal interplay. He assumed that such a representation results from the synchronization of activity in the hippocampus and some parts of the cortex due to the time delays in the connections between these structures. Experimental work confirms that the hippocampus is involved in the modulation of classical conditioning (for a review see Schmajuk & DiCarlo, 1992). Nevertheless, the role of the hippocampus and the mechanism of its interaction with the cortex are still being debated.

This chapter presents two types of oscillatory neural networks. Networks of neural oscillators of a Wilson-Cowan type (described later) are used to solve the binding problem for low level information processing. We describe a two-layer neural network, where envelope oscillations can appear with an appropriate choice of parameters. This network is able to synchronize regions of oscillatory activity at both high and low frequencies according to whether stimulation is by a simple or a complex stimulus, respectively. Networks of phase oscillators with a central element are used to model the different types of behavior associated with formation and switching of attentional focus. For the input represented by two stimuli, we give a complete description of conditions when a specific attention focus can be formed. The results obtained are interpreted and discussed in terms of attention modeling. This includes the interpretation of psychological experiments on visual selective attention, the problem of the focus of attention formation, and the possibility of spontaneous attention switching.

2. PREATTENTION MODELING: FEATURE BINDING

Feature binding is one of the main characteristics of preattentive information processing. In this section we model feature binding by an oscillatory neural network and investigate the types of synchronization that appear in the network for different stimulations. We show that several (at least two) interacting cortical areas can solve a relatively difficult task of feature binding for both simple and complex stimuli.

In the case of a simple stimulus (which is represented by the activity of locally coupled cortical neurons), it has been shown that feature binding can be implemented through the synchronization of oscillations of neural populations (König & Schillen, 1991; Schillen & König 1991; Wang, Buhmann, & Malsburg, 1990). Strong local coupling is one of the possible ways to get synchronization. Another possibility is to use a common source of synchronization that simultaneously influences the neural populations included in the binding. Such an approach has been presented in Horn et al. (1991). The authors consider a network of excitatory and inhibitory neurons that is able to generate synchronous oscillations. As a common source for synchronization, noise was added to the input of all neurons representing a given stimulus. The network can simultaneously process several stimuli because each of the different stimuli is associated with different uncorrelated noise. Thus, the noise is used as a label to synchronize the activity of neurons representing one stimulus while the activity of neurons representing different stimuli is kept nonsynchronous.

In Strong and Whitehead (1989), a model of feature binding in visual perception was presented whereby groups of neurons representing pooled features bind together during learning according to their spatial co-occurrence in the display. After removal of the display, the groups continue to demonstrate binding by means of synchronized bursting. The groups of neurons representing a pooled feature contain spiking model neurons. With an appropriate architecture of spiking neurons multiple bindings are possible. Phase relations of spiking neurons can be regarded as a basis for creation of a new type of logic, phase logic (Strong, 1993).

In this chapter we present a different approach to feature binding. This approach is based on the hypothesis that feature binding is realized via multifrequency (envelope) oscillations. The high-frequency components of these oscillations are used to synchronize the activity of directly coupled neural populations. The low frequency components are used to obtain the synchronization between the regions that do not share direct mutual connections. As we mentioned earlier, in the case of a complex stimulus we would not expect to find synchronization between different regions at a high frequency.

Here the idea about a common source of synchronization appears again but now it is formed automatically. Its role is played by a region located in some higher area of the cortex that is coupled with the regions to be synchronized. To implement this idea, we consider a two-layer oscillatory neural network. The stimulation is modeled by activating some external inputs to the oscillators of the first layer. The oscillatory activity in the first layer is spread to the second layer through feedforward convergent connections. In the case of a complex stimulus the first layer contains several separate groups of working oscillators. These groups induce oscillations in a compact region of the second layer. This region is a common source of synchronization of these groups at a low frequency. Its influence on the oscillators of the first layer is realized through convergent backward connections. For simplicity, we consider below the case of two groups, A and B, of oscillators activated in the first layer. Let C be the group of oscillators in the second layer activated by A and B (Fig. 14.1).

According to our hypothesis, the network should function in the following way. The presentation of a simple stimulus results in the synchronization of a group of

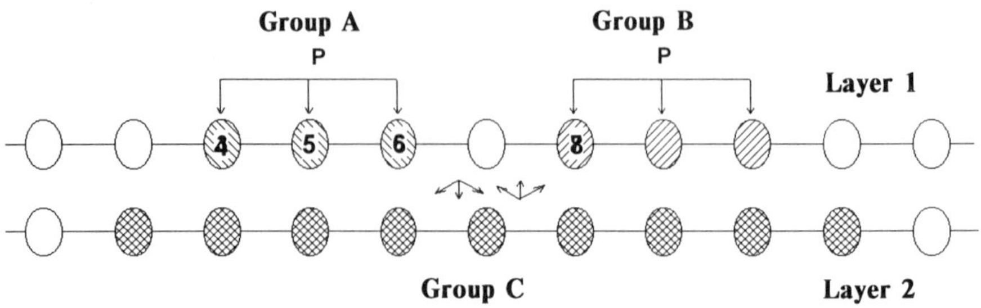

Fig. 14.1. Two-layer oscillatory neural network stimulated by a complex stimulus. *P* denotes external inputs to the oscillators with numbers 4, 5, 6 and 8, 9, 10 in the first layer. Shaded circles denote activated oscillators.

oscillators in the first layer at a high frequency. This is accomplished using local connections in the layer. The presentation of a complex stimulus produces:

1. synchronization of oscillators at a high frequency in each group *A* and *B*;

2. lack of synchronization between the oscillators of groups *A* and *B* at a high frequency; and

3. synchronization of oscillators of groups *A* and *B* at a low frequency.

Group *C* is a common source of synchronization at a low frequency for groups *A* and *B*. Still, its interaction with these groups is organized in such a way that the synchronization of all oscillators at a high frequency is absent.

To support the hypothesis, the following network has been developed (Fig. 14.2). The network consists of two layers. Each layer is represented by a chain of neural oscillators. The connections in a layer are local (i.e., each node is connected to two nearest neighbors; Fig. 14.2a). The feedforward and feedback connections between the layers are convergent; each oscillator is influenced by several oscillators from the local part of the other layer (Fig. 14.2b).

As an element of the network we use a Wilson-Cowan type of oscillator. The oscillator describes the average activities of excitatory and inhibitory populations of neurons. There is an external input to each element. The presentation of a stimulus increases the input signals of selected oscillators in the first layer. This induces oscillatory activity in the corresponding network elements. It is supposed that a simple

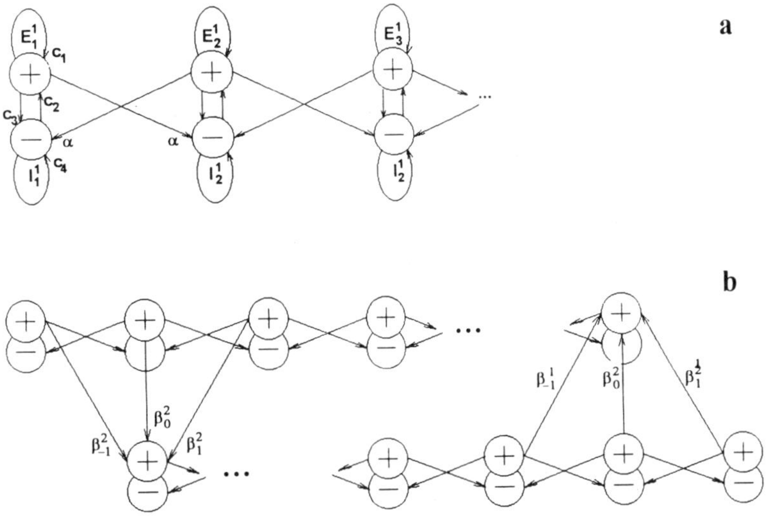

Fig. 14.2. Connections between Wilson-Cowan oscillators: (a) connections in a layer; (b) forward and backward convergent connection from excitatory to excitatory populations between layers.

stimulus elicits oscillatory activity in a locally connected group of oscillators. A complex stimulus, on the other hand, elicits oscillatory activity in separate groups of oscillators that are not locally coupled.

The dynamics of the network are described by the equations

$$\begin{cases} \dot{E}_n^1 = -E_n^1 + (k_e - E_n^1) S_e(c_1 E_n^1 - c_2 I_n^1 + P_n + R_n^1), \\ \dot{I}_n^1 = -I_n^1 + (k_i - I_n^1) S_i(c_3 E_n^1 - c_4 I_n^1 + W_n^1), \\ \dot{E}_n^2 = -E_n^2 + (k_e - E_n^2) S_e(c_1 E_n^2 - c_2 I_n^2 + R_n^2), \\ \dot{I}_n^2 = -I_n^2 + (k_i - I_n^2) S_i(c_3 E_n^2 - c_4 I_n^2 + W_n^2), n=1,\ldots,N. \end{cases}$$

Here $E_n^1(t)$, $I_n^1(t)$, $E_n^2(t)$, $I_n^2(t)$ are the activities of excitatory and inhibitory populations of the oscillator number n in the first and second layers, respectively (the superscript shows the layer, 1 or 2, to which the oscillator belongs); c_1, c_2, c_3, c_4 are positive parameters showing the coupling strengths between different types of populations; P_n is the value of the external input to the excitatory population of the oscillator n; $S_p(x) = S_p(x;b_p,\theta_p)$ are monotonically increasing sigmoid-type functions,

$$S_p(x) = 1/(1+\exp(-b_p(x-\theta_p))) - 1/(1+\exp(b_p\theta_p));\ p\in\{e,i\},$$

where b_e, θ_e, b_i, θ_i are constants; k_p is a constant, $k_p = 1/S_p(+\infty)$. The interaction of oscillators is given by

$$R_n^1 = \beta_{-1}^1 E_{n-1}^2 + \beta_0^1 E_n^2 + \beta_1^1 E_{n+1}^2,\ R_n^2 = \beta_{-1}^2 E_{n-1}^1 + \beta_0^2 E_n^1 + \beta_1^2 E_{n+1}^1,$$
$$W_n^1 = \alpha^1(E_{n-1}^1 + E_{n+1}^1),\ W_n^2 = \alpha^2(E_{n-1}^2 + E_{n+1}^2),$$

where α^1 and α^2 describe local coupling in the layers, β^1_{-1}, β^1_0, β^1_1, and β^2_{-1}, β^2_0, β^2_0, describe convergent connections between the layers. For the indices out of the range $[1, N]$ we use a reflection symmetry relative to the ends of the segment (thus, 0 means 2, -1 means 3, etc.). Such reflection symmetry is traditional as a boundary condition.

The particular choice of connections is important for our purposes. For a small coupling strength the local connections in the layers (from the excitatory population of an oscillator to inhibitory populations of the neighboring oscillators) lead to the synchronization of locally coupled oscillators (Borisyuk et al., 1995). Convergent connections between excitatory populations of the layers induce envelope oscillations. Appropriate dynamics of the network are observed, for example, with the following parameter values: $c_1 = 16$, $c_2 = 12$, $c_3 = 15$, $c_4 = 3$, $\theta_e = 4$, $b_e = 1.3$, $\theta_i = 2$, $b_i = 2$, $N = 13$.

A simple stimulus is coded in our modeling by the inputs

$$P_n = \begin{cases} 0, n = 1,\dots,L, \\ P^*, n = L+1,\dots,L+M, \\ 0, n = L+M+1,\dots,N, \end{cases}$$

where $P^* > 0$. The input distribution means that only M elements of the chain (beginning from the L+1 element) have non-zero inputs. With such stimulation (Fig. 14.3a), a connected region of excited oscillators working at a high frequency appears in the first layer. These oscillators are synchronous due to local connections in the layer (see Fig. 14.4a). This synchronous activity can be interpreted as the formation of a pattern relevant to a simple stimulus (the experimentally detected high-frequency synchronous oscillations are in the range of 40-70 Hz).

A complex stimulus is coded in our model by the inputs

$$P_n = \begin{cases} 0, n = 1,\dots,L_1, \\ P^*, n = L_1+1,\dots,L_1+M_1, \\ 0, n = L_1+M_1+1,\dots,L_2, \\ P^*, n = L_2+1,\dots,L_2+M_2, \\ 0, n = L_2+M_2+1,\dots,N \end{cases}$$

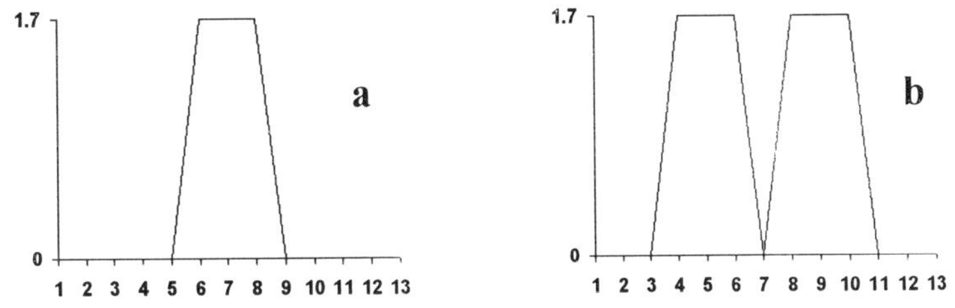

Fig. 14.3. Input P_n versus the oscillator number n ($n = 1, 2, ..., 13$): (a) Simple stimulus, $L = 5$, $M = 3$, $P^* = 1.7$; (b) Complex stimulus, $L_1 = 3$, $M_1 = 3$, $L_2 = 7$, $M_2 = 3$, $P^* = 1.7$.

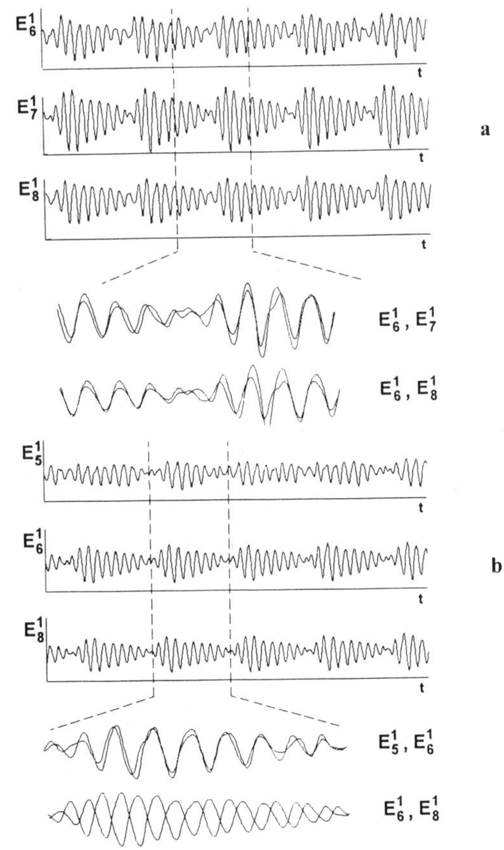

Fig. 14.4. Examples of dynamics of different oscillators in the first layer. (a) Simple stimulus. High-frequency synchronization of excitatory population. Zoom shows more clearly the synchronous dynamics of E_6(t), E_7(t), E_8(t). (b) Complex stimulus. Activities E_5(t) and E_6(t) belong to the excited area *A*, E_8(t) belongs to the excited area *B* (see Group *A* and Group *B* in Fig. 14.1). Note the envelope profile and synchronization between all shown oscillators at a low frequency. Zoom shows that E_5(t) and E_6(t) work in-phase at a high frequency and that E_5(t). E_6(t) work in antiphase with E_8(t).

Thus, two separate connected regions receive the input of a high level P^* while other oscillators receive zero input (Fig. 14.3b).

If connections between the layers were switched off, this stimulation would give synchronous oscillations within each region but there would be no synchronization between the regions. Due to convergent interlayer connections, the envelope oscillations appear in the network with an appropriate choice of parameters (in our experiments the modulation frequency was one order of magnitude lower than the main high frequency). Figure 14.4b shows the dynamics of oscillations in the first layer after the transitional period is over. These dynamics are exactly of the kind that we expected to get in the case of a complex stimulus. The populations E^1_5 and E^1_6 are synchronous at a high frequency because the oscillators are located at the same excited region. There is no synchronization at a high frequency between these populations and population E^1_8 because the latter population belongs to the other excitation region. Still, there is synchronization of all excited populations of oscillators at a low frequency. This synchronization can be interpreted as formation of a pattern relevant to feature binding of a complex stimulus.

3. ATTENTION MODELING: DYNAMICS OF NEURAL NETWORKS WITH A CENTRAL ELEMENT

To model attention, we use a network of phase oscillators. Such networks have been found helpful when a qualitative mathematical description of synchronization is needed (Kuramoto et al., 1992; Schuster & Wagner, 1990; Sompolinsky et al., 1990). A phase oscillator is described by one variable, the oscillation phase, and the interaction between oscillators is realized via phase locking. The basic theoretical results in this field were obtained by Kuramoto and Nishikawa (1987), Daido (1988, 1990), and Strogatz and Mirollo (1988).

We suppose that the set of POs is divided into two groups, namely A and B, each being activated by one of two stimuli simultaneously presented to the attention system. Let group A contain the POs whose natural frequencies ω^i_A are independently and randomly distributed in the interval (ω_A-1, ω_A+1), and let the POs of group B have natural frequencies ω^j_B that are independently and randomly distributed in the interval (ω_B-1, ω_B+1). Suppose that $\omega_B-\omega_A<21$ (the intervals do not overlap). Let $\theta^i_A(t)$ be the phases of POs of group A, $\theta^i_B(t)$ be the phases of POs of group B, $\theta_0(t)$ be the phase of the CO and ω_0 be its natural frequency. Then the dynamics of the network of phase oscillators with a central element is described by the equations

$$\begin{aligned}\dot\theta_0 &= \omega_0 + \frac{\alpha}{n}\sum_{i=1}^{n}\sin(\theta^i_A-\theta_0) + \frac{\beta}{n}\sum_{j=1}^{n}\sin(\theta^j_B-\theta_0)\\ \dot\theta_A &= \omega_A + \alpha\sin(\theta_0-\theta_A) \qquad\qquad (1),\\ \dot\theta_B &= \omega_B + \beta\sin(\theta_0-\theta_B)\end{aligned}$$

where n is the number of oscillators in each group, α and β are parameters that determine the interaction strengths between the CO and the oscillators of A and B, respectively. All natural frequencies of oscillators are chosen according to their distributions and then fixed. By definition, the derivatives of the phases in the right hand side of Equations (1) are the current frequencies of the oscillators. The architecture of the network is shown in Fig. 14.5.

The main problem considered next is the description of dynamic modes that may appear in the network for various values of these parameters. Three types of network dynamics are of interest to us:

- global synchronization (this mode is attributed to the case when the attention focus includes two stimuli);
- partial synchronization of the CO and a group of POs (this mode is attributed to the case when the attention focus includes one of two competing stimuli); or
- no-synchronization mode (this mode is attributed to the case when the attention focus is not formed).

Using analytical and computational methods, we find the boundaries of parameter regions where the above-mentioned types of dynamics take place.

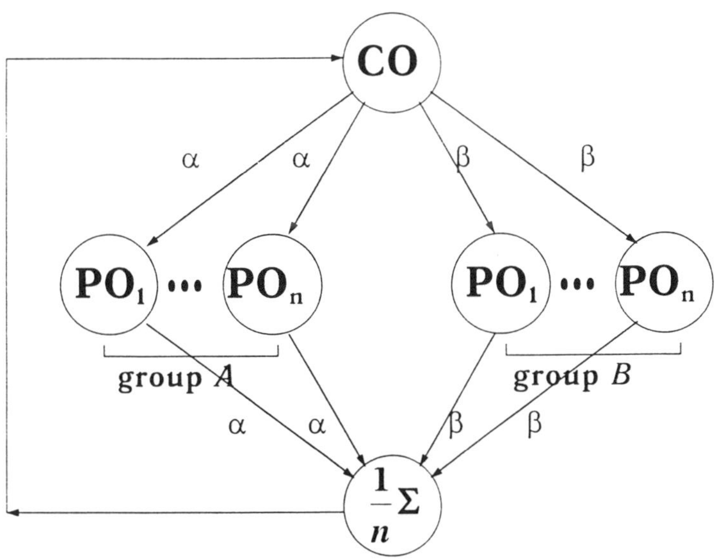

Fig. 14.5. Architecture of the network for attention modeling. CO is a central oscillator, representing the central executive of the attention system; POs are peripheral oscillators, representing cortical columns.

Note that by changing phases and time we can get arbitrary values of ω_A and ω_B. Hence, without loss of generality, we can restrict the consideration to any pair of fixed values ω_A and ω_B. We take the value of l one order lower than $\omega_B - \omega_A$. Thus, we study the dynamics of (1) as a function of three parameters ω_0, α, and β. Due to the symmetry of the role of groups A and B in the network, complete investigation of (1) can be restricted by the values of ω_0 satisfying the inequality $\omega_0 \geq (\omega_A + \omega_B)/2$. The results obtained in this case can evidently be reformulated for any other values of ω_0.

Let us say that the network is in a *global synchronization* mode if its dynamics is described by a stable solution of (1) such that all oscillators run with the same frequency Ω,

$$\Omega = \dot{\theta}_0 = \dot{\theta}^i_A = \dot{\theta}^j_B, i, j = 1, \ldots, n .$$

In this case the difference between the phases of a PO and the CO does not vary with time. Summing the right hand sides of (1), we find that

$$\Omega = \frac{\omega_0 + \overline{\omega_A} + \overline{\omega_B}}{3}, \tag{2}$$

where $\overline{\omega}_A$ and $\overline{\omega}_B$ are the average values of natural frequencies of POs in groups A and B, respectively,

$$\overline{\omega}_A = \frac{1}{n}\sum_{i=1}^{n} \omega^{i_A}, \quad \overline{\omega}_B = \frac{1}{n}\sum_{j=1}^{n} \omega^{j_B} .$$

Suppose that the network is not in the global synchronization mode. Let us say that the kth PO (that can belong to any group, A or B) is partially synchronous with the CO if the dynamics of the network is described by a stable (at least locally) solution of (1) such that the difference between the phases of this PO and the CO is restricted, that is, there exists such a constant C that for any moment t

$$|\theta_0(t) - \theta^k(t)| < C.$$

A group of oscillators (A or B) is called partially synchronous with the CO if all oscillators of the group are partially synchronous with the CO. In this case we say that the network is in the mode of *partial synchronization*. According to the given definition, the partial synchronization of a group does not necessarily require that all oscillators of the other group are out of partial synchronization with the CO. If all oscillators of one group are partially synchronous while none of the oscillators of the other group is partially synchronous, we say the network is in *strict partial synchronization* mode. If a stable dynamics of the network does not show either global or partial synchronization, we say that the network is in *no-synchronization* mode.

For a fixed value of ω_0 let us introduce the following notation for the regions on the plane (β, α) that correspond to various dynamic modes of the network:

- *GS* is the region where global synchronization takes place for some initial phases;

- PS_A, PS_B are the regions where partial synchronization of groups *A* and *B* takes place for some initial phases;

- *NS* is the region where the no-synchronization mode exists.

Note that these definitions imply that the regions may overlap because different types of dynamics can be conditioned by the choice of initial phases.

Consider a network with a large number *n* of oscillators in groups *A* and *B* and determine the boundaries of the regions *GS*, PS_A, PS_B, *NS*. Global synchronization implies that there exists a stable stationary solution of equations for the phase differences between the CO and POs. The necessary condition for global synchronization is

$$\left|\Omega - \omega^{i_A}\right| \leq \alpha, \left|\Omega - \omega^{j_B}\right| \leq \beta, \; i,j = 1,\ldots,n, \qquad (3)$$

where Ω is determined by (2). The corresponding boundary on the plane (β, α) is the right angle with the vertex $C = (\max_j |\Omega - \omega_B^{\,j}|, \max_i |\Omega - \omega_A^{\,i}|)$ and with arms parallel to the coordinate axes. Condition (3) is not sufficient because the region of parameters (β, α) defined by it may include subregions, where a stable stationary state is formed for special values of initial phases only.

Consider the boundary between the region of the no-synchronization mode and a region of partial synchronization. For definiteness, let it be the boundary between *NS* and PS_B. In fact, as computer experiments show, these regions are overlapping, but the overlapping takes place in a narrow strip whose width will be neglected in our approximation formulas. The following formulas are derived to approximate the boundary between *NS* and some subregion of PS_B, where strict partial synchronization takes place. It will be seen later that this boundary constitutes some part of the boundary between *NS* and PS_B.

The determination of this boundary is based on an equation that describes the time average of the current frequency of the CO as a function of interaction parameters. Denote this average value by

$$\langle\omega\rangle = \frac{1}{T}\int_{t_0}^{t_0+T} \dot{\theta}_0(\tau)\,d\tau,$$

where the time interval (t_0, t_0+T) is supposed to be sufficiently large.

As computer experiments show, if n is large and l is not too small relative to $<\omega>$, the deviation of the current frequency of the CO from $<\omega>$ under strict partial synchronization (after some moment t_0) is relatively small. This follows from the fact that under the formulated conditions the current frequencies of the oscillators from A vary more or less independently from each other (this independence is lost if l is small). Therefore, their integral influence on the CO is averaged and changes only a little with time. The oscillators from B have current frequencies that are quite near the frequency of the CO, hence these frequencies also change little. An example showing the time evolution of the current frequencies of the CO and POs is given in Fig. 14.6.

Thus, we can assume that $\dot{\theta}_0$ is approximately constant and is equal to $<\omega>$. This assumption allows us to consider a pair interaction between each PO and the CO independent of interaction with other POs. Then the strict partial synchronization condition for group B becomes equivalent to

$$\left|<\omega> - \omega_B^j\right|, \; j = 1,\ldots,n, \tag{4}$$

$$\left|<\omega> - \omega_A^i\right|, \; i = 1,\ldots,n. \tag{5}$$

The equation for $<\omega>$ is derived by the averaging technique presented in Kazanovich and Borisyuk (1999). The equation has the form

$$3<\omega> \; = \; h(<\omega>,\alpha) + \omega_0 + \omega_A + \omega_B, \tag{6}$$

where

$$h(<\omega>,\alpha) \; = \; g(<\omega> - \omega_A + l) - g(<\omega> - \omega_A - l),$$
$$g(x) \; = \; \frac{1}{4l}\left[x\sqrt{x^2 - \alpha^2} - \alpha^2 \ln(x + \sqrt{x^2 - \alpha^2})\right].$$

From (6) we find $<\omega>$ as a function of α using a continuation technique implemented in the program LOCBIF (Khibnik et al., 1993).

Following from (6), for $\alpha = 0$,

$$<\omega> \; = \; \frac{\omega_0 + \omega_B}{2}.$$

If α increases, $<\omega>$ monotonically approaches ω_A. Let $\bar{\alpha}$ be the maximal value of α for which the inequality $|<\omega> - \omega_A| \geq l + \alpha$ holds. For $\alpha < \bar{\alpha}$, (5) is fulfilled. Under this condition the equation for the boundary between NS and PS_B follows from (4) and has the form

$$\beta \; = \; \max_j \left|<\omega> - \omega^{j_B}\right|, \; j = 1,\ldots,n,$$

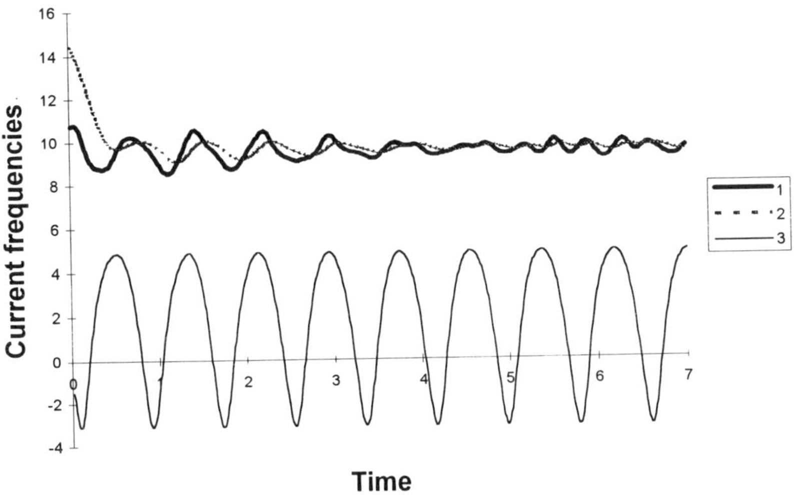

Fig. 14.6. Example of time evolution of current frequencies of the CO (1) and two POs from groups ***A*** (3) and ***B*** (2), $\omega_0 = 10$, $\alpha = 4$, $\beta = 5$, $n = 50$.

where $<\omega>$ is given by (6). If $\alpha > \overline{\alpha}$, (6) cannot be used because partial synchronization involves oscillators of both groups A and B. The boundaries of the regions of strict partial synchronization found according to the described procedure are shown in Fig. 14.7 by solid curves.

Now let us describe how the boundaries of the regions of various synchronization modes have been determined by computer simulation. The integration of (1) has been made according to a Runge-Kutta method with an adaptive time step and the integration error lower than 10^{-5}. In computations we put $n = 50$ and choose the initial phases of oscillators to be randomly and uniformly distributed in the range $(0, 2\pi)$. During the simulation a track has been kept of the phase differences between the CO and POs. The following types of network behavior have been found in the computer experiments:

- For all POs the phase difference between the CO and PO is gradually stabilizing. This corresponds to global synchronization.

- After some time, the phase difference between the CO and a PO changes in a range of the width not greater than 2π. This corresponds to the partial synchronization of this PO with the CO.

- The absolute value of the phase difference of the CO and a PO is gradually increasing. This increase can be either permanent or stepwise. In the latter case the difference is oscillating for some time around a fixed value, then it abruptly changes due to phase slipping and oscillates around another

> value which is shifted by 2π relative to the previous one. This implies that there is no synchronization between the CO and the PO.

The dynamic modes were determined for fixed values of α and β in 50 identical experiments, which only differed by a random choice of natural frequencies and initial phases of the oscillators. After 50 iterations the boundaries of the regions can be determined reproducibly with an accuracy not less than 0.1.

The computed boundary of *NS* is shown in Fig. 14.7 by filled circles. The boundaries of the regions PS_A and PS_B are located inside the region *NS* close to its

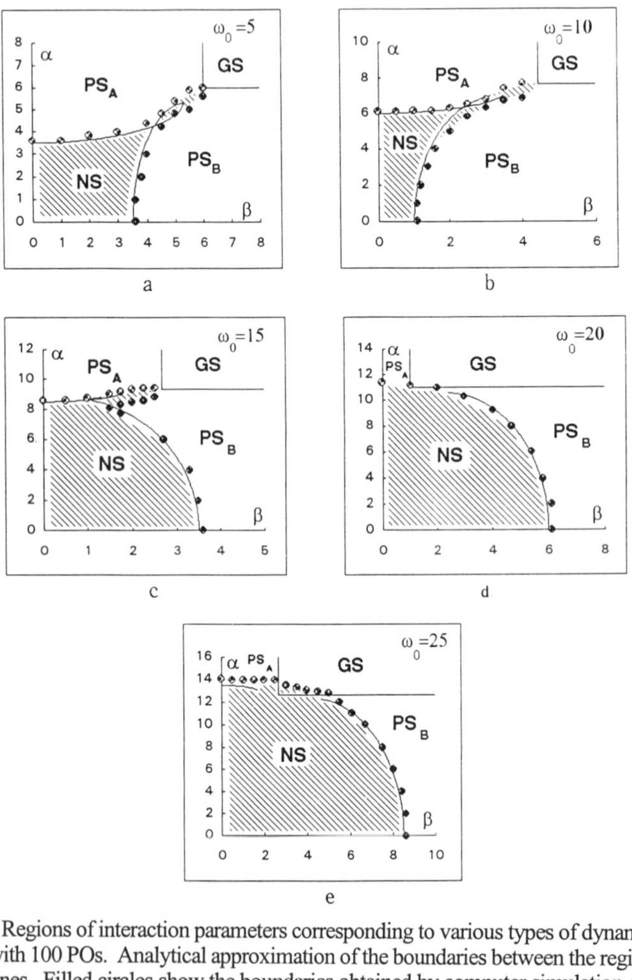

Fig. 14.7. Regions of interaction parameters corresponding to various types of dynamic modes in a network with 100 POs. Analytical approximation of the boundaries between the regions are shown by solid lines. Filled circles show the boundaries obtained by computer simulation of the network dynamics. Figures (a)-(e) correspond to different values of the natural frequency of the CO. *GS* is the region of global synchronization; PS_A and PS_B are the regions of partial synchronization of groups *A* and *B*; *NS* is the region of no synchronization.

boundary. Thus, the regions of partial synchronization and the region of no-synchronization mode overlap over narrow strips of multistability. In particular, in the "narrow" parts of *NS* (such narrow parts can be seen in Fig. 14.7a-c), where the regions PS_A and PS_B come close to each other, the partial synchronization of both groups *A* and *B* as well as no-synchronization mode can be found with the same values of network parameters.

As can be seen from Fig. 14.7(a)-(d), for $\omega_0 \leq 20$ the boundary between *GS* and *NS* consists of a single point *C*. If $\omega_0 > 20$, some region near the point *C* simultaneously belongs to *NS* and *GS* (Fig. 14.7e). This region also overlaps with PS_A and PS_B. No other overlapping of PS_A , PS_B and *NS* has been found.

Figure 14.7 shows that analytically obtained boundaries between the regions of strict partial synchronization and no-synchronization region are in good agreement with the results of computer simulation. For those values of interaction parameters, which make (6) sensible, the computer experiments show that the boundaries of the regions of partial synchronization and strict partial synchronization are identical. Relatively poor results in analytical determination of the boundary can be seen for $\omega_0 = 25$ in the boundary of PS_A. This inaccuracy is caused by the fact that for the given parameter values the variance of the natural frequencies of the oscillators from *A* becomes too small when compared to $\langle\omega\rangle$. This results in the violation of our assumption about the independent influence of the oscillators from *A* on the CO.

4. DISCUSSION

Our work has been devoted to the development and analysis of oscillatory neural networks that model binding and attention. The models are different in the choice of oscillatory units and in architecture, but both models are based on the same mechanism of synchronization of neural activity that we consider as a general principle of information processing in the brain at both the preattention and attention levels. The two-layer network of neural oscillators used in solving the binding problem shows that binding can be achieved through synchronization of multifrequency oscillations. The model of attention is designed as a network of phase oscillators with a central element. Its analysis shows that attention focus formation and switching can be explained in terms of synchronization of oscillations between the central oscillator and peripheral (cortical) oscillators. We discuss these models in more detail next.

4.1. Feature Binding

In this chapter we consider a simple version of the network for feature binding. This network can bind the features of a complex stimulus in the case when neural populations representing these features in the cortex are connected through a common region in a higher cortical structure. In fact, the processing of a stimulus may be more complex requiring more than two layers to bind the features that are significantly different. Each layer may be responsible for some level of abstraction. Then, to achieve a higher level of abstraction in representation of a complex stimulus in the brain, more than two frequencies should be used for feature binding. If this is the case, each layer in the pyramid-structure of Damasio's convergent zones can be associated with the main frequency which is used to bind the features at this layer. The higher one goes up this pyramid, the lower the frequencies. Thus, the model explains the necessity of a wide range of frequencies used in the cortex and predicts that lower frequencies can participate in feature binding at higher levels of abstraction.

An interesting question related to this scheme arises: How many different frequencies really participate in the binding of the most abstract features? From general consideration based on the complexity of information processed by humans, about 4-7 frequencies would be enough. We hope that better results will appear in future experiments.

4.2. Attention Modeling

Our analysis of the attention model fully describes the necessary conditions for various types of synchronization, global or partial, between the central oscillator and peripheral oscillators in the case when the natural frequencies of POs form two nonoverlapping clusters. The main results are presented in Fig. 14.7. The figure shows some interesting peculiarities in how the dynamics can change with the variation of network parameters. In particular, the transition from *GS* to *NS* is possible in one point if the natural frequency of the CO is relatively low, and the boundary curve appears between these regions in both cases if the natural frequency of the CO becomes greater than a critical value (Fig. 14.7e).

For some parameter values the model demonstrates multistability: depending on initial phases a network has various types of synchronization or its absence. Multistability takes place everywhere near the boundaries of *NS* with the regions *GS*, PS_A, and PS_B.

Note that our "rigid" definition of partial synchronization applied to all members of a group has been chosen mostly to simplify the presentation of the results. One could consider a "weaker" criterion of partial synchronization, for example, one which should be fulfilled for a given part of oscillators in the group. The mathematical results can be easily extended to this case. In fact, the regions in the parameter space near the boundaries are transient regions, where one mode of synchronization is gradually changed by the other.

Finally, let us discuss the possible implications of the results obtained for attention modeling. Suppose that two stimuli are inputted to the attention system. The stimuli are represented by their features that elicit the activity of peripheral oscillators associated with these features. We suppose that each stimulus is represented by a group of oscillators (groups *A* and *B*) whose natural frequencies form a cluster. The stimulation of the attention system also activates a central oscillator. The natural frequency of the CO is conditioned by the earlier evolution of the attention system and the interaction parameters between the CO and POs are assumed to be formed in previous learning.

In terms of the model the formation of the attention focus is related to the synchronization between the CO and some groups of POs. As the model shows, the focus of attention can combine both stimuli in a complex pattern (global synchronization), or the focus can be formed by the features of one of two competing stimuli, one of them representing a target and the other representing a distracting object (partial synchronization), or the stimuli can be ignored by the attention system (the no-synchronization mode).

The model predicts that depending on the relations between natural frequencies of the CO and POs, a distracting stimulus can either improve or impair attention focusing on the target stimulus. Suppose that *B* represents a target stimulus and *A* represents a distracting stimulus, that is, the interaction parameters are chosen to provide the partial synchronization of *B*. If $\omega_A < \omega_0 < \omega_B$ (this case is represented by Fig. 14.7a), the partial synchronization of *B* can be achieved for a smaller value of the interaction parameter β when *A* is silent ($\alpha = 0$) than when it is active ($\alpha > 0$). If $\omega_A < \omega_B < \omega_0$ (this case is represented by Fig. 14.7c-e), there is an interval of the values of β such that if we gradually increase α starting from 0, the system will be in the no-synchronization mode for the low values of α but will move into the region of partial synchronization with *B* if α becomes big enough. Thus, the presence of *A* allows the use of smaller values of β to achieve partial synchronization of *B*.

We think the difference between these two cases can be used to explain the results of psychological experiments that revealed the significance of a cue for attention focusing on a target (Posner, 1988). A typical experiment of this kind is organized in the following way. A person is trying to focus attention in the middle point of the visual field and should react to target stimuli that randomly appear in the left or in the right part of the visual field. A target stimulus can be preceded by a cue (a flash of light) in the left or right part of the visual field. The difficulty of the task is measured by the reaction time. It has been shown that the reaction time is lower (greater) than in the experiments without a cue if the cue appears in the same (in the opposite) part of the visual field relative to the target. In terms of the model we consider the cue as a distracting stimulus. Our hypothesis is that different locations of the cue correspond to different relations between natural frequencies of oscillators representing the stimuli and the central executive. Suppose that concentration of attention in the central portion of the visual field makes the central oscillator natural frequency equal to Ω_0. Suppose also that the natural frequencies of the POs are distributed so that those activated by a stimulus in the left part of the field have natural frequencies lower than Ω_0, and those activated by a stimulus in the right part of the visual field have natural frequencies greater than Ω_0. Note that, due to a short time lag between the cue and the target, there is a period of simultaneous activity of the two groups of POs representing the cue and the target in the cortex. Then, the presentation of the cue in the same, or in the opposite, part of the field corresponds to one of the above-mentioned cases when an additional stimulus can improve attention focusing on the other stimulus or make it more difficult.

Another important consequence of modeling is illustrated by Fig. 14.7e and states that decreasing the interaction of the CO with the oscillators representing one of two stimuli that form the attention focus may lead not to focusing attention on the other stimulus but to complete destruction of the attention focus. In this case the boundary between *GS* and *NS* has such a form that the transition between these regions can be realized by changing only one of the interaction parameters α or β.

The dependence of the dynamics of the model on initial conditions that is found for some parameter values provides for the possibility of a spontaneous shift of the attention focus. The necessary change in phase relations leading to attention switching can be caused by noise or by a special signal. Moreover, the abrupt shift of partial synchronization from one group to the other can be observed in the dynamics of the network without any additional signals. An example of such dynamics is represented in Fig. 14.8.

4.3. General Scheme of Information Processing in the Brain

Preattention and attention are important components of a general scheme of information processing in the brain. Here, we offer a sketch of this scheme because it has been a basis for developing our models and it may be helpful in the choice of future investigations.

The information from different modality receptors spreads by specific paths and reaches the nuclei of the thalamus. After the thalamus the information sequentially flows through convergent zones of the cortex (Damasio, 1989). Simple features detected in the early cortical areas are combined into more complex patterns in the higher areas finally giving patterns that include different modalities. The long-term memory is activated by associations with the input signal in the form of a constellation of active centers which represent information classes. The "distances" between the signal and the classes are estimated and used to control information processing through backward connections. Thus, the complex dynamics of neural activity appears as a result of interaction of convergent zones. This dynamics includes oscillations, envelope oscillations, chaotic activity, and various types of synchronization.

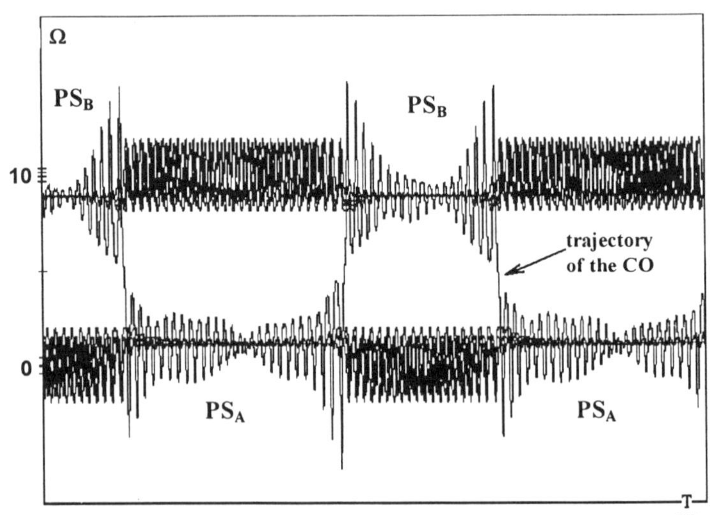

Fig. 14.8. Spontaneous shift of attention. The trajectories of current frequencies of oscillators show partial synchronization switching between groups ***A*** and ***B***; $\omega_0 = 5$; $\alpha = \beta = 1.5$; $n = 4$.

The hippocampus is considered as a central executive in the scheme of information processing. There are two main inputs to the hippocampus: (a) from the entorhinal cortex that delivers the main information about the stimulus (this input receives the information processed by sequential convergent zones); (b) from the septal theta-rhythm generator.

The interaction between these inputs determines the dynamics of hippocampal activity. The main functions of the hippocampus which we take into account in modeling are:

- the hippocampus is a central oscillator (central executive) of the attention system;

- the hippocampus contains a short-term memory system.

Note that the scheme presents two main streams of information flow:

- from receptors to the hippocampus (early information processing, features extraction, classification, information preparation for memorizing in the long-term memory).

- back from the hippocampus to convergent and motor zones of the cortex (synthesis, feature binding to create a complex pattern, forming an appropriate reaction on a stimulus etc.).

5. CONCLUSIONS

The results obtained here should be considered as only preliminary steps in understanding the neural mechanism of feature binding and attention. These results demonstrate a qualitative proximity to some experimental evidence and suggest the hypotheses for further experimental investigation. The next steps should be to improve the models and to reach a quantitative agreement with experimental data, for example, with reaction times registered in experiments with and without attraction of attention.

Another important and difficult problem is to combine the models of preattention and attention with the models of memory and learning. Such unification would give the possibility to describe the main functions of the brain basing on general facts of oscillatory neural networks theory. Hopefully, this theory will also provide new approaches to designing new types of computational devices, “attentional neuro-computers,” which will optimally combine parallel and serial information processing.

ACKNOWLEDGMENTS

This work was supported by Grants 94-01-01270-a and 99-04-49112 from the Russian Foundation of Fundamental Research.

REFERENCES

Basar, E., & Bullock, T. H. (Eds.). (1992). *Induced Rhythms in the Brain.* Boston: Birkhauser.

Borisyuk, G. N., Borisyuk, R. M., & Khibnik, A. I. (1992). Analysis of oscillatory regimes of a coupled neural oscillator system with application to visual cortex modeling. In J. G. Taylor, E. R. Caianiello, R. M. G. Cotterill, & J. W. Clark (Eds.), *Neural Networks Dynamics, Proceedings of the Workshop on Complex Dynamics in Neural Networks. Perspectives in Neural Computing* (pp. 208-225). New York: Springer-Verlag.

Borisyuk, G. N., Borisyuk, R. M., Khibnik, A. I., & Roose, D. (1995). Dynamics and bifurcations of two coupled neural oscillators with different connection type. *Bulletin of Mathematical Biology, 57*, 809-840.

Borisyuk, R. M., Borisyuk, G. N., Kazanovich, Y., & Strong, G. (1994). Modeling of binding problem and attention by synchronization of multilayer neural activity. In *IMACS International Symposium on Signal Processing, Robotics, and Neural Networks* (pp. 602-605). Lille, France.

Cowan, N. (1988). Evolving conceptions of memory storage, selective attention, and their mutual constraints within the human information-processing system. *Psychological Bulletin, 104*, 163-191.

Daido, H. (1988). Lower critical dimension for populations of oscillators with randomly distributed frequencies: A renormalization-group analysis. *Physical Review Letters, 61*, 231-234.

Daido, H. (1990). Intrinsic fluctuations and a phase transition in a class of large populations of interacting oscillators. *Journal of Statistical Physics, 60*, 753-800.

Damasio, A. (1989). The brain binds entities and events by multiregional activation from convergence zones. *Neural Computation, 1*, 123-132.

Eckhorn, R., Bauer, R., Jordan, W., Brosch, M., Kruse, W., Munk, M., & Reitboeck, H. J. (1988). Coherent oscillations: A mechanism of feature linking in the visual cortex? *Biological Cybernetics, 60*, 121-130.

Gray, C. M., König, P., Engel, A. K., & Singer, W. (1989). Oscillatory responses in cat visual cortex exhibit inter-columnar synchronization which reflects global stimulus properties. *Nature, 338*, 334-337.

Gray, C. M., & Singer, W. (1989). Stimulus-specific neuronal oscillations in orientation columns of cat visual cortex. *Proceedings of National Academy of Sciences, 86*, 1698-1702.

Horn, D., Sagi, D., & Usher, M. (1991). Segmentation, binding and illusory conjunctions. *Neural Computation, 3*, 510-525.

Kazanovich, Y. B., & Borisyuk, R. M. (1999). Dynamics of neural networks with a central element. *Neural Networks, 12*, 149-161.

Khibnik, A. I., Kuznetsov, Yu. A., Levitin, V. V., & Nikolaev, E. V. (1993). Continuation techniques and interactive software for bifurcation analysis of ODEs and iterated maps. *Physica D, 62*, 360-371.

König, P., & Schillen, T. (1991). Stimulus dependent assembly formation of oscillatory responses: I. Synchronization. *Neural Computation, 3*, 155-166.

Kryukov, V. I. (1991). An attention model based on the principle of dominanta. In A. V. Holden & V. I. Kryukov (Eds.), *Neurocomputers and Attention I. Neurobiology, Synchronization and Chaos* (pp. 319-352). Manchester: Manchester University Press.

Kuramoto, Y., Aoyagi, T., Nishikawa, I., Chawanya, T., & Okuda, I. (1992). Neural network model carrying phase information. *Progress in Theoretical Physics, 87*, 1119-1126.

Kuramoto, Y., & Nishikawa, I. (1987) Statistical macrodynamics of large dynamical systems. Case of a phase transition in oscillator communities. *Journal of Statistical Physics, 49*, 569-605.

Malsburg, C. von der (1981). The correlation theory of brain function. *International Report 81-2.* Goettingen: Max-Planck-Institute for Biophysical Chemistry.

Miller, R. (1991). *Cortico-Hippocampal Interplay and the Representation of Contexts in the Brain*. Berlin-Heidelberg-New York: Springer-Verlag.
Posner, M. (1988). Structures and functions of selective attention. In T. Boll & B. Bryant (Eds.), *Master Lectures in Clinical Neurophysiology* (pp. 173-202). Washington, DC: American Psychological Assocation.
Schillen, T. B., & König, P. (1991). Stimulus dependent assembly formation of oscillatory responses: II. Desynchronization. *Neural Computation*, *3*, 167-177.
Schmajuk, N., & DiCarlo, J. (1992). Stimulus configuration, classical conditioning, and hippocampal function. *Psychological Review*, *99*, 268-305.
Schuster, H. G., & Wagner, P. (1990). A model for neuronal oscillations in the visual cortex. 2. Phase description of the feature dependent synchronization. *Biological Cybernetics*, *64*, 83-85.
Sompolinsky, H., Golomb, D., & Kleinfeld, D. (1990). Global processing of visual stimuli in a neural network of coupled oscillators. *Proceedings of National Academy of Sciences, 87*, 7200-7204.
Strogatz, S. H., & Mirollo, R. E. (1988). Phase-locking and critical phenomena of coupled nonlinear oscillators with random intrinsic frequencies. *Physica D*, *31*, 143-168.
Strong, G. (1993). Phase logic is biologically relevant logic. *Behavioral and Brain Science, 168*, 472-473.
Strong, G., & Whitehead, B. A. (1989). A solution to the tag assignment problem for neural networks. *Behavioral and Brain Science*, *12*, 381-433.
Wang, D. L., Buhmann, J., & Malsburg, C. von der (1990). Pattern segmentation in associative memory. *Neural Computation, 2*, 94-106.
Zeki, S., & Shipp, S. (1988) The functional logic of cortical connections. *Nature*, *335*, 311-317.

15

Attentional Network Streams of Synchronized 40-Hz Activity in a Cortical Architecture of Coupled Oscillatory Associative Memories

Bill Baird
University of California at Berkeley

Todd Troyer
University of California at San Francisco

Frank Eeckman
Lawrence Berkeley Laboratory

ABSTRACT

We have developed a neural network architecture that implements a theory of attention, learning, and trans-cortical communication based on adaptive synchronization of 5-20-Hz and 30-80-Hz oscillations between cortical areas. It assigns functional significance to EEG, ERP, and neuroimaging data.

Using dynamical systems theory, the architecture is constructed from recurrently interconnected oscillatory associative memory modules that model higher order sensory and motor areas of cortex. The modules learn connection weights that cause the system to evolve under a 5-20-Hz clocked sensorimotor processing cycle by a sequence of transitions of synchronized 30-80-Hz oscillatory attractors within the modules.

The architecture employs selective "attentional" control of the synchronization of the 30-80- Hz oscillations between modules to direct the flow of communication and computation to recognize and generate sequences. The 30-80-Hz attractor amplitude patterns code the information content of a cortical area, whereas phase and frequency are used to "softwire" the network, since only the synchronized areas communicate by exchanging amplitude information; the activity of non-resonating modules contributes chaotic crosstalk noise.

Attentional control is modeled as a special subset of the modules with outputs that affect the resonant frequencies of other areas. They learn to control synchrony among these modules and direct the flow of computation (attention) to effect transitions of attractors within the areas to generate the strings of a Reber grammar. The internal crosstalk chaos is used to drive the required random transitions of the system that allow infinite nonrepeating sequences to be generated.

The system works like a broadcast network where the unavoidable crosstalk to all areas from previous learned connections is overcome by frequency coding to allow the moment to moment operation of attentional communication only between selected task-relevant areas. The behavior of the time traces in different modules of the architecture models the temporary appearance and switching of the synchronization of 5-20- and 30-80-Hz oscillations between cortical areas that is observed during sensorimotor tasks in monkeys and humans (Bressler & Nakamura, 1993; Gevins et al., 1989a, 1989b).

The architecture models the 5-20-Hz evoked potentials seen in the EEG as the control signals that determine the sensorimotor processing cycle. The 5-20-Hz clocks that drive these control signals in the architecture model thalamic pacemakers, which are thought by many physiologists to control the excitability of neocortical tissue through similar nonspecific biasing currents that cause the cognitive and sensory evoked potentials of the EEG (Elbert, 1993; Rockstroh, 1989). The 5-20-Hz cycles are thought to "quantize time" and form the basis of derived somatomotor rhythms with periods up to seconds that entrain to each other in motor coordination and to external rhythms in speech perception (Gray, 1982; O'Keefe & Nadel, 1978).

1. INTRODUCTION

Patterns of synchronized gamma band (30-80-Hz) oscillation have been observed in the large-scale activity (local field potentials) of vertebrate olfactory cortex (Freeman & Baird, 1987) and visual neocortex (Engel, König, Gray, & Singer, 1990; Freeman & van Dijk, 1987; Gray, König, Engel, & Singer, 1989) and shown to predict the olfactory, visual, auditory, and somatosensory pattern recognition responses of a trained animal (Barrie, Freeman, & Lenhart, 1996). Similar observations of gamma oscillation in auditory and motor cortex (in primates), and in the retina, thalamus, hippocampus, reticular formation, and EMG have been reported. Furthermore, gamma activity has been also found in insects, invertebrates, amphibians, reptiles, and birds. This suggests that gamma oscillation may be as fundamental to neural processing at the network level as action potentials are at the cellular level.

Additional evidence in monkeys and humans shows that this synchronized activity is most prominent in tasks requiring attention and that changing patterns of interarea synchronization correlate with the stages of sensorimotor tasks (Bressler, Coppola, & Nakamura, 1993; Bressler & Nakamura, 1993; Gevins et al., 1989a, 1989b). There is further evidence that although the oscillatory activity appears to be roughly periodic, it is actually chaotic when examined in detail (Freeman, 1987).

This suggests that oscillatory network modules form the actual cortical substrate of the diverse sensory, motor, and cognitive operations now studied in nonoscillatory networks. It remains to be shown how networks with more complex dynamics can perform these operations and what possible advantages are to be gained by such complexity. Our challenge is to accomplish real tasks that brains can do, using ordinary differential equations, in networks that are as faithful as possible to the known anatomy and dynamics of cortex. We have therefore constructed an architecture with interacting sensory and motor areas whose features can be mapped onto the known structure and dynamics of cerebral cortex, and applied it to a task that human brains can do — grammatical inference. We show how a set of novel mechanisms utilizing these complex dynamics can be configured to solve attentional and perceptual processing problems, and how associative memories may be coupled to recognize and generate sequential behavior.

Because we have developed a class of mathematically well-understood associative memory networks with complex dynamics, we can take a constructive approach to building a cortical architecture, using these networks as modules, in the same way that digital computers may be designed from well behaved flip-flop circuits. The construction views higher order cortex as a set of coupled oscillatory associative memories, and is also guided by the principle that attractors must be used by macroscopic systems for reliable computation in the presence of noise. This system must function reliably in the midst of noise generated by crosstalk from its own activity.

Present day digital computers are built of flip-flops which, at the level of their transistors, are continuous dissipative dynamical systems with different attractors underlying the symbols we call "0" and "1." In a similar manner, the network we have constructed can act as a symbol processing system and solve a grammatical inference problem. Even though it is constructed from a system of continuous nonlinear ordinary differential equations, the system can operate as a discrete-time and discrete state symbol processing architecture, but with analog input and oscillatory subsymbolic representations.

An important element of intracortical communication in the brain, and between modules in this architecture, is the ability of a module to detect and respond to the proper input signal from a particular module, when inputs from other modules that are irrelevant to the present computation are contributing crosstalk noise. We demonstrate that selective control of synchronization, which we hypothesize to be a model of "attention," can be used to solve this coding problem and control program flow in an architecture with dynamic attractors.

The crosstalk noise from the chaotic activity in unsynchronized modules supplies an input that is actually essential to the random choice of output attractors required for the search process of reinforcement learning and the generation of the strings of a grammar. We argue that chaos in the dynamics of neural ensembles at the network level is required as a noise source of sufficient magnitude to perturb network dynamics for an unbiased search process.

In future work, we intend to model specific cortical areas of known function so as to simulate and investigate the mechanisms of the various aphasias, apraxias, and dyslexias caused by cortical lesions in humans. We hope to explain how the uniform circuitry of cortex learns to self-organize its interconnections to become such a powerful processor of such diverse functionality. With the rapid evolution of new cortical probes such as VLSI electrode arrays, functional MRI, and fast optical dyes, there promises to be a wealth of new data on neural and cognitive processes that can refine the model and lead to a detailed understanding of high level neural processing.

The model cortical architecture is designed to demonstrate and investigate the computational capabilities of the following possible mechanisms and features of neural computation:

- Sequential sensorimotor computation with coupled associative memories.
- Combined use of attractor neural networks and connectionist map learning networks.
- Computation with attractors for reliable operation in the presence of noise.
- Operation of associative memories near multiple self-organized critical points for bifurcation control of attractor transitions.
- Discrete time and state symbol processing arising from continuum dynamics by bifurcations of attractors.
- Hybrid analog and symbolic computation.
- Attentional networks of synchronized "cognitive processing streams" controlling intercortical communication.
- Broad spectrum intercortical communication by synchronization of chaotic attractors.
- Chaotic search — chaotic crosstalk driving random choice of attractors in network modules.

2. BIOLOGICAL AND PSYCHOLOGICAL FOUNDATIONS

2.1. Attentional Networks of Synchronized Activity

There is abundant evidence for our claim that synchronized 30-80 Hz gamma band activity in the brain accomplishes attentional processing, because it appears in cortex where attention is required. For example, it is found in motor and premotor cortex of monkeys when they must pick a raisin out of a small box, but not when a rote lever press delivers the reward (Murthy & Fetz, 1992). In human attention experiments, 30-80-Hz activity in auditory cortex goes up when subjects are instructed to pay attention to their ears instead of reading (Tiitinen et al., 1993). Gamma activity declines in the dominant hemisphere along with errors in a learnable target and distractors task, but not when the distractors and target vary at random on each trial (Sheer, 1989). Anesthesiologists use the absence of 40-Hz activity as a reliable indicator of unconsciousness (Galambos, Makeig, & Talmachoff, 1981). Recent work has shown that cats with convergent and divergent strabismus who fail on tasks where perceptual binding is required also do not exhibit cortical synchrony (König et al., 1993). This is evidence that gamma synchronization is perceptually functional and not epiphenomenal.

The architecture illustrates the notion that synchronization of gamma band activity not only preattentively "binds" the features of inputs in primary sensory cortex into "objects," but further binds the activity of an attended object to oscillatory activity in associational and higher-order sensory and motor cortical areas to create an evolving attentional network of intercommunicating cortical areas that directs behavior. For example, consider that two sensory objects in the visual field are separately bound in primary visual cortex by synchronization of their components at different phases or frequencies. One object may be selectively attended to by its entrainment to oscillatory processing at higher levels such as V4 or IT, as von der Malsburg originally suggested (Malsburg & Schneider, 1986). These in turn are in synchrony with oscillatory activity in motor areas to select the attractors there which are directing motor output.

This is a model of "attended activity" as that subset that has been included in the selectively attended processing of the moment by synchronization to this network. This involves both a simultaneous spatial grouping of activity and a binding of two most recent steps of a sequence — a "sequential" grouping. Only inputs that are synchronized to the internal oscillatory activity of a module can effect the proper learned *transitions* of attractors within it.

2.1.1. Auditory and Cognitive Attentional Streams. The binding of sequences of attractor transitions between modules of the architecture by synchronization of their activity is similar to the "sequential binding" of perceptual and cognitive "streams" investigated by Bregman (1978), Jones and Boltz (1989), and others. In audition, successive events of a sound source are bound together into a distinct sequence or "stream" and segregated from other sequences so that one pays attention to only one sound source at a time (the cocktail party problem). Subjects presented with alternating tones of different frequency hear a single sequence bifurcate into two separate sequences or streams of high and low tones as the rate of presentation goes up and the frequency separation of the tones increases. Only one stream can be attended at a time, as evidenced by a subject's inability to determine the order of events between streams (Bregman, 1978).

We view the attentional network as a stream because the synchronized cortical areas within it are moving through a sequentially bound series of attractors at the 10-Hz rate. If attractors representing words are sequencing in a synchronized sensorimotor "phonological loop" between Wernicke and Broca's areas, such a stream would be the physiological basis of "cognitive streams" of subvocalized language or thought.

Cognitive streams are in evidence when two stories are told in alternating segments and listeners are unable to recall the relative order of events between them. The model incorporates the hypothesis that a thalamically coordinated cognitive stream of this synchronized activity loops from primary cortex to associational and higher order sensory and motor areas through hippocampus and back to bind them into the evolving attentional network of coupled cortical areas that directs behavior. The feedback from higher-order to primary cortical areas allows top-down voluntary control to switch this attentional stream or "searchlight" (Treisman, 1984) from one source preattentively bound in primary cortex to another source separately bound at a nearby frequency or phase.

This hypothesis explains and is substantiated by the MEG tomographic observations showing large-scale rostral to caudal motor-sensory sweeps of coherent thalamocortical 40-Hz activity across the entire brain (Ribary et al., 1991; Steriade & Llinas, 1988). This technique with millimeter and millisecond resolution literally gives a picture of the inner attentional stream. The phase of this sweep cycle is reset by sensory input in waking, but not in dream states.

2.1.2. Perceptual and Motor Rhythms. There is considerable evidence from studies of motor and perceptual performance that motor and perceptual behavior is organized by neural rhythms with periods in the range of 100-1500 milliseconds, and that entrainment of these to external rhythms in speech and other forms of communication, and to internal rhythms in motor coordination is essential to effective human performance (Jones, 1976; Jones & Boltz, 1994; McAuley, 1994).

In this view, just as two cortical areas must synchronize to communicate, so must two nervous systems. Work using frame-by-frame film analysis of human verbal interaction (Condon & Ogston, 1966) shows evidence of synchrony of gesture and body movement *changes* and EEG of both speaker and listener with the onsets of phonemes in speech at the level of a 10-Hz "microrhythm" — the base clock rate of our models. Infants are said to synchronize their spontaneous body flailings at this 10-Hz level to the mothers voice accents or to a recording of her voice, whereas autistics show no such synchrony and schizophrenics do not even self-synchronize.

In the "active touch" of rats exploring objects, their fast (10-Hz) paw palpitations will synchronize with an object vibrating at nearly this frequency (Glassman, 1994). In our model, these behavioral rhythms are also external reflections of internal cortical control rhythms, and should therefore be visible in the EEG. In fact, recent work by Bressler and Kelso shows prominent 1-3-Hz rhythms over most of cortex in phase with 1-3-Hz finger tapping behaviors (Bressler & Nakamura, 1993).

Experiments on bimanual tasks by Treffner and Turvey (1993) and Kelso, de Gutzman, and Holroyd (1991) show that human motor performance is constrained by physical law such that very high dimensional motor systems can be modeled by simple low dimensional dynamical systems with attractors. They demonstrate that coordination of rhythmic tasks such as the unconscious synchronizing of a right hand-held pendulum to auditory clicks (Treffner & Turvey, 1993), or to another pendulum in the left hand (Kelso et al., 1991) which is passively driven, follows the laws of entrainment of coupled nonlinear oscillators. It is characterized by the bifurcation diagram of Arnold tongues and the Farey tree of resonances (ratio of periods $\omega_1:\omega_2$) at which the two systems may synchronize (Treffner & Turvey, 1993). These experiments suggest the operation of automatic synchronization of rhythmic cycles within the cerebellar-striatal-thalamo-cortical system. We hypothesize next that interacting cortical cycles and thalamic clocks as captured in our model are the basis of this phenomenon.

Not only are these rhythms evident in motor behavior, but there is considerable evidence that perceptual attention itself has temporal rhythms (Jones, 1976). Expectation rhythms that support Jones' theory have been found in the auditory EEG. In experiments where the arrival time of a target stimulus is regular enough to be learned by an experimental subject, it has been shown that the 10-Hz activity *in advance of the stimulus* becomes phase locked to that expected arrival time (Basar, 1980). The same has been shown for hippocampal theta in rats, which is also found to be entrained to the speed of locomotion. This fits our model of rhythmic expectation where the 10-Hz rhythm is a fast base clock that is shifted in phase and frequency to produce a match in timing between the stimulus arrival and the output of longer period cycles derived from this base clock.

Evidence showing activation of 10-Hz oscillation in thalamus and cortex by a first stimulus in cortical evoked potential studies in auditory and sensorimotor cortex and phase resetting by a second stimulus lends further physiological support to this picture of adapting thalamo-cortical cycles (Kopecz, Schoner, Spengler, & Dinse, 1993; Schoner, Kopecz, Spengler, & Dinse, 1992). There is abundant evidence (Basar, 1980) that cortical rhythms from 3 to 100 Hz in visual, auditory, and somatosensory areas as well as the reticular system will entrain to periodic inputs. Steady stimulation at either 10 or 40 Hz in audition, vision, or somatosensation causes entrainment of 10- or 40-Hz activity in corresponding cortical areas. 20-Hz stimulation entrains the 40-Hz activity at a 1:2 resonance ratio and has been used medically as a diagnostic for proper function of cortical areas (Sheer, 1989).

2.2. Cortical Cycles

In our models, the 10-Hz sensorimotor cycles form the natural basis of these rhythms and can be employed to generate and entrain rhythmic motor output or temporal perceptual expectancies ("dynamic attention"); (Baird, 1997). We propose that the associative networks of the neocortex are clocked to change oscillatory attractors at a 5-20-Hz "framing rate" under thalamic control — much as the olfactory system appears to be clocked to change attractors between 40-Hz "bursts" by the 3-8-Hz respiratory rhythm (Baird, 1990b). Psychological experiments suggest the existence of multiple adaptive clocks whose periods can be modulated by input, arousal, neurotransmitters, and drugs (Jones, 1976; Meck, 1983, 1991).

In the brain, we hypothesize these cycles to be adaptively controlled by septal and thalamic pacemakers which alter excitability of hippocampal and neocortical tissue through nonspecific biasing currents that appear as the cognitive and sensory evoked potentials of the EEG. The cortical evoked potential is a roughly 10-Hz signal whose peaks and troughs are well known to correlate with stages of cortical information processing in sensorimotor tasks. It exhibits different topographic patterns of positivity in some cortical areas and negativity in others for different tasks (Gevins et al., 1989a, 1989b). We hypothesize that these are biasing currents reflecting the reciprocal action of thalamic clocking on different cortical areas to control the transmission of information between them. As in our model, some areas are opened to receive information and change attractors whereas others are clamped at their attractors to transmit their states to other areas (without disturbance from feedback connections as the receiving areas change state).

A number of studies now show that the famous "desynchronization" of EEG by reticular formation stimulation is actually a potentiation of the 40-Hz activity relative to the 10-Hz alpha activity (Galambos et al., 1981; Matthais, Roelfsema, König, Engel, & Singer, 1996). "Binding" by 40-Hz synchronization is also shown to be increased by reticular stimulation during visual stimulus presentation, without altering the stimulus specificity of the synchronization (Matthais et al., 1996). The 10-Hz activity is still present but it is masked by the gamma activity and must be averaged to be detected. Recent evidence shows that 40-Hz amplitude in primary auditory cortex is indeed modulated by the 10-Hz cycle — being boosted on the surface negative phase and attenuated on the positive phase (Galambos et al., 1981; Makeig & Galambos, 1989).

We hypothesize, for example, that CNV represents the clamping for "broadcast" at high amplitude of a cortical attractor state representing the expected stimulus. Then the P300 response to an oddball stimulus is indeed an "updating" to change that cortical attractor, as Donchin originally hypothesized (Donchin & Coles, 1988; Galambos et al., 1981), which is allowed by the unclamping due to the biasing currents visible as the P300 wave.

The schematic alternation of sensory and motor states in the model is inspired by the structure of cerebral cortex, with its segregation and pairing of functionally related sensory and motor areas across the central sulcus, and because it accomplishes the task of "quantizing time" (Gray, 1982; O'Keefe & Nadel, 1978) and distinguishing temporal order by "action-reaction." This allows the implementation of sequence learning weight changes between time steps without requiring that neurons somehow "store" their last activation states while engaging in new activity.

We do not assume that all cortical areas are associative memories — especially primary cortical areas where no categorical learning is in evidence. We hypothesize that attractors in higher order and associational areas (parietal, inferotemporal, cingulate, frontal, premotor, hippocampal, and entorhinal) feed back to lower levels to bias and categorically stabilize perception or direct motor output.

We subscribe to the modular view of Kosslyn and Koenig (1995), where the higher order areas contain modality specific representations that output back to primary areas. These feedback connections serve to check their states against input and filter primary inputs with their expectations or generate activity corresponding to mental images in the absence of input activity. The association areas then contain stereotyped modality independent pointers to these higher order representations, which can be manipulated as symbols in language in a highly abstract fashion (Hummel & Holyoak, 1997). These are just the roles suited to the attractors of our symbol processing system on both associative and higher order levels.

The categorical input and output modules of our model architecture are intended to correspond to higher order sensory and premotor areas, where categories of input and output are formed, and the context and hidden layer modules perhaps model patches of parietal and frontal association cortex respectively. The attentional control modules could be thought of as parts of posterior parietal and prefrontal cortex, as suggested by PET and lesion studies. In the interpretation of our model, these areas control 40 Hz synchrony in other areas through abundant layer VI outputs to thalamus (e.g., to pulvinar for visual areas); (Ribary et al., 1991; Steriade & Llinas, 1988).

Temporal transitions may not always be between officially sensory and motor areas, but between any reciprocally clocked and connected areas. For example, premotor and primary motor areas may cycle, as suggested by PET evidence of mutual activity during complex sequencing of finger movements (Roland, Larsen, Lassen, & Skinhoj, 1980). The fact that the language sensory association cortex is destroyed in Wernicke's aphasia, yet speech production is fluent, suggests that this motor output does not require cycling between the language sensory and motor association areas (Damasio & Geschwind, 1984). Modulation by that cycle however appears to be required for *meaningful* speech.

Similarly, perceptual cycles may occur between posterior parietal and primary sensorimotor cortex in tactile object recognition. The model requirement is only that activations preceding any new state are available in the reciprocal cortical area that drove it to change states. Then Hebbian sequence learning weight changes may be used during reinforcement learning.

2.2.1. Cycle Timing and Coordination. The mechanisms found in neocortex must have more rudimentary precursors in the reptile's brain containing only three layered paleocortex. A primary example of a cortical sensorimotor cycle is found in the hippocampus — which may be thought of as the highest level association cortex for reptiles, and which connects only to higher order neocortical areas and above in mammals. The hippocampus is thought to be a system wherein time is “quantized” (Gray, 1982; O'Keefe & Nadel, 1978) by the theta rhythm, to pace the steps of a motor program, and to separate Time t from Time t-1 so that predictions of the resulting sensory and motivational states held in the subiculum can be compared with input presently arriving in entorhinal cortex. There is a 90-180 degree phase shift in the peaks of the theta rhythm between the dentate- CA3 input areas and the CA1-subiculum output region (Winston, 1975). This supports our notion that the theta rhythm controls the processing cycle by reciprocal clocking of these areas.

The cerebellum is thought to compute timing in motor and perceptual processing, and evidence shows increased variability of motor timing and perceptual time judgments with lateral neocerebellar lesions or cooling of the dentate output (Ivry, 1996). Cerebellar output from the dentate nucleus can only affect *perceptual* timing through its output to the frontal, premotor, and motor areas. This suggests that higher-order sensorimotor loops are involved in such timing, and dense connections exist between auditory higher-order sensorimotor areas (Broca/Wernicke) to allow this. Inasmuch as the powerful climbing fiber input to the cerebellum is strongly synchronized to appear on the beat of a 10-Hz cycle by gap junctions in the inferior olive (Welsh, Lang,

Sugihara, & Llinas, 1995), it seems likely that this rhythm produces a strong temporal reference for the Purkinje cell output of processing in the cerebellum.

We predict that the dentate output will be in synchrony with the thalamic 5-20-Hz rhythm through which that output must pass to impact on frontal motor areas. Even if this system is learning temporal intervals as some suggest (Ivry, 1996), it must participate in the time warping available through adapting the phase and frequency of the basic sensorimotor cycle, or no relative timing invariance will be possible. We hypothesize that absolute memory intervals, like absolute clocks, are too rigid to be of use in motor timing.

The basal ganglia are another prominent subcortical system that receives input from all of cortex and sends feedback to the frontal half through the thalamus. Like cerebellum, they are thought to modulate and perhaps initiate frontal motor action within the context of the last complete brain state. Like the inferior olive, the substantial nigra pars compacta is seen to convey training signals to the striatum (Houk & Wise, 1995), but of expected reward in a given sensorimotor context instead of actual and expected motor and timing errors of that same context. In both cases these signals are prominent during learning and fade as habit takes over. The work of Meck (1983) and others suggests a roughly 10-Hz driving action from the substantia nigra like that from the inferior olive, and they believe parts of striatum act as accumulators for time intervals of up to minutes in duration. This might be the more reasonable temporal range for expectations of reward, versus the seconds range for timing in immediate action and perception.

The thalamus sends strong output to the striatum as well as mediating its output from the globus pallidus. The pallidum, like the dentate of the cerebellum, receives inhibitory output from the striatum. The thalamus is also reciprocally connected to the septo-hippocampal system, sending input to septum from the centromedian nucleus, and to the hippocampus through the perforant path. It receives strong output in turn from the fornix through the hypothalamic mammillary bodies on the way to cingulate cortex in the Papez circuit.

In all these systems there is an adaptive 5-20-Hz rhythmic context within which behavior is coordinated. We predict that temporary synchrony or resonance must occur between 5-20-Hz activity in cortical areas, thalamus, substantia nigra, inferior olive, reticular formation, and the septo-hippocampal system at certain phases of many sensorimotor tasks, for normal coordinated function. The thalamus is the central hub of all these networks, and should be the master coordinator of much activity. Recent work shows synchronized 10-Hz activity in the reticular system, thalamus, and somatomotor cortex during exploratory "whisking" in rats (Nicolelis, Baccala, Lin, & Chapin, 1995). Data in the inferior olive, substantia nigra, or septum were not taken at that time, but other work has shown 10-Hz synchrony of the olive and vibrissae during whisking (Welsh, Lang, Sugihara, & Llinas, 1995).

2.3. Chaotic Search

In cortex there is an issue as to what may constitute a source of randomness of sufficient magnitude to perturb the behavior of the large ensemble of neurons involved in neural activity at the cortical network level. It does not seem likely that the well-known molecular level of fluctuations that is easily averaged within a single neuron or small group of neurons can do the job.

The architecture here models the hypothesis that deterministic chaos in the macroscopic dynamics of a network of neural populations (the crosstalk noise from the chaotic activity of unsynchronized modules), which is the same order of magnitude as the coherent activity, can serve this purpose. In our architecture, this chaos serves the function of creating information, as discussed by Freeman (1992). It supplies uncertainty in the choice of attractors so that the actual choice learned by the system after reinforcement becomes a gain in information. In the architecture using synchronized chaotic instead of oscillatory attractors, we see the kind of intermittent "broadband" synchrony found by Bressler et al. (1993), where the coherence accross *a set of frequencies* rises and falls simultaneously.

3. THE MODEL ARCHITECTURE

3.1. Associative Memory Modules

In this section, we describe the "mechanics" of the operation of the higher-order cortical system as illustrated by the grammatical inference problem. The network modules of this architecture were developed previously as models of olfactory cortex, or caricatures of "patches" of neocortex with a well specified mapping of model features to known physiology (Baird, 1990a, 1990b, 1992). A particular subnetwork is formed by a set of neural populations whose interconnections also contain higher order synapses. These synapses determine attractors for that subnetwork independent of other subnetworks. Each subnetwork module assumes only minimal coupling justified by known anatomy (Baird, 1990b).

The mathematical foundation for the construction of network modules is contained in the normal form projection algorithm (Baird, 1990c; Baird & Eeckman, 1993). This is a learning algorithm for recurrent analog neural networks that allows associative memory storage of periodic and chaotic attractors. An N-node module can be shown to function as an associative memory for up to $N/2$ oscillatory and $N/3$ chaotic memory attractors (Baird, 1989; Baird & Eeckman, 1993).

By analyzing the network in the polar form of these "normal form coordinates" (Guckenheimer & Holmes, 1983), the amplitude and phase dynamics have a particularly simple interaction. When the input to a module is synchronized with its intrinsic oscillation, the amplitudes of the periodic activity may be considered separately from the phase rotation, and the network of the module may be viewed as a static network with these amplitudes as its activity. We further show analytically that the network modules we have constructed have a strong tendency to synchronize as required.

Previously we have shown how the discrete-time "simple recurrent" network algorithm (Elman, 1991) can be implemented in a network completely described by continuous ordinary differential equations (Baird & Eeckman, 1992; Baird, Troyer, &

Eeckman, 1993). We have also shown that the system can function as the 13-state finite automaton that generates the infinite set of six symbol strings that are defined by the Reber grammar described in Cleeremans, Servan-Schreiber, and McClelland (1989).

3.1.1. A Competing Oscillator Module. To illustrate the behavior of individual network modules, we examine a binary (two attractor) module; the behavior of modules with more than two attractors is similar. Such a unit is defined in polar normal form coordinates by the following equations of the Hopf normal form:

$$\dot{r}_{1i} = u_i r_{1i} - c r_{1i}^3 + (d - b\sin(\omega_{clock} t)) r_{1i} r_{0i}^2 + \sum_j w_{ij}^+ I_j \cos(\theta_j - \theta_{1i})$$

$$\dot{r}_{0i} = u_i r_{0i} - c r_{0i}^3 + (d - b\sin(\omega_{clock} t)) r_{0i} r_{1i}^2 + \sum_j w_{ij}^- I_j \cos(\theta_j - \theta_{0i})$$

$$\theta_{1i} = \omega_i + \sum_j w_{ij}^+ (I_j / r_{1i}) \sin(\theta_j - \theta_{1i})$$

$$\theta_{0i} = \omega_i + \sum_j w_{ij}^- (I_j / r_{0i}) \sin(\theta_j - \theta_{0i})$$

The clocked parameter $b \sin(\omega_{\mathrm{clock}} t)$ controls the level of inhibitory coupling or *competition* between oscillatory modes within each module. It is used to control attractor transitions in the Elman architecture discussed later. It has lower frequency (1/10) than the intrinsic frequency of the unit ω_i. When the oscillators are synchronized with the input, $\theta_j - \theta_{1i} = 0$, and the phase terms $\cos(\theta_j - \theta_{1i}) = \cos(0) = 1$ disappear. This leaves the amplitude equations $\dot{r}_{1i}$ and $\dot{r}_{0i}$ with static inputs $\Sigma_j w_{ij}^+ I_j$ and $\Sigma_j w_{ij}^- I_j$.

Examination of the phase equations shows that a unit has a strong tendency to synchronize with an input of similar frequency. Defining the phase difference, $\phi = \theta_0 - \theta_I = \theta_0 - \omega_I t$ between a unit θ_0 and its input θ_I we can write a differential equation for the phase difference ϕ,

$$\dot{\phi} = \omega_0 - \omega_I + (r_I / r_0) \sin(-\phi),$$

so the steady state value of ϕ is

$$\hat{\phi} = -\sin^{-1}[(r_0 / r_I)(\omega_I - \omega_0)].$$

There is an attractor $\hat{\phi}$ at zero phase difference $\phi = \theta_0 - \theta_I = 0$, and a repellor at 180 degrees in the phase difference equations $\dot{\phi}$ for either side of a unit driven by an input of the same frequency, $\omega_I - \omega_0 = 0$. In simulations, the interconnected network of these units described later synchronizes robustly within a few cycles following a perturbation.

If the frequencies of attractors in some modules of the architecture are randomly dispersed by a significant amount, $\omega_I - \omega_0 \neq 0$, phase-lags appear first, then synchronization is lost in those units. An oscillating module therefore acts as a band pass filter for oscillatory inputs.

Thus we have network modules that emulate static network units in their amplitude activity when fully phase-locked to their input. Amplitude information is transmitted between modules, with an oscillatory carrier as in Freeman's (1975) notion of the "wave packet."

3.1.2. Attractor Transitions by Bifurcation. For fixed values of the competition, in a completely synchronized system, the internal amplitude dynamics define a gradient dynamical system for a fourth order energy function. Figure 15.1 shows this energy landscape with no external input for high and low levels of competition. External inputs that are phase-locked to the module's intrinsic oscillation simply add a linear tilt to the landscape.

For low levels of competition, there is a broad circular valley. When tilted by external input, there is a unique equilibrium that is determined by the bias in tilt along one axis over the other. Thinking of r_{1i} as the "activity" of the unit, this activity becomes a monotonically increasing function of input. The module behaves as an analog connectionist unit whose transfer function can be approximated by a sigmoid. We refer to this as the "analog" mode of operation of the module. With high levels of competition, the unit will behave as a binary (bistable) digital flip-flop element. There are two deep potential wells, one on each axis. Hence the final steady state of the unit is determined by which basin of attraction contains the initial state of the system in the analog mode of operation before competition is increased by the clock. At high competition this state is "clamped." It changes little under the influence of external input because a tilt will move the location of the attractor basins only slightly.

Hence the module performs a winner-take-all choice on the coordinates of its initial state and maintains that choice independent of external input. This is the "digital" or "quantized" mode of operation of a module. We use this bifurcation in the behavior of the modules to control information flow within the network described next.

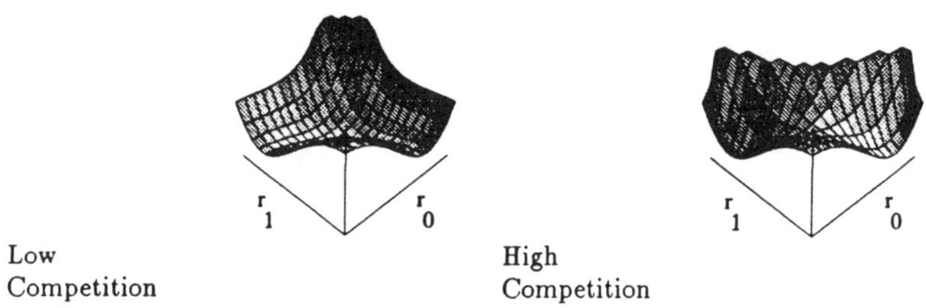

Fig. 15.1. Energy landscape of amplitudes of binary oscillatory unit with no external input. For low levels of competition, there is a broad circular valley. With high levels of competition, there is a deep potential wells on each axis. Phase-locked external inputs simply add a linear tilt to the landscape which will shift a single attractor across the circular valley at low competition, but cannot move it from a potential well at high competition.

3.2. Sensorimotor Architecture

To explore the use of these capabilities and demonstrate how sequential behavior might be learned by coupling these associative memories, we constructed a system that emulates the larger 13 state automata similar (less one state) to the one studied by Cleeremans, Servan-Schreiber, and McClelland (1989) in the second part of their paper. The graph of this automaton consists of two subgraph branches each of which has the graph structure of the automaton learned in the previous work mentioned earlier (Baird et al., 1993), but with different assignments of transition output symbols (see Fig. 15.2). We used two types of modules in implementing the Elman network architecture shown in Fig. 15.3. The input and output layer each consist of a single associative memory module with six oscillatory attractors (six competing oscillatory modes), one for each of the six symbols in the grammar. The hidden and context layers consist of the binary "units" above composed of two oscillatory attractors. We think of one mode within the unit as representing "1" and the other as representing "0."

The architecture consists of 13 binary modules in the hidden and context layers — three of which are special frequency control modules. The hidden and context layers are divided into four groups: the first three correspond to each of the two subgraphs plus

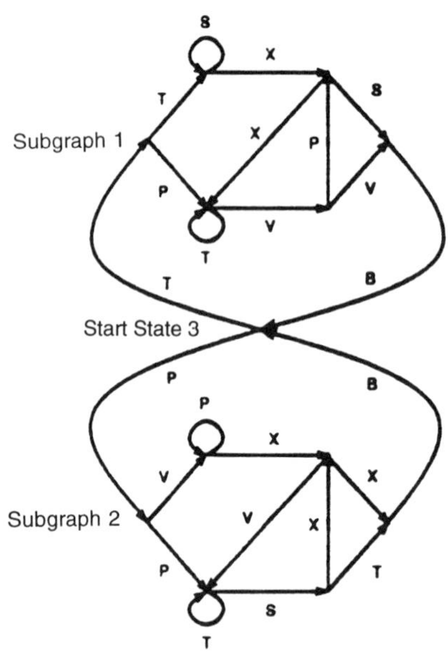

Fig. 15.2. Graph diagram of the automaton emulated by the network to generate the symbol strings of a grammar. It is composed of two subgraphs joined by a start/end state. At each node (network state), one of two symbols (output module attractors) is chosen at random (by crosstalk noise) and fed back as input to the network to direct the next transition of state as shown by the arrows of the diagram.

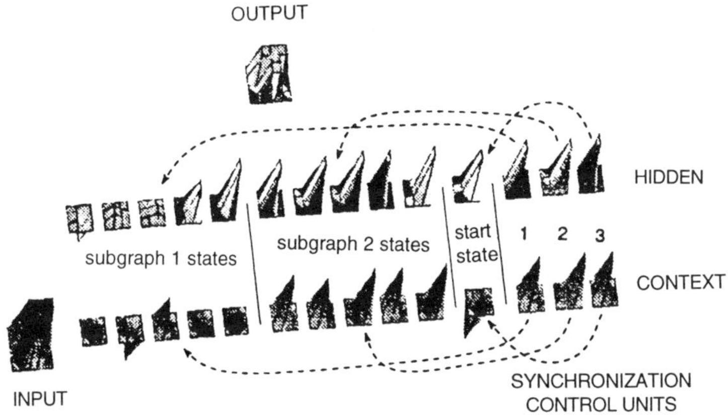

Fig. 15.3. Sensorimotor architecture: The input and output layer each consist of a single associative memory module with six oscillatory attractors, one for each of the six symbols in the grammar. The hidden and context layers consist of binary "units" composed of two oscillatory attractors. Activity levels oscillate up and down through the plane of the paper. Dotted lines show control outputs from the attention modules. Control unit 2 is at the one attractor (right side of the square active) and the hidden units coding for states of subgraph 2 are in synchrony with the input and output modules. Here in midcycle, all modules are clamped at their attractors.

the start state, and the fourth group consists of three control modules, each of which has only a special control output that perturbs the resonant frequencies of the modules of a particular state coding group when the control unit is in the zero state, as illustrated by the dotted control lines in Figure 15.3.

3.2.1. Sensorimotor Cycles. The time steps (sensorimotor cycles) of this discrete time recurrent (Elman) architecture system are controlled by rhythmic variation (clocking) of a bifurcation parameter. As shown earlier, this parameter controls the level of inhibitory coupling or "competition" between oscillatory modes within each module. It determines the depth of the potential wells for attractors in the Liapunov function for the amplitudes of oscillation in the "digital mode" of operation, and is lowered to allow attractor transitions to be determined by input in the "analog mode" of operation.

At the beginning of a sensorimotor cycle, the input and context layers are at high competition and their activity is clamped at the bottom of deep basins of attraction. The hidden and output modules are at low competition and therefore behave as a traditional feedforward network free to take on analog values. Then the situation reverses. For a Reber grammar there are always two equally possible next symbols being activated in the output layer, and we let the cross-talk noise break this symmetry so that the winner-take-all dynamics of the output module can chose one. Meanwhile high competition has now also "quantized" and "clamped" the activity in the hidden layer to a fixed binary vector.

Competition then is lowered in the input and context layers, freeing these modules from their attractors. An identity mapping from hidden to context loads the binarized activity of the hidden layer into the context layer for the next cycle. If the architecture is in generation mode, an additional identity mapping from the output to input module places the generated output symbol into the input layer. *We view this alternation and feedback of the information flow as an abstract model of sensory and motor interaction as described earlier*. It is the bifurcation in the phase portrait of a module from one to two attractors that contributes the essential digitization of the system in time and state. A bifurcation is a *discontinuous* change in the dynamical possibilities of a system, such as the appearance or disappearance of an attractor in this case, as the bifurcation parameter (competition) changes. We can think of the analog mode for a module as allowing input to prepare its initial state for the binary *decision* between attractor basins that occurs as competition rises and the double potential well appears. This ability to "clamp" a cortical network at an attractor is essential to the operation of this architecture. If competition is lowered in all units at once, the system soon wanders from its learned transitions, because feedback from units changing state perturbs the states of the units driving the state change. The feedback between sensory and motor modules is effectively cut when one set is clamped at high competition, because its state is then unaffected by that feedback input. The system can thus be viewed as operating in discrete time by alternating sets of transitions between finite sets of attracting states.

This kind of alternate clocking and buffering (clamping) of some states while other states relax is essential to the reliable operation of digital architectures. The clock input on a flip-flop clamps its state until its signal inputs have settled from previous changes and the choice of transition can be made with the proper information available. It is believed that 50-200 msec is about the time required in the brain for all relevant inputs to arrive at a cortical area before it can change state (Miller, 1991). In our view the existence and the rate of the 5-20-Hz sensorimotor processing cycle follows from this neural architectural constraint, just as the clock speed that is possible in a digital computer architecture follows from its buss transmission delays.

When the input and context modules are clamped at their attractors, and the hidden and output modules are in the analog operating mode and synchronized to their inputs, the network approximates the behavior of a standard feedforward network in terms of its amplitude activities. Thus a real valued error can be defined for the hidden and output units and standard learning algorithms like backpropagation and reinforcement learning can be used to train the connections. This is now a symbol processing system, but with analog input and oscillatory subsymbolic representations. The ability to operate as an finite automaton with oscillatory/chaotic "states" is thus an important benchmark for this architecture, but only a subset of its capabilities. At low to zero competition, the suprasystem reverts to one large continuous dynamical system and loses its learned trajectories. We expect that this kind of variation of the operational regime, especially with chaotic attractors inside the modules, though unreliable for habitual behaviors, may nonetheless be very useful in other areas such as the search process of reinforcement learning.

3.2.2. Attentional Control of Synchrony. As already described, an oscillatory network module has a passband outside of which it will not synchronize with an oscillatory input. Modules can therefore easily be desynchronized by perturbing their resonant frequencies, just as thalamic clock frequencies can be perturbed by neural and humoral inputs. Furthermore, only synchronized modules communicate by exchanging amplitude pattern information; the activity of nonresonating modules contributes incoherent crosstalk or noise. The flow of communication between modules can thus be controlled by controlling synchrony. By changing the intrinsic frequency of modules in a patterned way, the *effective* connectivity of the network is changed. The same hardware and connection matrix can thus subserve many different computations and patterns of interaction between modules without crosstalk problems. This control of frequency is our model of *selective attention*.

The attentional controller itself is modeled in this architecture as a special set of three hidden modules with outputs that affect the resonant frequencies of the other corresponding three subsets of hidden modules. The control modules learn to respond to a particular input symbol and context to set the intrinsic frequency of the proper subset of hidden units to synchronize with the input and output layer oscillation. Unselected modules are desynchronized by randomizing the resonant frequencies or applying antiphase inputs so that coherence is lost and a chaos of random phase relations results. This set is no longer communicating with the rest of the network. Thus the flow of communication (attention) within the network can be switched. The system in operation can be made to jump from states in one subgraph of the automaton to an other by desynchronizing the proper subset of hidden modules. The possibilities for transition of the system can thus be controlled by selective synchronization.

When either exit state of a subgraph is reached, the “B” (begin) symbol is then emitted and fed back to the input where it is connected by weights to the attention control modules to turn off the synchrony of the hidden states of the subgraph and allow entrainment of the start state to begin a new string of symbols. This state in turn activates both a “T” and a “P” in the output module. The symbol selected by the crosstalk noise and fed back to the input module is there connected to the control modules to desynchronize the start state module and synchronize in the subset of hidden units coding for the states of the appropriate subgraph and establish there the start state pattern for that subgraph.

In summary, varying levels of intramodule competition control the large-scale *direction* of information flow *between* layers of the architecture. To direct information flow on a finer scale, the “attention” mechanism selects a subset of modules *within* each layer whose output is effective in driving the behavior of the system. Coherent information flows from input to output only through one of the three channels representing subgraphs of the automaton. This is the “stream" or loop of synchronized activity.

The attention control modules thus effect the proper transitions between subgraphs of the automaton. Viewing the automaton as a behavioral program, the control of synchrony constitutes a control of the program flow into its subprograms (the subgraphs of the automaton).

ACKNOWLEDGMENTS

This work was supported by ONR grant N00014-95-1-0744. It is a pleasure to acknowledge the invaluable assistance of Morris Hirsch and Walter Freeman.

REFERENCES

Baird, B. (1989). A bifurcation theory approach to vector field programming for periodic attractors. *Proceedings of the International Joint Conference on Neural Networks, Washington, DC* (Vol. 1, pp. 381-388). Piscataway, NJ: IEEE.

Baird, B. (1990a). Associative memory in a simple model of oscillating cortex. In D. S. Touretzky (Ed.), *Advances in Neural Information Processing Systems 2* (pp. 68-75). San Mateo, CA: Morgan Kaufman.

Baird, B. (1990b). Bifurcation and learning in network models of oscillating cortex. In S. Forest (Ed.), *Emergent Computation* (pp. 365-384). Amsterdam: North Holland. Also in *Physica D*, Volume *42*.

Baird, B. (1990c). A learning rule for CAM storage of continuous periodic sequences. *Proceedings of the International Joint Conference on Neural Networks, San Diego*. (Vol. 3, pp. 493-498). Piscataway, NJ: IEEE.

Baird, B. (1992). Learning with synaptic nonlinearities in a coupled oscillator model of olfactory cortex. In F. H. Eeckman (Ed.), *Analysis and Modeling of Neural Systems* (pp. 319-327). Norwell, MA: Kluwer.

Baird, B. (1997). A cortical network model of cognitive attentional streams, rhythmic expectation, and auditory stream segregation. In J. Bower (Ed.), *Computational Neuroscience `96* (pp. 67-74). New York: Plenum Press

Baird, B., & Eeckman, F. H. (1992). A hierarchical sensory-motor architecture of oscillating cortical area subnetworks. In F. H. Eeckman (Ed.), *Analysis and Modeling of Neural Systems II* (pp. 96-104). Norwell, MA: Kluwer.

Baird, B., & Eeckman, F. H. (1993). A normal form projection algorithm for associative memory. In M. H. Hassoun (Ed.), *Associative Neural Memories*. New York: Oxford University Press.

Baird, B., Troyer, T., & Eeckman, F. H. (1993). Synchronization and grammatical inference in an oscillating Elman network. In S. Hanson, J. Cowan, & C. Giles (Eds.), *Advances in Neural Information Processing Systems 5* (pp. 236-244). San Mateo, CA: Morgan Kaufman.

Barrie, J., Freeman, W. J., & Lenhart, M. D. (1996). Spatiotemporal analysis of prepyriform, visual, auditory, and somesthetic surface EEG's in trained rabbits. *Journal of Neurophysiology*, *76*, 520-539.

Basar, E. (1980). *EEG-Brain Dynamics*. Amsterdam: Elsevier/North Holland Biomedical Press.

Bregman, A. S. (1978). Auditory streaming: Competition among alternative organizations. *Perception and Psychophysics*, *23*, 391-398.

Bressler, S., Coppola, R., & Nakamura, R. (1993). Cortical coherence at multiple frequencies during visual task performance. *Nature*, *366*, 153-156.

Bressler, S., & Nakamura, R. (1993). Inter-area synchronization in macaque neocortex during a visual pattern discrimination task. In F. Eeckman & J. Bower (Eds.), *Neural Systems: Analysis and Modeling* (p. 515). Norwell, MA: Kluwer.

Cleeremans, A., Servan-Schreiber, D., & McClelland, J. (1989). Finite state automata and simple recurrent networks. *Neural Computation*, *1*, 372-381.

Condon, W. S., & Ogston, W. D. (1966). Sound film analysis of normal and pathological behavior patterns. *Journal of Phonetics*, *3*, 75-86.

Damasio, A. R., & Geschwind, N. (1984). The neural basis of language. *Annual Review of Neuroscience*, *7*, 127-147.

Donchin, E., & Coles, M. G. H. (1988). Is the p300 a manifestation of context updating? *Behavioral and Brain Sciences*, *11*, 357-374.

Elbert, T. (1993). Slow cortical potentials reflect the regulation of cortical excitability. In W. C. McCallum & S. H. Curry (Eds.), *Slow Potential Changes in the Human Brain* (pp. 235-251). New York: Plenum.

Elman, J. (1991). Distributed representations, simple recurrent networks, and grammatical structure. *Machine Learning*, *7*, 91-103.

Engel, A. K., König, P., Gray, C., & Singer, W. (1990). Synchronization of oscillatory responses: A mechanism for stimulus-dependent assembly formation in cat visual cortex. In R. Eckmiller (Ed.), *Parallel Processing in Neural Systems and Computers* (pp. 105-108). Amsterdam: Elsevier.

Freeman, W. J. (1975). *Mass Action in the Nervous System*. New York: Academic Press.

Freeman, W. J. (1987). Simulation of chaotic EEG patterns with a dynamic model of the olfactory system. *Biological Cybernetics*, *56*, 139-147.

Freeman, W. J. (1992). Tutorial on neurobiology: From single neurons to brain chaos. *International Journal of Bifurcation and Chaos*, *2*, 451-482.

Freeman, W. J., & Baird, B. (1987). Relation of olfactory EEG to behavior: Spatial analysis. *Behavioral Neuroscience*, *101*, 393-408.

Freeman, W. J., & van Dijk, B. W. (1987). Spatial patterns of visual cortical EEG during conditioned reflex in a rhesus monkey. *Brain Research*, *422*, 267-276.

Galambos, R., Makeig, S., & Talmachoff, J. (1981). A 40-Hz auditory potential recorded from the human scalp. *Proceedings of the National Academy of Sciences*, *78*, 2643-2647.

Gevins, A. S., Bressler, S. L., Morgan, N. H., Cutillo, B. A., White, R. M., Greer, D. S., & Illes, J. (1989a). Event related covariances during a bimanual visuomotor task: I. Methods and analysis of stimulus- and response-locked data. *Electroencephalography and Clinical Neurophysiology*, *74*, 58-75.

Gevins, A. S., Bressler, S. L., Morgan, N. H., Cutillo, B. A., White, R. M., Greer, D. S., & Illes, J. (1989b). Event related covariances during a bimanual visuomotor task: II. Preparation and feedback. *Electroencephalography and Clinical Neurophysiology*, *74*, 147-160.

Glassman, R. B. (1994). Active touch. *Experimental Neurology*, *125*, 134-141.

Gray, C., König, P., Engel, A., & Singer, W. (1989). Oscillatory responses in cat visual cortex exhibit intercolumnar synchronization which reflects global stimulus properties. *Nature (London)*, *338*, 334-337.

Gray, J. A. (1982). *The Neuropsychology of Anxiety*. Oxford: Oxford University Press.

Guckenheimer, J., & Holmes, D. (1983). *Nonlinear Oscillations, Dynamical Systems, and Bifurcations of Vector Fields*. New York: Springer.

Houk, J. C., & Wise, S. P. (1995). Outline for a theory of motor behavior: Involving cooperative actions of the cerebellum, basal ganglia, and cerebral cortex. *Cerebral Cortex*, *5*, 95-110.

Hummel, J. E., & Holyoak, K. J. (1997). Distributed representations of structure: A theory of analogical access and mapping. *Psychological Review*, *111*, 357-374.

Ivry, R. (1996). The many manifestations of the cerebellar timing system. In J. Schmahmann (Ed.), *The Cerebellum and Cognition*. New York: Academic Press.

Jones, M. R. (1976). Time, our lost dimension: Toward a new theory of perception, attention, and memory. *Psychological Review*, *83*, 323-355.

Jones, M. R., & Boltz, M. (1989). Dynamic attending and responses to time. *Psychological Review*, *96*, 459-491.

Kelso, J. A. S., de Gutzman, G. C., & Holroyd, T. (1991). The self-organized phase attractive dynamics of coordination. In A. Babloyantz (Ed.), *Self-Organization, Emergent Properties, and Learning* (pp. 41-62). New York: Plenum Press.

König, P., Engel, A., Lowel, S., & Singer, W. (1993). Squint affects synchronization of oscillatory responses in cat visual cortex. *European Journal of Neuroscience*, *5*, 501-508.

Kopecz, K., Schoner, G., Spengler, F., & Dinse, H. (1993). Dynamical properties of cortical evoked (10-Hz) oscillations: Theory and experiment. *Biological Cybernetics*, *65*, 463-473.

Kosslyn, S. M., & Koenig, O. (1995). *Wet Mind — the New Cognitive Neuroscience*. New York: Free Press.

Makeig, S., & Galambos, R. (1989). The cerp: Event-related perturbations in steady state responses. In E. Basar & T. H. Bullock (Eds.), *Brain Dynamics* (pp. 375-400). Berlin: Springer.

Malsburg, C. von der, & Schneider, W. (1986). A neural cocktail party processor. *Biological Cybernetics*, *54*, 29-40.

Matthais, H., Roelfsema, P., König, P., Engel, A., & Singer, W. (1996). Role of reticular activation in the modulation of intracortical synchronization. *Science*, *272*, 271-274.

McAuley, J. D. (1994). Finding metrical structure in time. In M. C. Mozer, P. Smolensky, D. S. Touretzky, & A. S. Weigand (Eds.), *Proceedings of the 1993 Connectionist Models Summer School* (pp. 219-227). Hillsdale, NJ: Lawrence Erlbaum Associates.

Meck, W. H. (1983). Selective adjustment of the speed of internal clock and memory processes. *Journal of Experimental Psychology: Animal Behavior Processes*, *9*, 171-201.

Meck, W. H. (1991). Modality-specific circadian rhythmicities influence mechanisms of attention and memory for interval timing. *Learning and Motivation*, *22*, 46-62.

Miller, R. (1991). *Cortico-Hippocampal Interplay and the Representation of Contexts in the Brain*. Berlin: Springer-Verlag.

Murthy, V., & Fetz, E. E. (1992). Coherent 25- to 35-Hz oscillations in the sensorimotor cortex of awake behaving monkeys. *Proceedings of the National Academy of Sciences*, *89*, 2643-2647.

Nicolelis, M., Baccala, L., Lin, R., & Chapin, J. (1995). Sensorimotor encoding by synchronous neural ensemble activity at multiple levels of the somatosensory system. *Science*, *268*, 1353-1358.

O'Keefe, J., & Nadel, L. (1978). *The Hippocampus as a Cognitive Map*. Oxford: Oxford University Press.

Ribary, U., Joannides, K., Singh, K., Hasson, R., Bolton, J., Lado, F., Mogliner, A., & Llinas, R. R. (1991). Magnetic field tomography of coherent thalamocortical 40-Hz oscillations in humans. *Proceedings of the National Academy of Sciences*, *88*, 11037-11041.

Rockstroh, B. (1989). *Slow Cortical Potentials and Behavior*. Urban and Schwartzenburg.

Schoner, G., Kopecz, K., Spengler, F., & Dinse, H. (1992). Evoked oscillatory cortical responses are dynamically coupled to peripheral stimuli. *NeuroReport*, *3*, 579-582.

Sheer, D. E. (1989). Sensory and cognitive 40-Hz event related potentials: Behavioral correlates and clinical applications. In E. Basar & T. H. Bullock (Eds.), *Brain Dynamics* (pp. 339-374). Berlin: Springer.

Steriade, M., & Llinas, R. R. (1988). The functional state of the thalamus and the associated neuronal interplay. *Physiological Review*, *68*, 649-742.

Tiitinen, H., Sinkkonen, J., Reinikainen, K., Alho, J., Lavikainen, J., & Näätänen, R. (1993). Selective attention enhances the auditory 40-Hz transient response in humans. *Nature*, *364*, 59-60.

Treffner, P. J., & Turvey, M. T. (1983). Resonance constraints on rhythmic movement. *Journal of Experimental Psychology: Human Perception and Performance*, *19*, 1221-1237.

Treisman, M. (1984). Temporal rhythms and cerebral rhythms. In J. Gibbon & L. Allan (Eds.), *Annals of the New York Academy of Sciences: Timing and Perception* (Vol. 423, pp. 542-565). New York: New York Academy of Sciences.

Welsh, J., Lang, E., Sugihara, I., & Llinas, R. R. (1995). Dynamic organization of motor control within the olivocerebellar system. *Nature*, *374*, 453-457.

Winston, J. (1975). The theta mode. In R. L. Isaacson & K. H. Pribram (Eds.), *The Hippocampus, Volume 2: Neurophysiology and Behavior* (pp.169-183). New York: Plenum.

IV
Applications of Synchronized and Chaotic Oscillations

16
Foraging Search at the Edge of Chaos

George E. Mobus
Western Washington University

Paul S. Fisher
University of North Texas

ABSTRACT

Many animal species are faced with the problem of finding sparsely distributed resources that occur (and disappear) dynamically in a huge space. Furthermore the dynamics of these resources are stochastic and probably chaotic in terms of both spatial and temporal distribution. But they are not completely random. The search strategy is called foraging. It involves two interrelated phases that dominate the behavior of the animal based on the amount of knowledge it has regarding the location and timing of the resource. In the absence of knowledge or cues foraging animals adopt a stochastic search pattern that will have a reasonably high likelihood of bringing them into encounters with the resource. With knowledge or cues, the animal switches to a more directed search behavior.

Autonomous agents such as mobile robots may need to have these capabilities in order to find mission–critical objects yet no current algorithmic or heuristic search method adequately addresses this problem. The serendipitous discovery of a quasi-chaotic oscillating neural circuit used to generate motor signals in a mobile robot has led to the development of an autonomous agent search method that resembles foraging search in a number of details.

An oscillator circuit, based on the concept of a central pattern generator (CPG) in biology, is described qualitatively. Its role in controlling the motion of a mobile robot and the effects it has on search efficiency are presented. Constraining search to potentially fruitful paths *before* any useful heuristics are available to the searcher is a problem of general interest in artificial intelligence. Foraging search based on chaotic oscillators may prove useful in a more general way.

1. INTRODUCTION

Quite typically, mobile robots that search for objects in their environment are programmed to scan the vicinity and, if they spot what they are seeking, plan a movement path to the object. If they do not sense their target object, they plan a movement path that will position them at a new observation point. Most often, these programs seek an optimal path between the two points. These approaches are computationally expensive. In stark contrast, many animals, when searching for food or other resources, exhibit seemingly nonoptimal movements. They can be seen to weave and wander, sometimes erratically, through their search space. Animals are, however, generally successful in finding the resources they seek in spite of this seeming nonoptimal pattern of search behavior.[1]

Many animal species forage for critical survival resources such as food, water, and shelter, as well as what might be called mission resources such as mates or nesting material. Foraging is a search strategy that is employed when the subject knows what object is being sought but doesn't necessarily know where, in a usually vast space, to look. Further characteristics that make this search problem of general interest is that the resources often are sparsely distributed and may have chaotic dynamics with respect to their location, duration, and timing. Foraging for resources in a chaotic[2] world may be the quintessential task for any autonomous agent, natural or artificial.

We have been developing an artificial agent that is strongly inspired by biological models, an embodied (Brooks, 1991) Braitenberg (1984) vehicle, which is designed to learn how to perform a basic search mission in a nonstationary environment. The "robot" is called MAVRIC (Mobile, Autonomous Vehicle for Research in Intelligent Control); (Mobus & Fisher, 1993, 1994). The motivation for this objective comes directly from the observation that the "real" real world is open from the point of view of any realizable agent. Extending Brooks' (1991) notion of situatedness as a precondition for the successful demonstration of intelligence in artificial systems, we believe that ongoing real–time adaptation is an open–ended process that must extend over the life of an agent. In other words, we do not subscribe to the notion that artificial agents will be trained on some fixed set of patterns (even if only trained on some subset of the universe of patterns) and then be ready to survive in the real world. Things change too much even in environments that we know fairly well. Or in worlds we have not even adequately explored, things may be too different from our expectations to allow us to choose adequate training sets.

In foraging, animals may start with little or no knowledge of the organization of the environment. That is, they are not familiar with cue–resource relationships (situational heuristics) initially.[3] As they conduct their unguided search and then encounter the sought resource, they learn which cues (or landmarks) can be reliably

---

[1] This follows from the "Darwinian" argument that were they not successful, they would not survive.

[2] Here we are using the word in the sense of organized uncertainty, as in deterministic chaos. The world is organized within broadly determined "laws" but, owing to nonlinear interactions and lack of precision in determining initial conditions, becomes less predictable as the time horizon lengthens.

[3] In our system, a cue is a sensory gradient that extends over a much wider area than the sensory gradient of the resource object — for example, a visual cue (the sight of a landmark) may be seen from a greater distance than the scent of food.

counted on to lead to the sought resource and so they tend to improve their performance on subsequent searches. As they gain knowledge of these situational heuristics, they can use them to guide their searches. Should conditions change and the learned cue–resource relations no longer hold, animals revert to their *uninformed* search strategy and begin the process of learning the new cues. Our work centered on a neuromimic adaptive processor that allows an agent to learn the cue–resource relationships in a nonstationary environment such as this. The adaptive element of the neuromime, taking the place of a traditional synaptic weighting function, is called an Adaptrode (Mobus, 1994a, 1994b).

An adaptrode models the multiple time-scale memory trace mechanisms operative in the postsynaptic compartment of neurons (Alkon, 1987). Mathematically it is a cascaded, modified exponential smoothing function for pulse–coded primary input signals. Each level in the adaptrode corresponds to a longer time scale so that the adaptrode captures moving average activity over short–, intermediate–, and long–term periods. The smoothing functions at each level are gated into the next longer time scale by the receipt of a second, temporally ordered,[4] correlated signal to achieve associative learning. The adaptrode response to primary input (specifically the cue signal) is, thus, dependent on the history of inputs with higher weight given to more recent activity and longer–term weighting dependent on correlation with other signals (specifically resource detection signals that come some short time after excitation of the cue signal). Adaptrode response to input is effectively an estimate of the salience of the current input. It takes the place of the traditional weighted input signal in conventional neural network models. Thus weights in an adaptrode–based neuron are dynamic. They forget to the extent that recent inputs are not repeated and reinforced over time. As such they enable life-long learning networks. In previous work, Mobus (1994b) has shown that a simple two–cell network of competitive, adaptrode–based neurons can learn orthogonal associations so long as they separate in time domains. This is one solution to the destructive interference problem known to plague many conventional neural networks.

In MAVRIC, we wanted the robot to learn situational heuristics in which the detection of a cue, which is causally related to a resource event, could be used as a predictor of the location and timing of the event. Resource–cue associations in natural environments abound. Color, shape of plants, existence of a watering hole; all of these are exploited by numerous animals as cues to the potential presence of food. In our lab we arranged that light sources would be associated with (physically near) various resource objects. MAVRIC's task was to learn to find these resources by first learning the association and thereafter using the occurrence of a light as a predictor of the occurrence of the resource. Adaptrode-based neurons learn these relations in real–time and on–line. All that would be needed would be a way to get MAVRIC to experience the association a sufficient number of times so that the learning could take place.

---

[4] The temporal ordering observed is generally strict and requires that the primary signal arrives some time prior to the arrival of the secondary signal. The time interval required depends on the time–domain level being gated. In the case of gating the transfer of the short–term memory trace into the intermediate–term trace this may only require a few time steps. The ordering, however, ensures that a proper causal correlation is encoded.

We faced an early problem in terms of how to get the process started. It turns out that the strategy of motion of the agent before it has learned any useful relationships can have a significant impact on how quickly it is exposed to instances of successfully finding a resource and, consequently, learning the associated cues. MAVRIC, in classic Braitenberg style, uses fixed, semidirectional sensors. As a result, simply having MAVRIC move along in a straight line would severely restrict its ability to sample the space and, unless a resource (and its associated cues) happened to occur directly in its path, it would never find a resource, let alone learn cues that would lead to resources.

As an obvious starting point then, we provided MAVRIC with a random walk motor program in order to introduce some "novelty" into the search path. In this approach MAVRIC would move for a randomly chosen interval and then turn in a randomly chosen direction a randomly chosen number of degrees. It is possible to show that a random walk search is guaranteed to cover the entire space — but it may take an infinite amount of time to do so. From the standpoint of increasing the number of successful finds and subsequent learning, this method would work if we didn't care how long it took MAVRIC to find resources. The adaptrode learning mechanism is very fast at encoding associations (Mobus, 1994a, 1994b), so that after five or six encounters MAVRIC became quite good at finding the resource based on following cues. However, it might take MAVRIC several days to even locate the first such encounter by chance, let alone the five needed to get it to start following cues. Under those circumstances we followed a program of "training" MAVRIC on cue–resource relationships in which we placed the objects sufficiently close to MAVRIC so that it was guaranteed at least five encounters in a short time (Mobus & Fisher, 1991a, 1991b). Thereafter, the robot would reliably follow the learned cues *if* they were detected.

However, this was not a "good" solution for two reasons. First, the required training was not the same as allowing MAVRIC to learn from naturally occurring experience. We were trying to achieve the same level of autonomy that animals possess in the wild. Every time conditions changed we would have to retrain the robot. This initial approach resembled conditioned learning experiments conducted in animal learning (e.g., classical or Pavlovian conditioning); (Mackintosh, 1983), but this was not what we wanted.

Second, unless the density of resources spread throughout the environment were sufficiently high, the random walk search might still cause MAVRIC to fail to find that for which it was looking for long periods. Animals seeking food in the wild are under time and energy constraints that necessitate finding *some* instances of food every so often. Evolution works to match the species' search procedure–sensory apparatus and the resource density (both space and time) provided by the environment (niche). Grazing animals that are virtually surrounded by their food can accommodate nearly any strategy. Bacteria that swim in a medium relatively rich in nutrients employ a tumbling mechanism not unlike the random walk until they sense the chemical gradient leading to their food (Koshland, 1980). Sheep flocks tend to graze in "straight" lines until something (like a sheepdog) redirects their movements. Grazers do not rely on cue signals to find their food. Animals that hunt (forage) for a living rely on very different mechanisms.

Foraging is a complex behavior in most species. However the search phase can be characterized in two subphases depending on the animal's possession of knowledge or cues that would lead it to the resource. In the absence of knowledge or cue an animal tends to "wander" along novel paths as it attempts to perform a sensory sweep of the area. This can be observed directly by watching scout ants walking over a sidewalk or driveway. The ant does not wander aimlessly as in a random walk, rather it takes a weaving pattern, generally leading in some given direction. The path is novel (stochastic) yet follows some general pattern. Or observe a hound dog trying to pick up the scent of a prey. It will tend to weave back and forth over the area with a minimum of crossing back over its own path.

Once an animal has either acquired knowledge (e.g., honeybee workers observe the dance of a worker that has found a source of nectar) or senses the nearness of the resource (e.g., odor of food), the search becomes more directed, bringing the animal sufficiently close to the resource that the final stages involve direct sensory contact. Even with cues and/or knowledge there is still some uncertainty associated with the actual location of a resource due to imprecision in sensory measurements in navigation and communication (as in the case of the bees). Animals can be seen to continue a weaving motion, though with much lower amplitude, as they "home in" on the resource. This motion may be needed to obtain triangulation or gradient information necessary for computing the location of the object. But the existence of the motion as a gradation of that used in stochastic search is an important clue to understanding the underlying motor program generating the search patterns.

Another problem with using programmatic motor control models was interfacing the program with the neural decision process. As our robot acquired the sensory detection of a cue, how should it switch from nondeterministic search mode to directed mode? The neural network itself provided information for following gradients, but it wasn't clear how to best integrate the output of the neural net with the motor control program.

As we had done in looking for solutions to the learning mechanism by turning to biological models, we started looking for neurological mechanisms that might help solve this problem. A class of neural circuits, called central pattern generators (CPGs) are oscillators that are responsible for a number of rhythmic motor functions in a wide variety of animals. We were inspired by the way a relatively simple network of neurons could produce oscillatory outputs of the (intuitively) right form. The fact that these circuits are known to be modulated by other neural inputs, hence allowing the shaping of output waveform, was another attractive feature. We decided to investigate artificial CPG circuits constructed from adaptrode neurons. It turned out to be a useful approach.

2. CENTRAL PATTERN GENERATORS

Motion in animals involve opponent processes such as opposing muscleclature or muscle–hydrostatic pressure opponents as in arachnid limb movement or cardiac pumping. Such opponent forces are mediated by neural control signals that convey the appropriate phase and amplitude information such that the direction and force of the motion achieve the desired result without overstraining the motor elements themselves. These motions often involve some degree of tension between the motors but are always coordinated so as to protect the "machinery" from undue stress. Many movements in animal behavior repertoires as well as internal functions such as cardiac pumping and digestive tract movement are oscillatory in nature.

The undulatory swimming motion of a leech, the escape swimming of the mollusk *Tritonia diomedea*, and the heartbeat of the lobster are known to be controlled by a type of neural circuit called a central pattern generator or CPG. In fact, such circuits are known to control a wide variety of rhythmic motions such as breathing, walking, and swimming (Kleinfeld & Sompolinsky, 1989).

A number of heterogeneous architectures have been described that have similar kinds of behavior. In swimming control circuits where opponent muscle groups are alternately stimulated, the architectures involve two output groups, each of which generates bursts of pulses in alternating fashion (Selverston & Mazzoni, 1989). Thus the opposing muscle groups alternately contract and relax in approximately 180 degree phase shift from each other.

The general architecture of these circuits involves multiple groups or clusters of neurons, some of which excite other groups or clusters and some of which inhibit. Feedback inhibition, in which one group excites another and the later inhibits the former, is often seen. This pattern is seen when one or both clusters involve cells with tonic activity (self-excitation). Figure 16.1 shows a two-cell CPG of this form. Far more complicated circuits with many connections are seen in many animals.

An important feature of these circuits is the temporal behavior of connections, or synaptic dynamics. Slow and fast synapse responses are known. Thus, as in Fig. 16.1, the excitatory synapse from A to B may operate quickly to cause B to fire, whereas the feedback inhibition on A may be slow, thus allowing B to continue being excited (and hence firing) for some time before shutting A down. The output from such a circuit appears as a half-wave.

Another extremely important aspect of many CPGs is the way in which external inputs to the circuit can cause the output form to be modulated in frequency or amplitude. Some circuits are turned on and off by outside inputs (Roberts, 1989). This feature gives these circuits considerable flexibility in responding to outside influences. Animals can change their rhythm (or gait), and speed with the same basic circuit. Such features are attractive when designing a control system.

3. AN ADAPTRODE-BASED CPG

Oscillatory motion would be a desirable approach to causing a fixed–sensor robot such as MAVRIC to perform a sensory "sweep" of its environment as it moves in a generally forward direction. This could be achieved by modulating the amplitudes of two output lines, one controlling the right stepper motor and the other controlling the left motor in an alternating fashion. The net effect from the two motors would simultaneously determine the degree of turning and the forward speed of the vehicle.

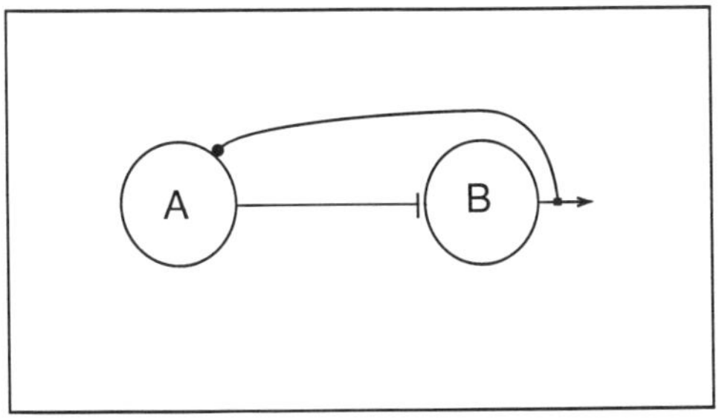

Fig. 16.1. A simple CPG circuit showing feedback inhibition. Cell A may be a tonically firing (self–excitatory) one that excites (flat terminal) cell B to fire. The latter then inhibits (circular terminal) cell A. Output from the circuit (pointed arrow) shows an episodic burst pattern.

Getting (1989) describes the simulation of a small CPG network based on the escape swimming control circuit of the mollusk *Tritonia diomedea*. The methods employed, namely continuous systems modeling, were appropriate for the purpose of explicating some aspects of the mechanisms of a biological network. These were quite different from our own purposes — to emulate behavior with a discrete system model. Nevertheless, certain features of these models and those of adaptrode–based neurons that we had been using to mediate nonadaptive dynamical functions in MAVRIC's brain, suggested the possibility of obtaining behavioral results similar to those inferred from continuous models.

We were led to the notion of building a CPG circuit for MAVRIC's motor control using adaptrode–based neurons because of the similarities between the time-course behavior of some synapses (i.e., fast and slow connections) in biological models and that of nonassociative adaptrodes having different valued control parameters (Mobus, 1994a). Adaptrodes with slowly or rapidly rising or falling response curves can easily be constructed. Additionally, as noted by Getting (1989), some types of interneurons participating in CPG circuits demonstrate an habituating–like behavior in that they cease firing after some period of continued stimulation even though the stimulus remains. This is modeled in adaptrode-based neurons by using a special adaptrode, the input to which is actually the output of the neuron, to up-modulate the threshold of that neuron so that, after a burst of activity, the neuron's firing rate diminishes and eventually ceases. Using the basic description of the simulated tadpole swimming circuit (Roberts, 1989) we constructed a simple four-cell model CPG (Fig. 16.2).

The circuit in Fig. 16.2 reflects the bilateral symmetry of the vehicle and the opponent process used to steer. It is composed of two "tonic" cells, which spontaneously fire at a relatively constant low rate, and two "feedback" cells. In operation the right tonic cell is given a boost in firing rate by an input from the "left bias" neuron (to get things started). In turn, the right tonic cell stimulates the right feedback cell which undergoes a transient increase in its output. This cell provides inhibitory feedback to the tonic cell, thus dampening its output, but it also provides excitatory input to the left tonic cell, increasing its output. Subsequently, the left tonic cell excites the left feedback cell which inhibits the left tonic cell and excites the right tonic cell, thus starting the cycle over again. Once set in motion, the contralateral excitation, unilateral inhibition cycle will continue indefinitely.

Output from the tonic cells is used to excite the right and left motor cells (these generate the stepper motor pulses) on their respective sides. When the right tonic cell is active (and the left tonic cell is relatively quiet by comparison) the right motor cell generates many more pulses per unit time and thus causes the right stepper motor to rotate faster. This produces a net left turning motion in the robot. Similarly, when the left tonic cell is more active, a right turning motion is made. The net effect of this alternating activity between right and left motor cells is to cause the robot to follow a weaving course, first turning leftward, then rightward, as it moves in a generally forward direction.

Excitatory synapses are implemented using relatively fast–response, slow decay nonassociative adaptrodes, while inhibitory synapses are implemented with slow–response, fast decay nonassociative adaptrodes. In addition, the threshold of the feedback

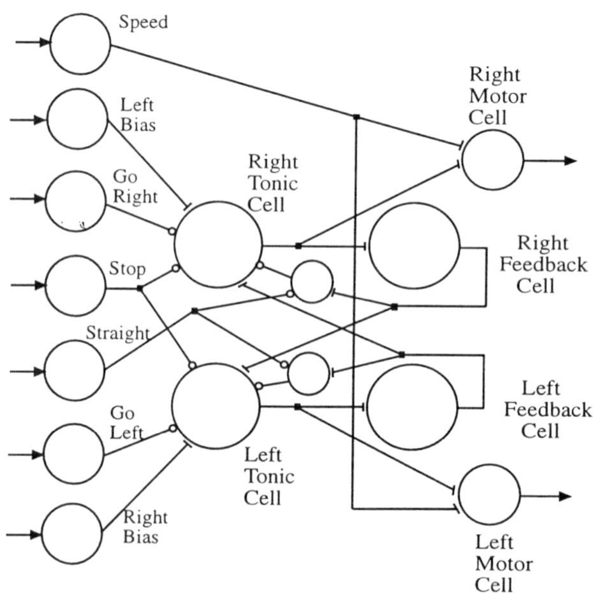

Fig. 16.2. The Central Pattern Generator (CPG) motor control circuit is comprised of four "core" neurons that generate a quasi–chaotic sinusoidal signal (left motor minus right motor). Additional neurons provide signal distribution for externally applied control signals that are used to modulate and shape the output signals. Pointed arrows indicate signals from/to the external environment. Flat terminals indicate excitatory connections while circular terminals indicate inhibitory ones.

cells are modulated, slowly, by an adaptrode which gets its input from the output of those cells. The modulation pushes the threshold of the cell lower than its resting level, thus making it easier for the net input to the cell to cause the cell to fire. Because adaptrodes continue to provide a decaying response after the input signal ceases, the effect is to cause the feedback cells to act as bursters. That is, they fire a volley of pulses that continues for a time after the offset of the excitatory input from the corresponding tonic cell. The length of time that this burst continues then determines the time that the corresponding tonic cell will be inhibited and the contralateral tonic cell will be excited. Clearly, the slowness of the inhibitory synapse from the feedback cell to the tonic cell must match the duration of the burst.

Additional inputs to the circuit (shown in Fig. 16.2 as pointed arrows) provide a convenient method of modulating the oscillator in a manner reminiscent of the biological CPGs described earlier. These inputs are distributed by a layer of neurons that provide a means of overriding, through inhibition (not shown), the effect of the primary signal. The input labeled "Speed" does not directly effect the oscillator circuit. It merely increases the firing rate of the two motor output cells as shown. Other inputs change the form of the output as depicted in the histogram in Fig. 16.3. The "Straight" signal can be seen to provide inhibitory input to two cells that supply the inhibitory feedback signal to the tonic cells. This action induces the two tonic cells to become more synchronous leading to a nearly zero net output and the robot moves in a somewhat straight line. When the "Straight" signal is removed or just reduced, the signal returns to its oscillatory behavior with a peak amplitude proportional to the level of the "Straight" signal.

Similarly, the "Go Right" or "Go Left" signals dampen their respective tonic cells which in turn dampens the contralateral excitation feedback. This allows the undamped tonic cell to provide a more or less steady output to its respective motor cell and results in the robot making a smooth and sustained turn. A weaker signal at one of these inputs results in a weaker turning with a small oscillatory wave superimposed.

The "Left Bias" and "Right Bias" signals perform a slightly different function when used. If the "Right Bias" cell is active (it is actually a tonic cell also), the net output signal to the motor cells is essentially the same in form but tends to favor the left motor output. The robot will move in the same weaving pattern but has a tendency to move in a diverging spiral. The capacity to make turns or go straight is not seriously hampered. The modulatory inputs to the CPG circuit come from the cue recognition and direction determining networks of MAVRIC's brain (Mobus & Fisher, 1994).

As originally conceived, this circuit was expected to produce a sinusoidal net output (between left and right motor cells). Indeed, the weaving pattern that the robot followed when run with the new neural oscillator controller was roughly sinusoidal. However we noted certain peculiarities in the pattern. Far from producing a fixed sinusoid, the weave pattern of the robot showed erratic deviations from a sine curve. Sometimes it would make short right or left turns followed by long, sweeping turns. Other times it would make short turns one way and long turns the other causing it to veer dramatically from a given course. Our first conjecture on this behavior was that this was simply the result of slippage of the wheels, a notorious problem in conventional robotics. However, after looking at the pulse counts being sent to the motors it was clear that the

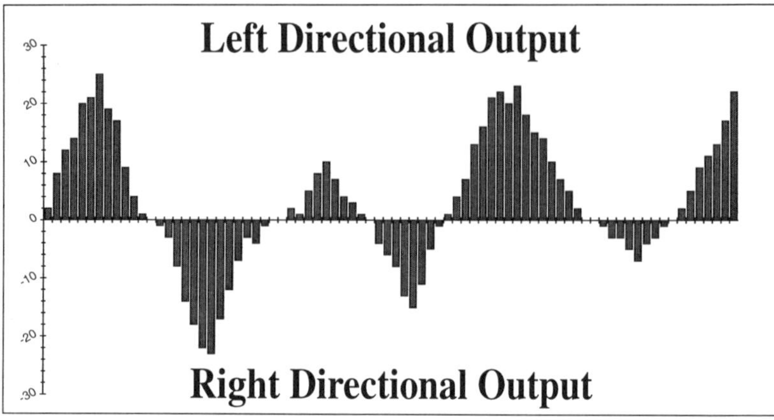

Fig. 16.3. A histogram of the CPG net (of right and left motor signal) output shows that the direction of the robot varies in a roughly sinusoidal pattern with nondeterministic characteristics of amplitude and wave length. The amplitude of each bar represents the degree of turning that the robot does per second. Negative values represent turns to the right, positive values indicate turns to the left.

erraticness was due to the output of the oscillator. Subsequently we collected and analyzed the raw count data from the oscillator and were surprised to discover that it generated a more complicated signal. As seen in the histogram in Fig. 16.3, the oscillation appears to have a complex waveform.

Following a suggestion by Bruce West, we decided to look at this data from the perspective of chaos theory. Specifically we undertook to reconstruct the attractor dynamics from a large sample of the time series as shown in the histogram. Figure 16.4 shows a plot of a two-dimensional attractor based on plotting a reconstructed phase space from two points in the time series separated by a specified number of time points — in this case 2. As can be seen in the plot, some kind of nonperiodic attractor is associated with the oscillator process. To claim that the system is chaotic, in the sense of deterministic chaos, would be premature from this one form of evidence. However, several observations might be made. First, it is clear that the system is bounded in phase space — hence some kind of attractor is operative. Second, it appears to be the case that the system does not repeat itself — that it is not merely a quasi-random number generator. A final piece of evidence comes from mapping the course taken by the robot (unstimulated by external cues) over a number of runs. This plot (Fig. 16.5), showing divergence as the search time increases, strongly suggests that the path taken is sensitive to initial conditions.

We have not pursued a more rigorous analysis of this process with respect to its apparent chaotic nature for the simple reason that it isn't terribly important to our main

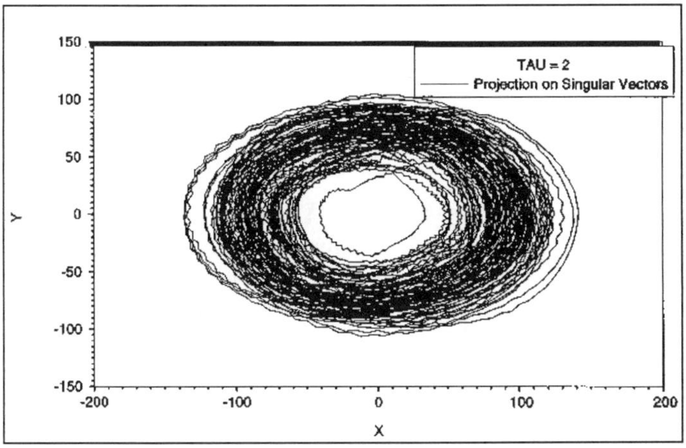

Fig. 16.4. Plot of a reconstructed, two-dimensional phase space showing the attractor dynamics of the CPG oscillator. This plots the behavior in a space defined by two points taken from the time series data as shown in Fig. 16.3. The two points are separated by two time ticks (TAU = 2). This plot was generated from 20,000 data points.

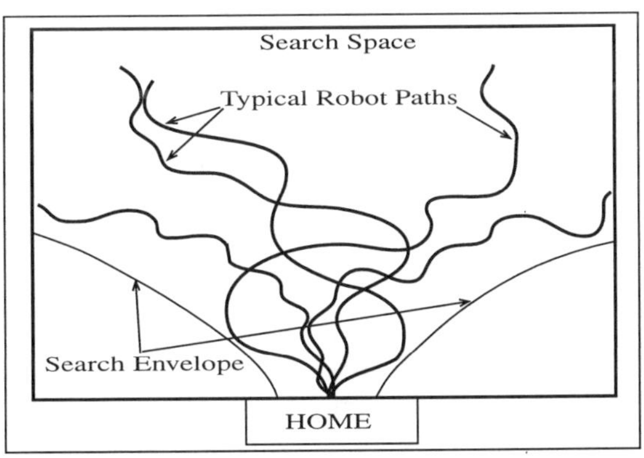

Fig. 16.5. Examples of typical search paths traversed by MAVRIC show the drunken weave pattern resulting from the OSC output as shown in Fig. 16.2. Also note the apparent bounded nature of the search envelope and the fact that each run takes a novel course.

line of work to show that the oscillator is chaotic in some strict sense. We were seeking a means of getting a robot to scan its environment while it moved, and to that end the oscillator provided a good solution. That it should introduce novelty into the search path was, from our perspective, a bonus. However, the form that this novelty takes, that is in not being a random walk, may have important consequences for the notion of foraging search.

4. RESULTS OBTAINED WITH MAVRIC

Our original objective had been to get MAVRIC to weave as it moved forward so that it would obtain a sensory sweep of its environment. We also required that the motor program allow for easy modulation so that the robot could shift to directed movement gracefully. To those ends the CPG oscillator network produced excellent results. In numerous test runs from a fixed starting point, (home), MAVRIC was able to sense and thus learn a sufficient number of cue–mission events that were placed in its workspace. Subsequent runs showed that MAVRIC was able to locate resources from cue information alone as described in Mobus and Fisher (1993, 1994). We had achieved the desired level of autonomy in that MAVRIC no longer needed to be "trained" on specific contingencies in order to succeed in finding its mission resources.

That the oscillator produced a novel search path each time the robot was started from its home did not seem to have any negative consequences[5] for the success of the robot, as had been the case with the random–walk novelty scheme. It did not immediately dawn on us that these paths might have a real beneficial impact on the capabilities of the robot.

When thinking about the nature of real-world environments we realized that many mission resources occur in stochastic episodes. Certainly the food resources of foraging animals appear and disappear in different locations. There may be a certain amount of regularity in these dynamics, for example, fruit may ripen in a given season or prey animals may always show up at a watering hole. Thus the nature of resource dynamics may, itself, be chaotic, and the timing and quality of the resource are subject to variations that make precise prediction impossible. Because the occurrence and location of resources might be indeterminate, it would be counterproductive for an agent to follow the same path on each iteration of searching. Rather, following a novel path will further ensure that the agent searches a larger volume of the space. Novel search paths would also provide an answer to the problem of occlusion of a resource behind fixed obstacles.

At the same time, search paths would seem to best be constrained in terms of a general direction. Random-walk search, while producing completely novel paths on each iteration, appears to cover too much of the volume. If, as we have speculated, resource dynamics in natural environments follow a chaotic pattern (at least in the

---

[5] Ironically, we spent a fair amount of time trying to smooth out the erraticness of the oscillations without increasing the complexity of the circuit — to no avail. Eventually, after seeing that the novel paths did not reduce the robot's ability to find resources, we decided to let well enough alone.

general case), then it makes sense that one should constrain the search volume to correspond with the spatial extent of the sought phenomena. A chaotic search pattern would thus provide constrained novelty to match that found in the sought resource.

To do a preliminary test of this notion, we projected part of the trajectory of a Lorenz attractor phase space map onto the plane. A series of points along the trajectory were chosen randomly to represent locations and times for the occurrence of mission–critical events. Within the sensory envelope of the event a second event, called a cue, was defined which would reliably associate with the mission event.[6] The result was that resources (and cues to their presence) appeared stochastically and episodically as the trajectory evolved (Fig. 16.6). MAVRIC was set on a series of iterative searches over the course of this evolution. The figure shows a single mission event and its relationship to the search envelope resulting from the chaotic weave pattern of MAVRIC's motion. Two paths, as shown, lead to finding the resource. The path labeled A shows the result of a coincidental discovery of the resource prior to learning the association between the

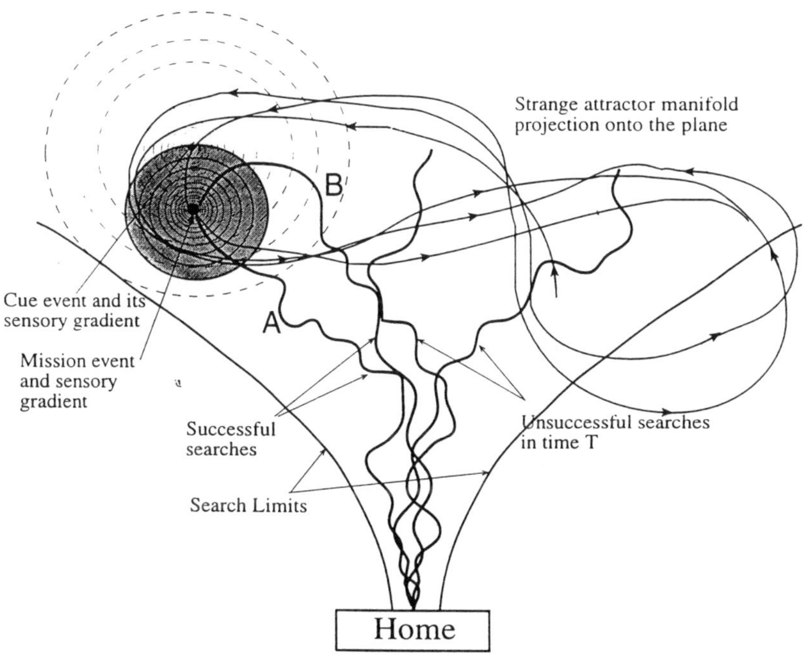

Fig. 16.6. Experimental layout for MAVRIC to search for a chaotic resource. A common chaotic attractor phase space map has been projected onto the plane of the lab floor. This trajectory is used to place and time the occurrence of resource (mission–critical) events and their associated cue events. Several representative MAVRIC search tracks are shown.

---

[6] Typical mission events would be the sounding of a specific tone the volume of which was varied to represent the gradient field. A cue event was the placement of a light near the speaker. The light would be dimmed so that MAVRIC had to be within a certain distance before it could detect the light.

resource and the cue event (a light source). MAVRIC's course is unaffected by the cue gradient, but as the robot encounters the resource gradient it transitions from the chaotic weave pattern to a gradient following pattern. This transition is effected via the modulation of the CPG oscillator by the directional input, "Straight," as shown in Fig. 16.2. This signal is supplied by a gradient detection network that increases the "Straight" signal in proportion to the difference between two successive samples of the stimulus.[7]

The path labeled B shows a path after learning the association in which MAVRIC follows the cue gradient, by the same mechanism as it follows a resource stimulus gradient, until it encounters the resource gradient, afterwhich it follows the latter to the source. In this model, the learned cue need not be contiguous with the resource object. The extent of the cue field should be greater than that of the resource so that it has the effect of enlarging the latter. Sensing the cue at a greater distance from the resource than it could sense the resource itself, the robot transitions from chaotic wandering and entering the cue field improves its chances of encountering the resource field.

Other paths depicted in the figure would lead to failure. Under additional assumptions regarding the average resource density, several mission (or resource) events might be present in the map of the trajectory at any given time. These would be spaced so that there would be no overlap in the resource gradient fields as detected by MAVRIC.

Thus MAVRIC was set to searching for its mission resources in what we believe represented a natural–like environment. As it had when the resource was set in the same location each time, MAVRIC was able to find its objective in a completely autonomous way—first finding the resource coincidentally and then learning how to improve its results by following the cue gradients that it encountered.

Because of its flexibility and ease of interfacing directional and speed controls with the other parts of MAVRIC's brain, the CPG oscillator proved to be an excellent, if not convenient, approach to solving the motor program problem for this class of robot. The injection of novelty in the absence of directed search has added additional, unanticipated, functionality to the process and, at least from the perspective of our initial experiences, has improved the actual performance of that process

5. SOME IMPLICATIONS AND OTHER APPLICATIONS

Searching a large, dynamic space for a consumable resource, within time constraints, presents some interesting challenges for robotics and autonomous agents in general. The nature of the dynamism of natural environments should in general be considered at best stochastic and possibly chaotic. This translates into some degree of

---

[7] This strategy emulates the tumbling search mechanism in swimming bacteria reported by Koshland (1980).

uncertainty as to the location of the resource each time a search is conducted. In the case of chaotic dynamics, traditional statistical-based prediction is probably inadequate.

Our experience with the chaotic oscillator motor drive network or artificial CPG has led us to consider the role of novelty in generating search paths in the absence of cue-directed searches. Novelty ensures that the search path selected on iterative searches will not lead the agent to the same places each time. In this regard it may be analogous to the use of simulated annealing (SA) to prevent gradient-following algorithms from getting stuck in local minima. Clearly, once a resource has been found at a given location, and consumed, the agent need not return to that location in a subsequent search. The degree of novelty (perhaps analogous to the temperature in SA) is important in that too much results in something like a random walk in which old territory may be explored repeatedly. Not enough results in a relatively narrow envelope of exploration relative to the total space.

That a simple circuit such as the CPG can generate novelty of the "right" form in motor control suggests other possibilities for the role of such circuits in exploration in general. The existence of oscillations in the cortex of vertebrate brains has been established. Is it possible that some of these are sufficiently chaotic to cause novel firing patterns of other neural circuits? Could such circuits give rise to creativity in human mental processing? One of the cornerstones of human level search in a high dimensional "thought" space is the role of creativity in finding novel paths to a solution. Do we not often "forage" (or hunt) for a solution to a problem? These are, of course, highly speculative musings and clearly far beyond the realm of investigating intelligent behavior in snail level artificial agents. However, such speculations may prove to be useful guides in exploring brain architectures for more complex robots in the future.

In the meantime, we have begun to think of the method of foraging, in the sense of coupling a chaotic path generator with a learning mechanism, as a solution to search problems in discrete domains such as computer memories. Exhaustive search of a discrete space, as represented, say, by a graph, is not overly burdensome, computationally, in that it is known to scale linearly with the number of nodes and edges. However, the problem of searching a large space for dynamically changing resources (graph labels) can be problematic if the rate of change in the labeling or topology of the graph is greater than the time needed to conduct the search. If one views the combined memory space of all computers tied into the Internet, for example, as a vast, dynamic search space, then it is possible that the method of foraging search may be brought to bear. We are thus beginning to look at the extrapolation of the methods that have proven useful in our physical robotics application to the cyberspace environment afforded in the Internet. Here a "knowbot" agent, or software robot (Etzioni & Weld, 1994), might forage through the network, looking for resources, such as documents containing specific key phrases. One such knowbot, under development, explores the World Wide Web for documents containing search terms. It looks also at significant words near URL links, storing those in short-term memory. If it takes that link and subsequently finds the sought terms, it transfers the remembered words to longer-term memory and they become cues. Such cues, if found in other documents near URL links will increase the likelihood that the knowbot will explore that link and find the sought terms. A chaotic oscillator is used to decide which link to follow when the knowbot does not find any cues.

ACKNOWLEDGMENTS

We would like to thank Manny Aparicio for his contributions to this work in discussions and collateral work with Mobus on foraging search in animals.

REFERENCES

Alkon, D. L. (1987). *Memory Traces in the Brain.* New York: Cambridge University Press.

Braitenberg, V. (1984). *Vehicles: Experiments in Synthetic Psychology.* Cambridge, MA: MIT Press.

Brooks, R. A. (1991). *Intelligence without reasoning* (Tech. Rep. A.I. Memo No. 1293). Cambridge, MA: MIT Artificial Intelligence Laboratory.

Durbin, R., Miall, C., & Mitchison, G. (Eds.). (1989). *The Computing Neuron.* Reading, MA: Addison–Wesley.

Etzioni, O., & Weld, D. (1994). A softbot-based interface to the internet. *Communications of the ACM, 37,* 72-76.

Getting, P. A. (1989). Reconstruction of small neural networks. In C. Koch & I. Segev (Eds.), *Methods in Neuronal Modeling: From Synapses to Networks.* (pp. 171–194). Cambridge, MA: MIT Press.

Kleinfeld, D., & Sompolinsky, H. (1989). Associative network models for central pattern generators. In C. Koch & I. Segev (Eds.), *Methods in Neuronal Modeling: From Synapses to Networks* (pp. 195–246). Cambridge, MA: MIT Press.

Koshland, D. E. (1980). *Bacterial Chemotaxis as a Model Behavioral System.* New York: Raven Press.

Mackintosh, N. J. (1983). *Conditioning and Associative Learning.* London: Oxford University Press.

Mobus, G. E. (1994a). *A Multi-Time Scale Learning Mechanism for Neuromimic Processing.* Unpublished doctoral dissertation. Denton, TX: University of North Texas.

Mobus, G. E. (1994b). Toward a theory of learning and representing causal inferences in neural networks. In D. S. Levine & M. Aparicio (Eds.), *Neural Networks for Knowledge Representation and Inference,* (pp. 339–374). Hillsdale, NJ: Lawrence Erlbaum Associates.

Mobus, G. E., & Fisher, P. S. (1991a). Conditioned response training of robots using adaptrode-based neural networks I: Continuous adaptive learning. In G. Mesnard & R. Swiniarsk (Eds.), *Proceedings of the International AMSE Conference on Neural Networks.* (pp. 171–182). San Diego: Association for the Advancement of Modeling and Simulation Techniques in Enterprises.

Mobus, G. E., & Fisher, P. S. (1991b). Conditioned response training of robots using adaptrode-based neural networks II: Simulation results. In G. Mesnard & R. Swiniarsk (Eds.) *Proceedings of the International AMSE Conference on Neural Networks.* (pp. 183–194). San Diego: Association for the Advancement of Modeling and Simulation Techniques in Enterprises.

Mobus, G. E., & Fisher, P. S. (1993). *A mobile autonomous robot for research in intelligent control* (Tech. Rep. CRPDC-93-12). Denton, TX: Center for Research in Parallel and Distributed Computing, University of North Texas.

Mobus, G. E., & Fisher, P. S. (1994). MAVRIC's Brain. In F. D. Anger, R. V. Rodriguez, & M. Ali (Eds.), *Proceedings of the Seventh International Conference, Industrial and Engineering Applications of Artificial Intelligence and Expert Systems* (pp. 315–322). Yverdon, Switzerland: Gordon and Breach Science Publishers.

Roberts, A. (1989). A mechanism for switching in the nervous system: turning on swimming in a frog tadpole. In R. Durbin, C. Miall, & G. Mitchison (Eds.), *The Computing Neuron* (pp. 229–243). Reading, MA: Addison–Wesley.

Selverston, A., & Mazzoni, P. (1989). Flexibility of computational units in invertebrate cpgs. In R. Durbin, C. Miall, & G. Mitchison (Eds.), *The Computing Neuron* (pp. 205–228). Reading, MA: Addison–Wesley.

17
An Oscillatory Associative Memory Analogue Architecture

Anthony G. Brown and Steve Collins
DRA(Malvern), Worcestershire

ABSTRACT

A model of an oscillatory associative memory is described which is an ideal candidate for implementation as a self-organising analogue information-processing system. The equations that represent a fixed point associative memory are modified to introduce oscillations and create a system that is capable of reproducing the input segmentation behaviour exhibited by similar oscillatory systems. Within this system phase locked oscillations are employed to represent correlations that can be reinforced via a Hebbian learning rule. Consideration of small systems demonstrates that these phase locked oscillations are based on cooperative interactions between nodes. The system's ability to segment a mixed input into its constituent components is enhanced by variations between nodes, which will be unavoidable in any analogue system.

1. INTRODUCTION

Results from several groups suggest that mimicking the oscillatory behaviour observed in biological systems may lead to novel information processing architectures with new capabilities (Andreou & Edwards, 1993; Horn & Usher, 1991; Wang, Buhmann, & von der Malsburg, 1990). Although digital computers can be used to model these systems, this approach may be too computationally expensive for some applications. Fortunately, analogue circuits offer a mature technology that could be exploited to implement this type of system. The aim of this chapter is to describe a model which is both easy to understand and potentially easy to implement as an array of analogue circuits (Brown & Collins, 1994).

It is the desire to eventually implement a model as an array of analogue circuit that constrains the types of model that can be considered. In particular, because each device has one input, complex connections with several inputs will require more devices, and therefore more area, than connections with one input. Thus the key criteria for selecting a model as the basis for an analogue architecture is the simplicity of the connections among individual circuits. Unfortunately, existing models, such as the one proposed by Wang, Buhmann, and Malsburg (1990), contain connections with multiple inputs that would be difficult to implement easily. The best starting point from which to develop a suitable model is the equations representing the circuits used to implement fixed point associative memories (Hertz, Krogh, & Palmer, 1991), modified to be equivalent to the model proposed by Horn and Usher (1991). This starting point leads to a model that will be easy to implement, while ensuring that it retains the interesting behaviours described by both Wang, Buhmann, and von der Malsburg and Horn and Usher.

Following a short discussion of the background to the proposed model in Section 2, its key features are described in Section 3. Simple systems containing a small number of nodes are then considered both to determine the relevant values of various model parameters and develop the intuitive understanding of the system behaviour.

Consideration of one and two node systems show that the self-sustained oscillations, representing previously learnt inputs or known states, arise from cooperative interactions between nodes. The desirable ability to decompose or segment a mixed input into its constituent parts is then shown to arise from phase separation of different groups of phase-locked oscillators. Furthermore, this behaviour is reliably observed only if the symmetry within the system is broken by explicitly introducing variations between equivalent components that naturally arise in analogue systems.

Consideration of these simple systems also leads to the identification of a parameter that can be used to control the existence of states that are equivalent to spurious states in a fixed point associative memory. The ability of this parameter to decrease the number of these states is then confirmed by simulation and a parameter value is selected, allowing the system to retain its ability to recognise incomplete inputs. Finally, the ability to distinguish novel inputs is demonstrated. Furthermore, these novel inputs lead to a transient response that can be exploited within the context of a simple learning rule to allow the system to create new known states.

The similarity between part of the proposed system and the Hopfield network then led to an investigation of the memory capacity of the system. Simulation results suggest that the memory capacity of this system is twice that of an equivalent size Hopfield network. However, this is the only disappointing result. In all other respects an oscillatory associative memory is an ideal means of creating an adaptive analogue system.

2. BACKGROUND

Analogue circuits are a natural medium in which to mimic the oscillatory behaviour observed in biological systems to create new information-processing architectures. One example of the type of system arising from this approach is the architecture constructed by Andreou and Edwards (1993). Within this imaging architecture each pixel is designed to have an activity that oscillates in response to a strong input. The oscillatory response of each pixel is then communicated to its nearest neighbours via predetermined connections. These connections are designed to cause phase-locking between pixels within the same object so that the architecture segments a scene into its constituent parts.

One way to extend the functionality of oscillatory systems is to use adaptive connections, or weights, to create a self-organising system. A key requirement when creating an adaptive system is a learning rule that determines how these weights change in response to activity within the system. Because our aim is to develop a model with a simple connectivity, which is easy to implement, the ideal learning rule is one in which weight changes are based on local information.

There is evidence that within some oscillatory biological systems, temporal correlations in the activity of a pair of neurons will cause changes in any synaptic connections between the pair which strengthen their interaction (Larson & Lynch, 1986). The result is a Hebb-like learning rule that could form the basis of an associative memory. This biological result suggests that temporal correlations could be used to create an adaptive associative memory, if the system is designed so that a known input or stimulus results in phase-locked oscillations.

Systems that combine a Hebb-like learning rule with oscillatory behaviour have been proposed previously by Wang et al. (1990) and Horn and Usher (1991). These groups have demonstrated that this type of oscillatory system has all the capabilities of an associative memory which represents known states as fixed points. Furthermore they have shown how the extra degrees of freedom introduced by using oscillations to represent known states allow the system to segment or separate a mixed input into its constituent parts.

Overall, there is some evidence from biological systems to suggest that temporal correlations within oscillatory systems can be exploited to create an associative memory. Furthermore, the systems investigated by Wang et al. (1990) and Horn and Usher (1991) show that this type of system will be capable of segmenting or decomposing a mixed input into its constituent parts. Our aim is to implement this type of system using analogue circuits to create an adaptive analogue architecture.

3. A MODEL FOR AN OSCILLATORY ASSOCIATIVE MEMORY

A good starting point for an analogue oscillatory associative memory is one of the various implementations of a Hopfield network (Hertz, Krogh, & Palmer, 1991). Oscillations can then be introduced into the system by either following the example of Horn and Usher (1991) and changing the neuron threshold or by introducing a conventional negative feedback loop. Although either of these two mechanisms could be employed, the intuitive understanding required to design an analogue system, is most easily achieved by considering a system containing negative feedback loops. The result is an associative memory whose dynamics are governed by

$$\begin{aligned} x_i &= -\alpha x_i - h_i x_i + \sum_j T_{ij} g(x_i) + I_i \\ y_i &= -\alpha y_i + \sigma(x_i) \end{aligned}$$

where α is the internal node decay constant, h_i is the linear inhibitory constant, g is a step function, σ is a sigmoidal function, and the weights (or connection strengths) can be calculated using a symmetric Hebbian learning rule

$$T_{ij} = \begin{cases} \frac{1}{n}\sum_s \xi_i^s \xi_j^s , i \neq j \\ 0, i = j \end{cases}$$

The most commonly used representation of the input to an associative memory ξ_i is as a vector whose components can take on the values +1 or −1. Unfortunately, when used in conjunction with the Hebb rule this representation correlates both active and inactive nodes. Because our aim is to create a system that correlates activity within the system, this representation has to be changed to one in which inputs are vectors with a value of 0 or 1. Unfortunately, this representation is unsuitable for use with a symmetric Hebb rule.

To understand the particular problem that arises, consider a four-node system with two known states, (1, 1, 0, 0) and (1, 0, 1, 0). These states overlap and there is one node that occurs in neither pattern. Clearly, for these patterns, an input to either node two or node three implies that there must be an input to node one. In contrast, an input to node one only implies an input to either node two or node three. Ideally, therefore, nodes two and three should have a stronger influence upon node one than node one has upon either node two or node three. Thus we need an asymmetric learning rule, based on local information, such as

$$T_{ij} = \begin{cases} \frac{1}{n}\sum_s (\xi_i^s - \kappa)\xi_j^s, i \neq j \\ 0, i = j \end{cases}$$

where κ is a constant.

Assuming for simplicity that the constant $\kappa = 1/4$ for the two known states (1, 1, 0, 0) and (1, 0, 1, 0), this modified learning rule leads to

$$T = \begin{bmatrix} 0 & \frac{3}{16} & \frac{3}{16} & 0 \\ \frac{1}{8} & 0 & -\frac{1}{16} & 0 \\ \frac{1}{8} & -\frac{1}{16} & 0 & 0 \\ -\frac{1}{8} & -\frac{1}{16} & -\frac{1}{16} & 0 \end{bmatrix}$$

Now, as required, the effects of nodes two and three on node one (T_{12} and T_{13}) are stronger than the effect of node one on either of them (T_{21} and T_{31}). Further, any activity in these three nodes inhibits node four, while node four has no effect on the other three nodes. This is consistent with the fact that node four is in neither known state and has the advantage that it prevents the system from being detrimentally affected by noise injected by the input of this node.

4. ANALYSIS AND SIMULATION

The desired behaviours of this system can be understood by considering simple models containing 1, 2, 4, and 12 pairs of nodes. Consideration of the single node pair shows how stimulation creates a decaying oscillatory response. Using a system containing only two pairs of nodes the self-sustained oscillations, which are required to represent known states, are then shown to arise from cooperative (excitatory) interactions. Furthermore, this simple system is sufficient to establish the conditions, relating the various parameters within the equations, which are required for these oscillations to occur.

The system's ability to segment or decompose a mixed input into its constituent parts is then investigated by considering a system containing 4 pairs of nodes. This small system both confirms the existence of this emergent behaviour and demonstrates that it occurs more readily in a system in which each pair of nodes has a slightly different natural frequency. Finally, a larger system of 12 nodes is used to demonstrate pattern completion and the ability of the system to detect novel inputs and adapt to create new known states.

4.1. One Node Pair

First, consider a single, isolated node pair (i.e., $T_{ij} = 0$). In this situation the dynamic equations become

$$\begin{aligned} \dot{x} &= \alpha x - hx + I \\ \dot{y} &= \alpha y + \sigma(x) \end{aligned}$$

Now assume that $\sigma(x)$ is a sigmoidal function that includes regions in which its value is relatively independent of x. In these regions there is no feedback within the equations and hence no oscillations.

Oscillations therefore only occur in the region over which $\sigma(x)$ varies. For simplicity, assume that $\sigma(x) = \sigma'(x)$ over this region of interest. The equations now represent transient oscillations with a frequency $\sqrt{h\sigma'}$ and decay constant α. Thus oscillations are only observed if $\alpha < \sqrt{h\sigma'}$ and the system eventually comes to rest at the fixed point (x_0, y_0), where x_0 and y_0 are

$$\begin{aligned} x_0 &= \alpha I/(\alpha^2 + \sigma' h) \\ y_0 &= \sigma' I/(\alpha^2 + \sigma' h) \end{aligned}$$

Because the fixed point depends on the input I, it is this input that must bias the pair of nodes into the region in which $\sigma(x)$ varies and oscillations may occur. Furthermore, because the fixed point for zero input is (0,0), the initial condition for subsequent simulations is assumed to be the origin.

4.2. Two Node Pairs

Because isolated nodes decay to a fixed point, the required self-sustained oscillatory behaviour must emerge from cooperative interactions between different pairs. This can be demonstrated by considering the dynamics of one of two pairs of nodes, (x_1, y_1) and (x_2, y_2). Assuming that the sigmoid σ is approximately linear in the region of interest, (x_1, y_1) has a fixed point $(\overline{x_1}, \overline{y_1})$, where $\dot{x}_1 = \dot{y}_1 = 0$. This fixed point is

$$\overline{x_1} = \alpha(I_1 + T_{12}g(x_2))/(\alpha^2 + \sigma' h_1)$$

$$\overline{y_1} = \sigma'(I_1 + T_{12}g(x_2))/(\alpha^2 + \sigma' h_1)$$

Because g is a step function, there are two possible fixed points for (x_1, y_1), depending on the value of $g(x_2)$. This means that if x_2 moves through the threshold of g the fixed point $(\overline{x_1}, \overline{y_1})$ will suddenly change. The effect of this sudden change in fixed point is to cause sustained oscillations. This can be seen in simulation results such as those in Fig. 17.1. The effect of the sudden change in fixed point is demonstrated in this figure which shows the activities of both an isolated pair of nodes and a pair of nodes interacting with a neighbouring pair. As expected, without any input from a neighbouring pair of nodes, the oscillations of the isolated node pair decay toward a fixed point. A behaviour represented by the spiral trajectory ending at a fixed point is shown in Fig. 17.1. In contrast to the trajectory of the isolated node the trajectory of the connected node is a closed orbit which represents a sustained oscillation. Inspection of the shape of this orbit reveals two kinks, indicating that this orbit is formed from two constituent parts. Each part of the orbit represents a period during which the activity of the node is decaying toward one of the two fixed points. However, because the two node pairs are oscillating at the same frequency there is a regular sudden shift in the position of the fixed point. It appears that, by disrupting the decay of (x_1, y_1), this sudden change in fixed point position gives rise to self-sustained oscillation.

Thus oscillations are sustained in one of a pair of nodes if the other pair cross through threshold. Inasmuch as this condition applies equally to each of the two pairs of nodes, self-sustained oscillations will only occur if both the pairs cross through the threshold. This suggests that oscillations will only occur if the fixed points of both pairs of nodes are close to the threshold of g. Assuming that the threshold of g is 0.5, this leads to the general condition

$$\overline{x_i} = \alpha(I_i + \sum T_{ij}g(x_j))/(\alpha^2 + \sigma' h_i) \approx 0.5 .$$

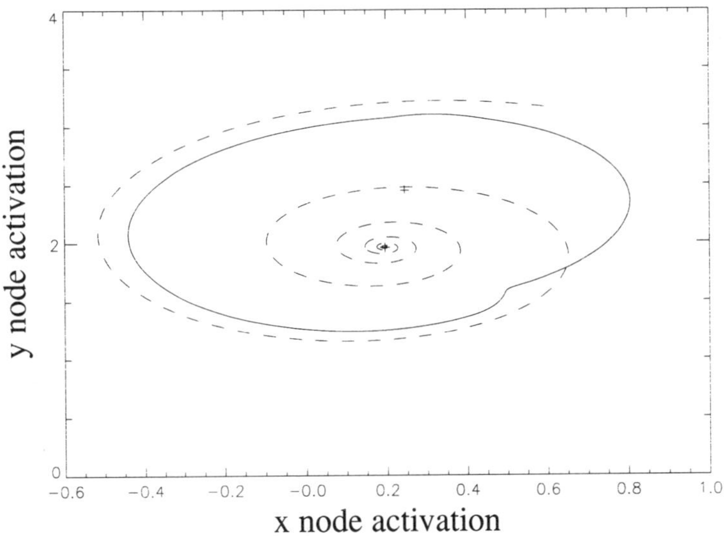

Fig. 17.1. A comparison of x_1 and y_1 without coupling (dashed line) and with coupling (solid line) showing that the change in position of the fixed point (crosses) gives rise to a complete orbit, indicative of self-sustained oscillation.

This expression can be simplified by assuming that the external input is dominant, so that $I_i = 1 \gg \sum T_{ij} g(x_j)$. Because oscillatory behaviour occurs if $\sqrt{\sigma h_i} > \alpha$, sustained oscillations only occur if $\alpha \approx \sigma' h_i / 2$.

4.3. Mixture Decomposition

An important emergent behaviour that can be understood by considering a simple system is segmentation or mixture decomposition (Horn & Usher, 1991; Wang et al., 1990). Consider a four-node system, adapted to store two orthogonal patterns, (1, 0, 1, 0) and (0, 1, 0, 1). The connection matrix for this system is

$$T = \begin{bmatrix} 0 & -\frac{1}{16} & \frac{3}{16} & -\frac{1}{16} \\ -\frac{1}{16} & 0 & -\frac{1}{16} & \frac{3}{16} \\ \frac{3}{16} & -\frac{1}{16} & 0 & -\frac{1}{16} \\ -\frac{1}{16} & \frac{3}{16} & -\frac{1}{16} & 0 \end{bmatrix}.$$

The system response to an input consisting of both patterns presented simultaneously is shown in Fig. 17.2a. Initially all nodes react to the stimulus by oscillating in phase. However, the cooperative effect between nodes within the same known state is almost cancelled out by the inhibition from the other pair of nodes. The oscillations therefore begin to decay away.

This observed decay does not occur if the two different groups oscillate out of phase. The change in the relative phase of the two groups required to prevent decay arises reliably and quickly if each pair of nodes has a different value of h_i, to represent variations between the equivalent devices within each circuit, which creates a difference in the natural frequencies of the nodes.

To understand how this creates the required change in the relative phase of the two groups consider a pair of nodes *i* and *j*. Without loss of generality we can assume that the phase of node *j* is slightly behind that of node *i*. If both nodes are in the same known state, then as node *i* passes through threshold it will increase the input to node *j* (since the connections between nodes in the same patterns are positive) thus advancing the phase of node *j*. Hence patterns within the same grouping will remain phase locked. However, if the nodes *i* and *j* are not in the same known state, then the extra input to node *j* when node *i* passes through threshold is negative and will retard the phase of node *j* still further. Therefore the nodes in a group will remain phase locked, while the phase of different groups will be forced apart.

The effect of this process can be seen in the simulation result shown in Fig. 17.2a. All nodes start in phase, but by the third period of oscillation the two groups are noticeably out of phase. By the fourth period the phase of the one group is sufficiently advanced with respect to that of the other group that total inhibition occurs. Half a period later the two groups are out of phase.

Once phase separation has occurred the inhibitory interaction between the two groups leads to a negative impulse at a time when the node amplitude is decreasing. This force is now in phase with the oscillatory motion and it therefore increases the amplitude of the oscillations. Hence the amplitude of the oscillatory groups will increase. The result is the self-sustained, out of phase, oscillations.

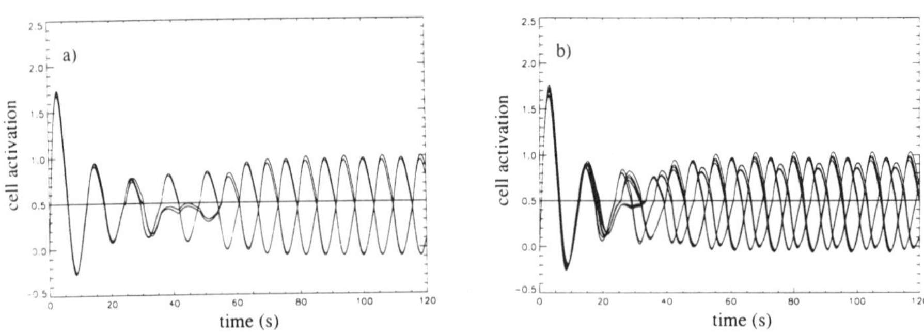

Fig. 17.2. Simulation results showing segmentation of inputs containing two (a) and three (b) constituents.

The occurrence of mixture decomposition has been confirmed by simulations of larger systems containing more nodes. These simulations indicate that larger systems can also deal with more complex inputs. One example of this type of behaviour, Fig. 17.2b, is a system of 12 pairs of nodes that is able to separate three known, orthogonal states presented simultaneously. Further simulations indicate that although it is possible to separate mixtures with more components, it becomes progressively more difficult to obtain reliable results. Usually, when a system is presented with an input containing a large number of known states, it is capable of separating out two or three dominant components. The combined inhibitory effect of these states suppresses the occurrence of the other components of the mixture. Thus for applications requiring the reliable separation of an input with a large number of constituents, the system should be modified to include an inhibitory input such as that used by Li (1990). This input can then be used to suppress a dominant response so that an input can be decomposed into its constituents parts sequentially.

4.4. Simulations on a Larger System

To confirm the other predicted behaviours of the oscillatory system, more simulations were performed using a system consisting of 12 pairs of nodes. Although relatively small, this system is large enough to give a good indication of the possible performance of large systems without becoming too computationally intensive.

One problem that may arise with larger systems is that the connections that arise from the correlations of several known states may lead to situations in which random inputs can lead to self-sustained oscillations. These inputs will then create spurious outputs that are indistinguishable from known states. They should therefore be prevented.

Our analysis of an isolated pair of nodes suggested that the fixed point about which the system oscillates is (x_0, y_0), where

$$x_0 = \alpha I/(\alpha^2 + \sigma' h)$$
$$y_0 = \sigma' I/(\alpha^2 + \sigma' h).$$

For small values of h the position of the fixed point is independent of h. Changing this parameter will therefore have little effect on the size of the impulse required to ensure that a node crosses through threshold to sustain oscillations. However, changing this parameter will increase the frequency of oscillation and reduce the amount of decay that occurs between impulses. Oscillations will therefore become easier to sustain. Eventually, when $\alpha^2 \approx \sigma' h$, changes in h will begin to move the fixed point away from threshold. Larger impulses are then required to sustain oscillatory behaviour and there will be fewer chance combinations of inputs that will led to self-sustained oscillations. The number of spurious states will therefore decrease. Unfortunately, for large values of h it will also become difficult to sustain oscillations even when an input corresponds to a known state. A value of h must therefore be selected which balances the desire to reduce the number of spurious states, with the need to ensure that known states are recognised and the pattern completion is possible.

In order to investigate the effect of these two competing mechanisms a series of simulations was undertaken to investigate the impact of changing $\langle h_i \rangle$ upon both known states and spurious states. The dynamical equations used were

$$\begin{aligned} x_i &= -\alpha x_i - h_i x_i + \sum_j T_{ij} g(x_j) + I_i \\ \dot{y}_i &= -\alpha y_i + \sigma(x_i) \end{aligned}$$

and for computational efficiency the form of σ was chosen to be as simple as possible, with the proviso that it be smooth everywhere:

$$\sigma(x) = \begin{cases} -1 & x \le -1 \\ (3x - x^3)/2 & |x| < 1 \\ 1 & x \ge 1 \end{cases} .$$

Finally, a value of $\kappa = 0.2$ was used to calculate the weight matrix to represent four known states.

The system response was then simulated for all possible binary inputs ((0, . . . , 0) through to (1, . . . , 1)) for a range of values of $\langle h_i \rangle$ around $\alpha \approx \sigma'\langle h_i \rangle/2$. The results showed that over this range as $\langle h_i \rangle$ increases it becomes increasingly difficult for spurious states to exist. As these states are destabilised their number falls dramatically, and more inputs are attracted toward the periodic orbits that represent known states. However, as expected, it eventually becomes difficult to sustain oscillations even for inputs corresponding to known states. The result is a peak in the number of known states retrieved which occurs close to $\alpha \approx \sigma'\langle h_i \rangle/2$. Thus by selecting $\langle h_i \rangle$ the number of known states retrieved can be maximised.

One of the desirable behaviours that could be lost when determining the value of $\langle h_i \rangle$ to minimise the number of spurious states is the ability to recognise incomplete inputs. Further simulations were therefore undertaken, with $\alpha = 0.16$ and $\langle h_i \rangle = 0.3$ (with standard deviation 0.02). The system ability to complete an input pattern is demonstrated in Fig. 17.3, where the activities of the 12 nodes are compared to the horizontal line that indicates the threshold of the step function g. Because this step function creates the system output only nodes that cross its threshold will be classified as active and included in the phase-locked group. Thus in the first part of Fig. 17.3 an extra input initially produces oscillation through threshold and would therefore form part of the recognised group. However, the cooperative inhibitory effect of the other nodes is sufficient to eventually suppress this node until it no longer crosses the threshold. This node is therefore excluded from the phase-locked group. In contrast, in the second part of this figure, positive weights are just sufficient to recruit a node to start to oscillate through threshold, thus correcting an initially inaccurate response.

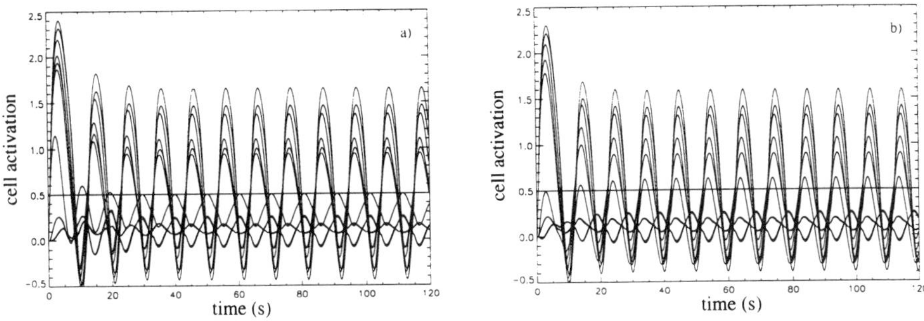

Fig. 17.3. The response of the system to a known input with an extra input (a) and one with a missing input (b), showing the ability of the system to perform pattern completion.

4.5. Novel Inputs and Learning

Another system behaviour demonstrated by these simulations is shown in Fig. 17.4. This figure shows a response to an input corresponding to a known state and the response to a novel input. As expected, the known input leads to self-sustained oscillations in which all the nodes cross the output threshold, resulting in phase-locked outputs from the excited nodes. In contrast, the response to the novel input is an oscillatory transient, which decays until none of the nodes cross the threshold and there is no output.

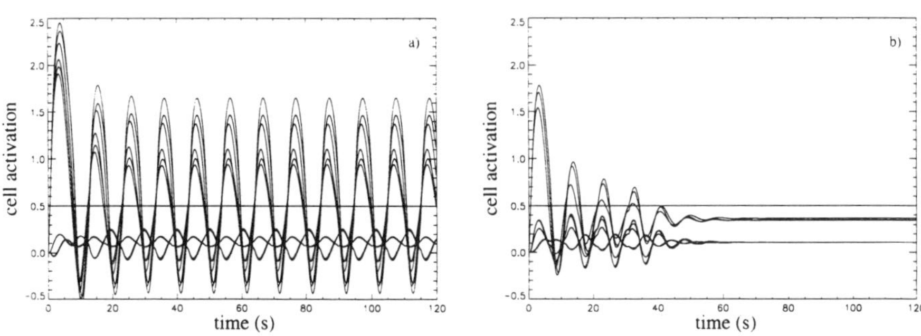

Fig. 17.4. The response of the system to a known input (a) and a random input (b) respectively.

Initially, the transient oscillations that arise in response to a novel input appear to be insignificant and possibly confusing. However, it is precisely this feature of the system behaviour that is required to create an adaptive system. In particular, these transient oscillations are required to indicate the correlations within novel inputs that must be reinforced so that a commonly occurring novel input can create a new known state.

The process by which a novel input becomes a known state has been demonstrated using a simple example in which the weight update rule

$$\Delta T_{ij} = \delta(x_i - \kappa)x_j ,$$

where δ is the learning rate, was used to change the weights during a simulation. The results, in Fig. 17.5, show that the weight changes that occur every time a particular new input is presented to the system gradually extend the period over which oscillations occur. Eventually, after several presentations, the response of the system to the initially novel input will be self-sustained oscillations. This demonstrates that even a simple learning rule, combined with the transient response to a novel input, could be used to create an adaptive system.

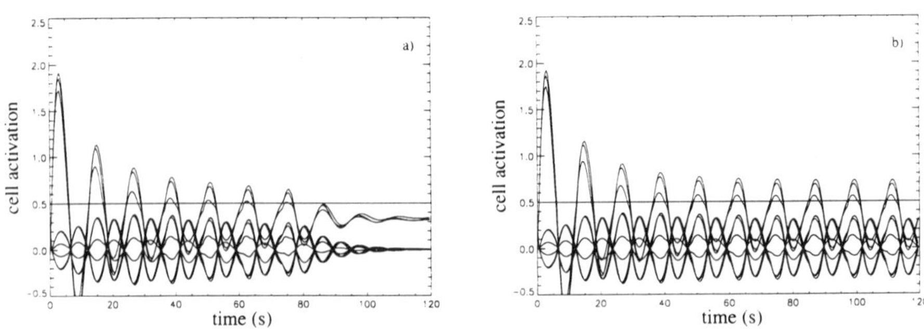

Fig. 17.5. The response of the system to the novel input in Fig. 17.4, with learning after 4 presentations (a) and 10 presentations (b) respectively.

5. COMPARISONS WITH THE HOPFIELD NETWORK

A special case of the proposed model occurs in the excitatory layer of the network if $h_i = \kappa = 0$. Under these conditions the equations governing the dynamics of the system become

$$x_i = -\alpha_i x_i + \sum_j w_{ij} g(x_j) + I_j$$

which are similar to those of the associative memory originally suggested by Hopfield and Tank (1986). A well-known problem associated with these systems is the limited memory capacity. It is therefore important to investigate the memory capacity of the oscillatory systems.

For a Hopfield network a formal derivation of the memory capacity in the limit for large numbers of nodes, N, has been obtained which is commonly approximated to $0.14N$ (Hertz et al., 1991). Unfortunately, the dynamics of the oscillatory system are considerably more complex than those of the standard Hopfield network and this appears to make the formal derivation of a limit to the memory capacity difficult, if not impossible. The memory capacity of an oscillatory network has been investigated by simulation. In particular a system with 12 nodes with $\langle h_i \rangle = 0.34$ and $\alpha = 0.15$ was investigated.

In order to measure the memory capacity of a system known states were chosen randomly from the set containing four, five or six inputs. The weight matrix was then calculated for this selection of states and then the system's ability to recall each known state was tested. If all the known states were recalled successfully, then another known state was added to the existing list and the weight matrix recalculated. This procedure was repeated until the system fails to respond correctly to at least one known state. The memory capacity is then the maximum number of states that can be stored correctly. However, because the memory capacity will depend on the known states being represented, this procedure was repeated 100 times to estimate the memory capacity of this system. Because the storage capacity of the system depended on the particular combinations of known states the result is a spread in the memory capacity of this system from 3 to 8, with a mean of 5.

One observation that could be exploited to increase the memory capacity of the network is that restricting the system to known states with only four active nodes increases the mean memory capacity to 5.71. The advantages of employing sparse coding schemes can be understood from a heuristic argument.

Consider the equations of motion of the system

$$
\begin{aligned}
\dot{x}_i &= -\alpha x_i - h_i x_i + \sum_j T_{ij} g(x_j) + I_i \\
\dot{y}_i &= -\alpha y_i + \sigma(x_i)
\end{aligned}
$$

where

$$
T_{ij} = \left\{ \begin{array}{ll} \frac{1}{n} \sum_s (\xi_i^s - \kappa) \xi_j^s & i \neq j \\ 0 & i = j \end{array} \right\}.
$$

As isolated pairs (i.e., where $T_{ij} = 0$) all of these units would decay to a fixed point and it is the extra periodic stimuli, given by the connections to the other nodes, that produce oscillations. For a known memory, $\Xi^\mu = (\xi_1^\mu, \ldots, \xi_n^\mu)$, the correct response is obtained if two conditions apply:

- For nodes that should oscillate through threshold, the weighted sum $\Sigma_j T_{ij}\xi_j^{\mu}$ must be strictly greater than zero, in order to create the periodic impulses that are large enough to sustain oscillations.

- For the nodes that should not oscillate, the weighted sum $\Sigma_j T_{ij}\xi_j^{\mu}$ must be small so that internal decay can prevent this node from oscillating through threshold.

The strength of the internal decay constant can be modified to ensure that this second condition is easily satisfied. Thus the significant condition required to create the desired behaviour is the one that applies to those nodes that oscillate through threshold. Reducing the number of these nodes, by using a sparse coding scheme, thereby makes this condition easier to satisfy. Sparse coding schemes will therefore increase the average number of states that can be stored before the above conditions no longer apply.

Although using a sparse coding scheme can increase the memory capacity of the system, the resulting mean, between 5 and 6, is small compared to the 4,096 possible states that could be chosen. However, this initially disappointing result must be judged in comparison with the Hopfield network. The experimental procedure used with the oscillatory system was also used with a Hopfield network. The results suggest that a 12-node Hopfield network has a mean storage capacity of 3.1. This suggests that the storage capacity of the oscillatory system is larger than that of a Hopfield network. Unfortunately, the increase in memory capacity may be insufficient to justify an implementation of the proposed system and techniques should be investigated that will allow further increases.

6. CONCLUSIONS

As the first step to creating an adaptive analogue architecture a simple model has been proposed. The model was developed by including negative feedback within the circuit equations of a fixed point system. This feedback creates oscillations that allow the system to perform signal separation and adaptation.

An intuitive understanding of the system, required to create an efficient implementation, has been developed by considering systems with a small number of nodes within the model. These considerations show that the self-sustained oscillatory behaviour required to represent a known input arises from cooperative interactions. Furthermore, one of the parameters within the model has been identified as a possible means of controlling the number of erroneous system responses. With the correct parameter values the system has several useful capabilities:

- it is able to recognise incomplete input patterns

- it can segment a mixed input into its constituent parts

- it can easily detect novel inputs

- it can reinforce the internal connections in response to novel inputs so that a commonly occurring input becomes a known state

Furthermore, features such as:

- a learning rule based on local information
- the need for device variations to ensure that spontaneous phase-locking does not persist

make the model ideally suited for implementation as an adaptive analogue architecture.

REFERENCES

Andreou, A. G., & Edwards, T. G. (1993). Phase locking architectures for feature linking in multiple target tracking systems. *Advances in Neural Information Processing Systems* 6 (pp. 866-873). San Mateo, CA: Morgan Kaufman.

Brown, A. G., & Collins, S. (1994). An oscillatory associative memory. *Proceedings of the Fourth International Conference on Micro-electronics for Neural Networks and Fuzzy Systems* (pp. 186-191). Los Alamitos, CA: IEEE Computer Society Press.

Hertz, J., Krogh, A., & Palmer, R. G. (1991). *Introduction to the Theory of Neural Computation.* Santa Fe: Addison-Wesley.

Hopfield, J. J., & Tank, D. W. (1986). Computing with neural circuits: A model. *Science, 233,* 625-633.

Horn, D., & Usher, M. (1991). Parallel activation of memories in an oscillatory neural network. *Neural Computation, 3,* 31-43.

Larson, J., & Lynch, G. (1986). Induction of synaptic potentiations in hippocampus by patterned stimulation involves two events. *Science, 232,* 985-988.

Li, Z. (1990). A model of olfactory adaptation and sensitivity enhancement in the olfactory bulb. *Biological Cybernetics, 62,* 349-361.

Wang, D., Buhmann, J., & Malsburg, C. von der (1990). Pattern segmentation in Associative Memory. *Neural Computation, 2,* 94-106.

18

Symbolic Knowledge Encoding Using a Dynamic Binding Mechanism and an Embedded Inference Mechanism

Nam Seog Park
General Electric Corporate Research and Development

Dave Robertson, and Keith Stenning
The University of Edinburgh

ABSTRACT

This chapter describes how synchronous activity between neuron elements can be used to build a dynamic binding mechanism and knowledge encoding mechanisms in a connectionist manner. The purpose of these mechanisms is to build a connectionist inference architecture that can replicate common symbolic styles of inference. To build such an inference architecture, an extended temporal synchrony approach (Park, Robertson, & Stenning, 1995) is used as a basic building block. This is a revision and extension of an approach to the dynamic binding problem in connectionist systems, proposed by Shastri and Ajjanagadde (1993). In addition, we introduce a set of algorithms that gives us a means of compiling a class of symbolic rules into a uniform inference network called a structured predicate network. This is used as a connectionist knowledge encoding mechanism which encodes symbolic rules and supports very fast inference.

1. INTRODUCTION

The study of oscillations in neural systems has attracted much attention from many researchers. Engel, König, Kreiter, Gray, and Singer (1991) observed that neurons in different parts of the brain oscillate in synchrony in response to certain stimuli. One hypothesised function for such synchronous activity is to solve the binding problem in human perception. Some researchers already have shown such a possibility in visual perception (Horn, Sagi, & Usher, 1991; Hummel & Biederman, 1992; Strong & Whitehead, 1989; Wang & Terman, 1995).

Using temporal synchrony in a connectionist model to support inference is found in the early work of Fahlman (1979) in which temporal synchrony is represented by the notion of marker passing. Each node in the network stores a small number of discrete markers. These markers propagate between nodes under the supervision of the network controller to achieve dynamic bindings and symbolic inference. Thus, nodes in his system were required to have high computational abilities, in order to store, match, and selectively propagate maker bits. Later, Clossman (1988) used synchronous activity to represent argument-filler bindings for a connectionist model of categorisation and learning, but without an efficient encoding mechanism for rules and facts. Recently, Ajjanagadde and Shastri (1991) and Shastri and Ajjanagadde (1993) proposed another connectionist model for reflexive reasoning called SHRUTI. It provides an efficient connectionist mechanism to represent dynamic bindings based on temporal synchrony and other mechanisms that encode rules and facts involving predicates with *n* arguments. However, SHRUTI's dynamic binding mechanism cannot properly represent a variable binding and Park et al. (1995) extended their dynamic binding mechanism to cope with this limitation.

The purpose of this chapter is to introduce a connectionist inference architecture which encodes symbolic rules into the corresponding networks and performs fast inference over them. To start with, we describe in Section 2 a type of symbolic knowledge and common styles of symbolic inference that we would like to replicate using the proposed connectionist inference architecture. Then, Section 3 explains the dynamic binding problem in connectionist systems and outlines the temporal synchrony approach and its extension. The emphasis is on how temporal synchronous activities among neuron elements can be used to support dynamic bindings. This section also deals with how subtasks involved in symbolic styles of inference can be represented in a connectionist manner. In Section 4, we propose a connectionist inference architecture that uses the extended dynamic binding mechanism and the connectionist equivalents to the symbolic inference subtasks. A rule encoding and a connectionist inference procedure by the proposed architecture is demonstrated using some example rules. Section 5 compares our inference architecture to other similar inference models currently available. Finally, Section 6 discusses the results and concludes this chapter.

2. A BASIC SYMBOLIC INFERENCE

Predicate calculus is a formally defined representation scheme that allows us to express the knowledge needed to solve a problem. Our chosen knowledge representation scheme is a subset of *first-order Horn clause expressions*, which is a set of universally quantified expressions in first-order predicate calculus of the form:

$$p_1(...) \wedge p_2(...) \wedge ... \wedge p_n(...) \rightarrow q(...)$$

where $p_i(...)$ and $q(...)$ are positive atomic expressions called *predicates*. The conjunction of $p_i(...)$ is called the *antecedent* and the $q(...)$ the *consequent*. An expression with no antecedent is called a *fact* and an expression that has both antecedent and consequent is called a *rule*. The symbol $\rightarrow$ is normally read as "implies" and called the *implication*. Some example sentences translated into facts and rules are:

"Adam is a man.": *man(adam);*
"For any X, if X is a man then X is mortal.": $man(X) \rightarrow mortal(X)$;
"John loves Mary.": *love(john,mary);*
"For any X and Z, if there is some Y such that X loves Y and Y loves Z, then X is jealous of Z.":
$love(X,Y) \wedge love(Y,Z) \rightarrow jealous(X,Z)$.

As can be seen, the basic structured component of rules and facts is a predicate. Each predicate having n arguments (n-ary predicate) is represented using a predicate symbol followed by n terms where terms are constant symbols or variable symbols.

If we translate the statement "Every man is mortal. Adam is a man." into first-order Horn clause expressions, the first statement is represented by the rule

$$\text{man}(X) \rightarrow \text{mortal}(X),$$

based on the notion that "X is a man" by the predicate $man(X)$, and "X is mortal" by the predicate $mortal(X)$. The two symbols *man* and *mortal* are called predicate names, and X's in the bracket are called *arguments* of the predicates.

The second sentence, "Adam is a man.", is then represented by the fact

man(adam).

In order to draw inference based on these expressions, we need inference rules. An inference rule is a mechanical means of producing a new expression from other expressions. Two inference rules frequently used are *universal instantiation* and *modus ponens* (Luger & Stubblefield, 1989):

- *universal instantiation* states that if any universally quantified variable in a true expression is replaced by any appropriate term from the domain, the result is a true expression. Thus, if a is from the domain of X, the $\forall X\, p(X)$ lets us infer $p(a)$. The meaning of the symbol $\forall$ is "for all," and it is called the *universal quantifier.*

- if the fact p and the rule $p \rightarrow q$ are known to be true, then *modus ponens* lets us infer q.

Because the X in the rule is universally quantified, we may substitute any value (also called a *filler*) in the domain for X and it still has a true statement under the inference rule of universal instantiation. Based on the known fact, *man(adam)*, we can substitute *adam* for X in the rule. As a result, we obtain the expression, $man(adam) \rightarrow mortal(adam)$. From this new expression and the known fact, *man(adam)*, we can now apply modus ponens and infer the conclusion *mortal(adam)*.

In order to apply the inference rule, modus ponens, an inference system must be able to determine when two expressions are the same or match. This requires a decision process for determining the variable substitutions under which two or more expressions can be made identical. In the example rule and fact, for instance, the antecedent of the rule *man(X)* and the fact *man(adam)* can be identical when we substitute *adam* for the variable *X*. This substitution is called a binding and represented by the notation {adam/X}. This binding is used later to substitute the value *adam* for all the occurrences of the variable *X* in the rule to obtain a new expression on which we can apply modus ponens inference rule. In summary, a step of forward chaining inference based on modus ponens is carried out by two subtasks, *matching* and *substitution*. For a given set of rules already known, when a fact is presented, the matching subtask tries to match between the presented fact and the antecedents of rules. If there is any match, it produces a set of bindings. The substitution subtask then uses these bindings to substitute all occurrence of variables in the rule matched. The resulting expression provides the conclusion of inference.

In some cases, a variable can be identified with another variable. For example, the sentence, "There is someone who is a man.", could be translated into the expression, *man(U)*, where *U* is a variable standing for someone. Matching this fact with the antecedent of the example rule produces the binding, {U/X}. Substituting *U* for all *X*'s in the rule generates the new expression, *man(U)* → *mortal(U)*. By applying modus ponens, we reach the conclusion "*U* is mortal."

Therefore, according to types of symbol names involved, there are two types of bindings: a constant binding and a variable binding. The term *constant binding* will be used to refer to the situation where a variable is bound to a constant, and *variable binding* the situation where a variable is bound to a variable. For instance, a binding between the constant *adam* and *X*, {adam/X}, is called a constant binding, and a binding between the variable *U* and *X*, {U/X}, a variable binding.

Any connectionist system which replicates this type of symbolic inference must provide ways of representing symbolic knowledge and inference rules as well as representing bindings in a connectionist manner. This requires us to represent in a connectionist style the basic components of symbolic rules, such as symbols and predicates having *n* arguments. Representing inference rules requires how to represent the subtasks involved in a step of symbolic inference.

3. REPRESENTING DYNAMIC BINDINGS

3.1. Dynamic Bindings and Symbolic Inference

Let us consider the sentence, "If someone owns something, she or he can sell it.", which may be represented by the following rule:

own(X,Y) → *can_sell(X,Y)*.

By being told the fact, "John owns Car21.", which may be translated into the predicate *own(john,car21)*, one can infer the conclusion, "John can sell Car21." In the same way, by being told the fact, "Mary owns Book42," one can infer the different conclusion, "Mary can sell Book42.", using the same rule. During these inference procedures, an inference system dynamically produces a different set of bindings between the arguments of the antecedent of the rule and their corresponding fillers to support each inference: {john/own:X, car21/own:Y} at the first time and {mary/own:X, book42/own:Y} at the second time. These dynamic bindings are used to generate new expressions

own(john,car21) → can_sell(john,car21),
own(mary,book42) → can_sell(mary,book42),

from which both conclusions are reached. The importance of a dynamic representation of bindings is therefore due to its ability to create a new temporal binding to apply inference rules.

However, the ability of a connectionist system to represent dynamic bindings has been doubted (Fodor & Pylyshyn, 1988; McCarty, 1988), because the expression "John owns Car21.", *owns(john,car21)*, cannot be represented dynamically by simply activating the nodes representing the arguments, *own:X* and *own:Y* and the nodes representing the fillers, *john* and *car21*. The problem is that the given expression does not merely express an association between the arguments and fillers, it expresses a specific relation in which each binding between an argument and a filler plays a distinct role in the expression (Shastri & Ajjanagadde, 1993). What is required is a connectionist representation of correct bindings between predicate arguments and their fillers, {john/own:X, car21/own:Y}, from which we can recognise the expression, *own(john,car21)*, dynamically.

3.2. A Temporal Synchrony Approach

One solution to this dynamic binding problem is a temporal synchrony solution proposed by Shastri and Ajjanagadde (1993). The basis of this solution is a separation of the period of the oscillation cycle into several phases and the use of phase-sensitive neuron elements. A *phase* is a minimum time interval in which a neuron element performs its basic computations — counting the number of spikes and comparing to a threshold. An *oscillation cycle* is a window of time in which neuron elements show their oscillatory behaviours.

The computational behaviours of the phase-sensitive neuron elements are as follows:

- ρ-btu elements become active on receiving one spike in an oscillation cycle. On becoming active, ρ-btu elements produce a train of spikes that are in phase with the driving inputs.

- τ-or elements become active on receiving one or more spikes within an oscillation cycle. On becoming active, τ-or elements produce an oscillatory pulse train whose pulse width spans the entire oscillation cycle.

- multiphase τ-or elements become active on receiving more than one inputs in different phases within an oscillation cycle. On becoming active, multiphase τ-or elements produce an oscillatory pulse train whose pulse width spans the entire oscillation cycle.

Their approach also uses a τ-and element that behaves as a temporal AND element. However, its computational behaviour is not discussed because this chapter will not need it for the purpose of presentation.

If one phase-sensitive element A is connected to another element B, a periodic activation of A leads to a periodic and in-phase activation of B. It is assumed that a neuron element can respond in this manner as long as the period of activation (oscillation cycle), π, lies in the interval $[\pi_{min}, \pi_{max}]$. This interval can be interpreted as defining the frequency range over which a neuron element can sustain a synchronised response. A threshold, n, associated with each element indicates that the element will be active only if it receives n or more synchronous inputs. Figure 18.1 graphically depicts neuron elements and their temporal characteristics.

The temporal synchrony approach uses these neuron elements to represent components of symbolic rules to build networks encoding them. Arguments of expressions and potential fillers for those arguments are represented using ρ-btu elements, and an n-ary predicate in a rule is represented by an assembly of n ρ-btu elements, where each element corresponds to each argument. The predicate *p(X,Y)*, for instance, is represented by using an assembly of two ρ-btu elements corresponding to the arguments *p:X* and *p:Y*. Figure 18.2a depicts this predicate and the two constant fillers *a* and *b*.

Based on this representation, the set of bindings, {*a*/*p*:X, *b*/*p*:Y}, which will be used to generate the new predicate *p(a,b)* is represented in the following ways:

- The constant binding between the argument *p:X* and the constant *a*, {a/p:X}, is represented by activating in the same phase the element representing *p:X* and that representing *a*. Similarly, the constant binding {b/p:Y} is represented by activating in the same phase the element representing *p:Y* and that representing *b*.

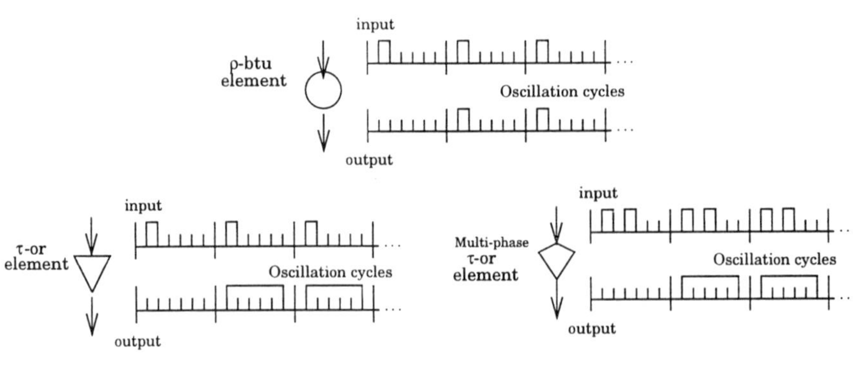

Fig. 18.1. Temporal behaviours of phase-sensitive neuron elements.

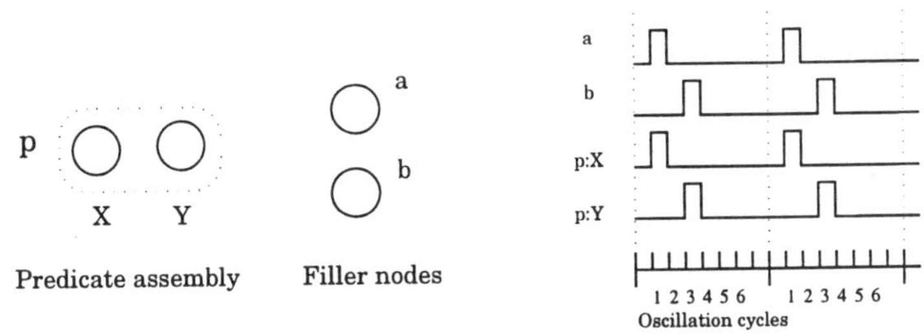

(a) Representing the predicate p(X,Y) and two constant a and b

(b) Representing dynamic bindings using a synchronous activities

Fig. 18.2. A representation of the predicate and dynamic bindings.

Figure 18.2b demonstrates these two constant dynamic bindings. Another set of dynamic bindings, {*c*/*p*:X, *d*/*p*:Y}, to produce the new predicate *p(c,d)* can also be represented simply activating two ρ-btu elements representing the new fillers, *c* and *d*, in-phase with the elements representing arguments, *p:X* and *p:Y*. Thus, the temporal synchrony approach can represent dynamic bindings very efficiently by using synchronous activity between neuron elements.

This solution, however, has limitations (Park et al., 1995). One important limitation is that it cannot represent variable bindings. This is because ρ-btu elements are used to represent only constant fillers in their mechanism. For instance, it cannot differentiate two variable bindings, {U/p:X, V/p:Y} because no ρ-btu element is used to represent the variable fillers *U* and *V*. Consequently, the ρ-btu elements representing *p:X* and *p:Y* remain inactive throughout inference. Connectionist systems that replicate symbolic inference should be capable of dealing with both constant and variable bindings dynamically without disrupting the structure of the network.

3.3. An Extended Temporal Synchrony Approach

Park et al. (1995) extended the temporal synchrony approach to overcome the limitation demonstrated in the previous subsection. This extension involves generalisation of ρ-btu elements and introduction of entity nodes.

3.3.1 Generalisation of ρ-btu Elements. Shastri and Ajjanagadde's system restricted their ρ-btu element to carrying only one spike per oscillation cycle. We generalise the ρ-btu element so that it can carry more than one spike per oscillation cycle.

The detailed temporal behaviour of the generalised element, which we call a π-btu element, is as follows:

A π-btu element becomes active on receiving one or more spikes in different phases of any oscillation cycle. On becoming active, a π-btu element produces oscillatory spikes that are in-phase with the driving inputs. A threshold, n, associated with each element indicates that the element will fire only if it receives n or more spike inputs in the same phase.

Figure 18.3 demonstrates the behaviour of π-btu elements.

This π-btu element allows multiple spikes per cycle and propagates these in synchrony with the driving inputs. This requires higher signal transfer rates than Shastri and Ajjanagadde's ρ-btu elements. Eckhorn (1993) observed that the signal transfer rates on biological neurons are much higher than those of ρ-btu elements. Such high rates in a single neuron are capable of signalling complex messages, including routing dynamic representations. This allows the possibility that there exists a type of neuron whose signal transfer ability is even higher than the π-btu element.

3.3.2. Representing Entities and Predicates. To represent symbolic entities, the extended approach introduces an entity node. An entity node is a pair of π-btu elements. The left element is used to represent a variable role of the entity and the right element a constant role. A symbolic entity name may be used as a label of an entity node. For convenience in discussion, we represent an entity node using the notation, *entity_name([0],[0])*, where the left square bracket represents the state of the left π-btu element and the right square bracket that of the right π-btu element. The symbol "0" denotes that the element is inactive. The notations, $entity\_name_{left}[0]$ or $entity\_name_{right}[0]$ are used to indicate each state of the left or the right π-btu element. When an entity node is used to represent a constant filler, only its right element is used. When the entity node is used to represent a variable filler, only its left element is used. However, when it is used to represent an argument of a predicate, either or both elements may be used at the same time. When an entity node is used simply to represent a constant or a variable filler, the notations, *var_name[0]* or *const_name[0]* is used to shorten the representation.

Using entity nodes, an n-ary predicate is then represented by an assembly of n entity nodes, labelled $A_1, A_2, ..., A_n$, where the entity node A_i represents the ith argument of the predicate. We use the notation,

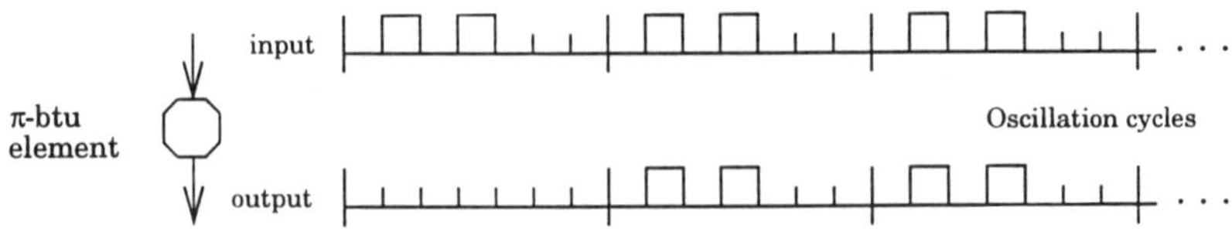

Fig. 18.3. Temporal behaviour of a π-btu element.

$$pred\_name{:}\{\, A_1([0],[0]),\ A_2([0],[0]),\ \ldots,\ A_n([0],[0])\},$$

to represent an n-ary predicate assembly symbolically. Figure 18.4a depicts a graphic representation of the predicate assembly representing $p(X,Y)$ and the two fillers a and U.

Because entity nodes are used to represent both fillers and arguments, dynamic bindings are represented using temporal synchronous activity between entity nodes. When the predicate $p(X,Y)$ and the two fillers a and U are represented as shown in Fig. 18.4a, the dynamic bindings, $\{a/p{:}X,\ U/p{:}Y\}$, between these fillers and the arguments of the p predicate assembly are represented in the following ways:

- the constant binding between a and $p{:}X$ is represented by activating the entity node representing a and the right element of the entity node representing $p{:}X$ in the first phase so that $a[0]$ becomes $a[1]$ and $p{:}X_{rightl}[0]$ becomes $p{:}X_{rightl}[1]$, where the number 1 stands for the first phase;

- the variable binding between U and $p{:}Y$ is represented by activating the entity node representing U and the left element of the entity node representing $p{:}Y$ in a new phase, the second phase for example, so that $U[0]$ becomes $U[1]$ and $p{:}Y_{leftl}[0]$ becomes $p{:}Y_{leftl}[2]$, where the number 2 indicates the second phase.

3.3.3. Representing Dynamic Bindings. Figure 18.4b depicts the phasic representation of these dynamic bindings. Basically the in-phase activation of two or more entity nodes represents bindings between them. Constant bindings or variable bindings are distinguished by the position of the activated element of the entity node. This is a feature absent in Shastri and Ajjanagadde's temporal synchrony approach.

(a) Representation of the predicate and fillers

(b) Representation of dynamic bindings

Fig. 18.4. The extended representation of the predicate and dynamic bindings.

3.4. Representing Inference Procedures

Even if we have a connectionist binding mechanism and a way of representing symbolic knowledge components, there still remains the problem of how to represent symbolic inference procedures in a connectionist manner. As described in Section 2, a step of symbolic inference involves two subtasks, matching and substitution. If we reconsider the following rule again

$$own(X,Y) \rightarrow can\_sell(X,Y).$$

Presenting the fact "John owns something." which may be represented by the predicate *own(john, U)*, to an inference architecture should result in the set of bindings {john/own:*X*, U/own:*Y*} to complete the matching subtask. If the predicate *own(X, Y)* and the two fillers, *john* and *U*, are represented using the following predicate assembly and entity nodes

$$own{:}\{X([0],[0]), Y([0],[0])\}, john[0],\ U[0],$$

the above situation can be represented easily by setting up dynamic bindings between argument nodes of the predicate assembly and the two filler nodes as follows:

$$own{:}\{X([0],[1]), Y([2],[0])\}, john[1],\ U[2],$$

where in phase oscillations between $own{:}X_{right}[1]$ and *john[1]* and between $own{:}Y_{left}[2]$ and *U[2]* represent the required bindings, {john/own:X, U/own:Y}.

Once a set of bindings are obtained, the substitution subtask substitutes these fillers for the arguments and this results in the new expression

$$own(john,U) \rightarrow can\_sell(john,U).$$

If the predicate *can_sell* is represented with the predicate assembly

$$can\_sell{:}\{X([0],[0]), Y([0],[0])\},$$

the effect of this substitution subtask may be achieved in a connectionist manner by activating $can\_sell{:}X_{right}[0]$ in the first phase and $can\_sell{:}Y_{left}[0]$ in the second phase as follows:

$$can\_sell{:}\{X([0],[1]), Y([2],[0])\}.$$

Then, the new oscillatory behaviour between the constant filler node *john[1]* and $can\_sell{:}X_{right}[1]$ represents the new constant binding {john/can_sell:X} and in-phase activation between the variable filler node *U[2]* and $can\_sell{:}Y_{left}[2]$ the new variable binding {U/can_sell:Y}. From the sets of dynamic bindings obtained from the *own* and *can_sell* predicate assemblies, a new expression $own(john,U) \rightarrow can\_sell(john,U)$ can be obtained to conclude *can_sell(john, U)*.

Observation of these subtasks and their connectionist representations suggests that common symbolic styles of inference can be achieved in a connectionist manner by the following procedure:

Step 1: When a rule is given, represent the antecedent and the consequent of the rule using predicate assemblies; The predicate assembly corresponding to the antecedent is called the antecedent predicate assembly, and that corresponding to the consequent of the rule the consequent predicate assembly.

Step 2: When a fact is presented, set up initial bindings between the fillers appearing in the presented fact and the argument nodes of the antecedent predicate assembly of the rule matched in the following way:

- represent each filler appearing in the presented fact using an entity node (let us call it a filler node);
- activate each filler node and its corresponding argument node of the predicate assembly matched in a unique phase in such a way that: if the filler is a constant, activate both the right elements of the filler and the argument nodes; if the filler is a variable, activate both the left elements of the filler and the argument nodes.

Step 3: To complete a step of inference, propagate the initial bindings from each argument node of the antecedent predicate assembly to its corresponding argument of the consequent predicate assembly (which share the same argument name).

The last step of inference is possible by setting up links between each argument node of the antecedent predicate assembly and the corresponding argument node of the consequent predicate assembly, after the antecedent and the consequent of the rule are represented using their predicate assemblies. However, care must be taken when establishing these links because this automatic propagation of initial bindings from the antecedent predicate assembly to the consequent predicate assembly can be affected by the type of rules involved.

3.5. Handling Difficult Issues

Until now a simple rule has been used to illustrate the extended dynamic binding mechanism and connectionist symbolic inference procedures. If the proposed mechanism has to deal with a more complex symbolic rule such as $p(X,X) \rightarrow q(X)$ which requires repeated arguments of the p predicate to get bound to the same constant filler or free variable fillers, an additional connectionist mechanism is needed to force this condition. This is because the initial binding instantiation mechanism simply sets up bindings without involving any consistency checking within a group of unifying arguments (the repeated arguments X's for p). Therefore, an additional connectionist submechanism is needed to detect a consistency violation when two different constant fillers are assigned to different occurrences of the same variable argument.

This requires an additional submechanism to be added apart from the links which connect the antecedent predicate assembly with the consequent predicate assembly. The role of this additional submechanism is to ensure consistency conditions that are enforced by the syntax of a rule and to block binding propagation from the antecedent predicate assembly to the consequent predicate assembly if there is any consistency violation.

Other types of rules which also require special treatment are

- rules having constant arguments: $p(a,b,X) \rightarrow q(b,X)$; If constant arguments appear in the antecedent of a rule, an additional submechanism has to perform consistency checking to ensure all the fillers assigned to the constant arguments are the same as the ones specified as constant argument names;

- rules requiring consistency checking across different groups of unifying arguments: $p(X,X,Y,Y) \rightarrow q(X,Y)$; This is more general case of the rule $p(X,X) \rightarrow q(X)$ but requires binding interaction across different groups of unifying arguments (between X's and Y's). Thus, it requires us to check any consistency violation occurring across these two groups of unifying arguments.

Because each type of rule requires a different structure for the additional submechanism, special algorithms are needed to decide a proper structure of the submechanism according to the type of the given rule. The algorithms for these tasks are described in greater detail in the next section.

4. A CONNECTIONIST INFERENCE ARCHITECTURE

Having introduced the extended connectionist dynamic binding mechanism and the connectionist symbolic inference procedures, the rest of the chapter describes how these mechanisms can be used as basic building blocks for a connectionist inference architecture.

4.1. A Structured Predicate Network

When a symbolic rule is encoded, representation of the antecedent and the consequent is easily done by creating their corresponding predicate assemblies. The main issue is how to build a proper intermediate mechanism between them because the intermediate mechanism has to be designed not only to provide a path for binding propagation but also to prevent incorrect substitution during unification. This needs to take into account consistency of bindings in the antecedent; correct propagation of bindings from antecedent to consequent; and consistency of bindings in the consequent after binding propagation. This suggests that each rule needs to be encoded into a special type of network which has a unique intermediate mechanism to support a target form of symbolic inference. This special type of network, which will be called a structured predicate network (SPN), can be defined as follows:

Definition: A structured predicate network (SPN) is a localist network which encodes a rule. Each SPN is composed of three parts, $SPN = \{P_a, M, P_c\}$, where P_a is a predicate assembly representing the antecedent, P_c is a predicate assembly representing the consequent, and M is the intermediate mechanism that connects them. The overall structure of an SPN looks like the network shown in Fig. 18.5.

Whenever a rule is encoded, the intermediate mechanism, M, for the rule will be implemented in such a way that it includes several submechanisms that carry out all the necessary subtasks to achieve the target symbolic inference.

4.2. Basic Definitions

This subsection defines some basic definitions that will be used to decide required submechanisms when a rule is encoded.

Definition: For a given predicate, $p(A_1, A_2, ..., A_n)$, a *unifying argument group* (UAG) of the predicate p, G_{Ai}, is a set of arguments that have an identical symbol name A_i. If there are repeated arguments in the predicate, a series of subscript numbers may be used to differentiate one from others. If the argument group is for a constant name, G_{Ai} is called a *constant UAG* and if the argument group is for a variable name, G_{Ai} is called a *variable UAG*. Because each rule has an antecedent and a consequent, we obtain two sets of UAGs from a rule. To distinguish a set of UAGs generated by the antecedent from that produced by the consequent, we use two symbols, S_a and S_c.

Definition: For two sets of UAGs corresponding to the antecedent and the consequent of a rule:

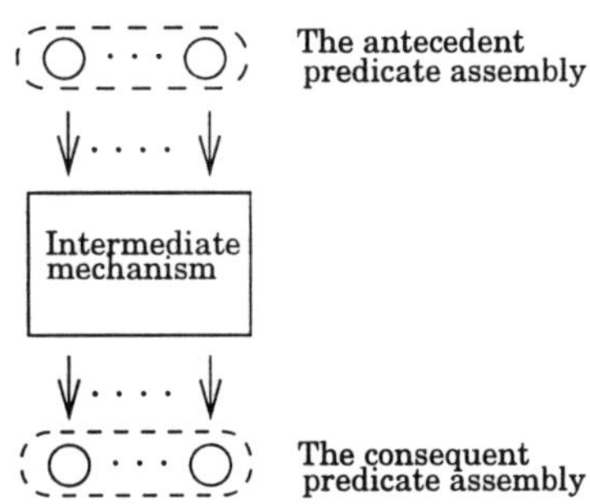

Fig. 18.5. The structure of a SPN.

$$S_a = \{G_{A1}, G_{A2}, \ldots , G_{An}\},$$
$$S_c = \{G_{A1}, G_{A2}, \ldots , G_{Am}\},$$

we say that G_{Ai} in S_a is *related* to G_{Aj} in S_c and vice versa if *Ai* and *Aj* refer to the same symbolic argument name, that is, $Ai = Aj$. In other words, two UAGs obtained from the antecedent and the consequent are related if they are obtained from the same symbolic argument name.

To illustrate these definitions, let us consider the following rule:

$$p(X, X, Y, Y) \rightarrow q(X, Y).$$

From the antecedent, *p(X, X, Y, Y)*, we get

$$S_a = \{G_X, G_Y\}, \text{ where } G_X = \{p{:}X_1, p{:}X_2\},\ G_Y = \{p{:}Y_1, p{:}Y_2\}.$$

Note that the subscript numbers in the argument names of G_X indicate the order of each argument repeatedly appearing in the predicate. This is simply to differentiate repeated arguments in different argument positions and does not affect the meaning of the original argument name.

From the consequent, *q(X, Y)*, we obtain:

$$S_c = \{G_X, G_Y\}, \text{ where } G_X = \{q{:}X\},\ G_Y = \{q{:}Y\}.$$

We say that G_X in S_a is related to G_X in S_c because they are obtained from the same argument name *X*. Also G_Y in S_a is related to G_Y in S_c.

Definition: The *size of* a set of UAGs is a number of UAGs in the set and the size of a UAG is a number of arguments in the UAG. If the size of a UAG is greater than 1, this means that the UAG was obtained from repeated arguments of a predicate.

If we consider the following rule

$$p(X, Y) \rightarrow q(X, Y, Z),$$

the S_a and S_c of the rule are

$$S_a = \{G_X, G_Y\}, \text{ where } G_X = \{p{:}X\},\ G_Y = \{p{:}Y\},$$
$$S_c = \{G_X, G_Y, G_Z\}, \text{ where } G_X = \{q{:}X\},\ G_Y = \{q{:}Y\},\ G_Z = \{q{:}Z\},$$

$size(S_a) = 2$ and $size(S_c) = 3$ and the sizes of all UAGs in S_a and S_c are 1.

4.3. Building an Intermediate Mechanism

When encoding each rule, a mechanical procedure is required to build the intermediate mechanism. This subsection describes such a procedure which determines the required submechanisms automatically based on the information about two sets of UAGs (S_a and S_c) obtained from the given rule.

4.3.1. Binding Collection For Each UAG. Any repeated arguments of the antecedent force the condition that they have to get bound to the same constant filler or free variable fillers during inference. This requires any bindings generated from the repeated arguments to be collected for consistency checking. A binding collection submechanism (*BCM*) is needed for this purpose. The group of UAGs which need a *BCM* can be determined by checking the size of each UAG in the antecedent:

$$BCM = \{G_{Ai} | \, G_{Ai} \in Sa \wedge size(G_{Ai}) > 1\}.$$

The structure of a *BCM* is demonstrated in Fig. 18.6. As can be seen, the *BCM* consists of one entity node, called a *binding node*, and associated links. The argument nodes representing the repeated arguments in G_{Ai} are connected to the binding nodes through the links. When the initial bindings are set up on these argument nodes, they propagate to the binding node automatically. The left element of the binding node then represents variable bindings of all argument nodes and the right element constant bindings. The consistency of these intermediate bindings is checked later by another consistency checking submechanism.

4.3.2 Binding Propagation for Each UAG. To achieve symbolic inference, the initial bindings that are set on the antecedent predicate assembly need to propagate to the consequent predicate assembly. Therefore, a binding propagation submechanism (*BPM*) is needed to provide paths for binding propagation from the argument nodes of any UAG in the antecedent predicate assembly to those of the related UAG in the consequent predicate assembly. The UAGs that need a *BPM* are determined by the following condition:

$$BPM = \{G_{Ai} \mid G_{Ai} \in S_a \wedge G_{Ai} \in S_c\}.$$

According to the type of a UAG, two different *BPM*s are required: A *BPM* for a variable UAG (BPM_v) and a *BPM* for a constant UAG (BPM_c). Figure 18.7 illustrates them.

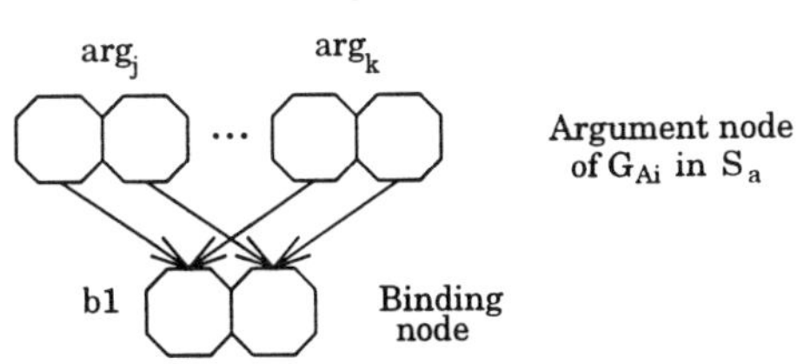

Fig. 18.6. The structure of a *BCM*.

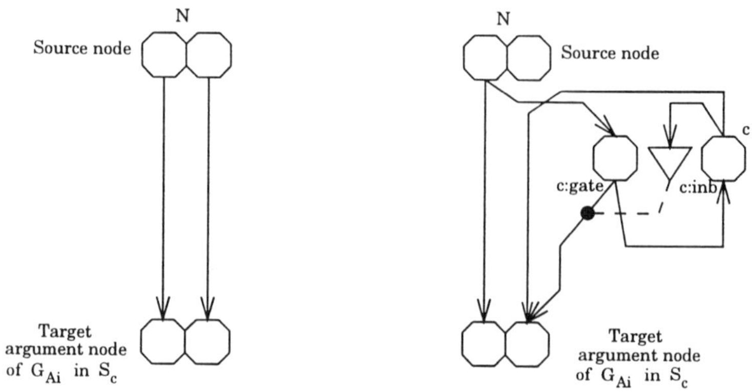

(a) A BPM for a variable UAG (b) A BPM for a constant UAG

Fig. 18.7. The structure of BPMs.

In the figure, the source node *N* is the binding node introduced as the *BCM* if the arguments of a UAG in S_a are repeated ones. Otherwise, it indicates the argument node of the UAG in S_a. As can be seen in Fig. 18.7a, the BPM_v for a variable UAG consists of simple links between the argument node of G_{Ai} in S_a and that of G_{Ai} in S_c. However, the BPM_c for a constant UAG is more complicated as shown in Fig. 18.7b. The constant argument of this example UAG is assumed to be *c* for the purpose of explanation. If a variable filler is assigned to the source node of the BPM_c, the variable binding propagates from N_{left} to the left element of the target argument node. At the same time, the same binding also propagates to the right element of the target argument node through the *c:gate* node to achieve unification between the variable filler and the constant argument. If the constant filler, *c*, is assigned to the source node, the right element of the target argument node receives the constant binding from the *c* node directly. The inhibitory link (drawn in a dashed line) from the *c:inb* node is used to block the binding propagation path from N_{left} to the right element of the target argument node through the *c:gate* node when the constant node *c* becomes active at the initial binding setup stage.

4.3.3. Consistency Checking for Each UAG. Two types of consistency checking submechanisms (*CCM*s) are required: consistency checking for a constant UAG (CCM_c) and consistency checking for a variable UAG (CCM_v) which has repeated arguments. A CCM_c forces the condition that all constant argument nodes in the UAG must get bound to the same constant specified as the constant argument or free variable fillers during inference. This condition should be forced whether or not the constant argument is repeated in the antecedent, that is, regardless of the size of the UAG. In the same way, a CCM_v forces all the repeated variable argument nodes in the UAG to get bound to the same constant filler or free variable fillers. The groups needing this treatment are determined by

$$CCM_c = \{G_{Ai} \mid G_{Ai} \in S_a \wedge const(Ai)\},$$
$$CCM_v = \{G_{Ai} \mid G_{Ai} \in S_a \wedge var(Ai) \wedge size(G_{Ai}) > 1\}.$$

Figure 18.8a illustrates a CCM_c for the constant UAG which has one constant argument, *c*, and Fig. 18.8b a CCM_v for a repeated variable UAG.

In Fig. 18.8a, the CCM_c is represented using a τ-or element labelled *to1*. This node will be activated whenever the right element of the source node is bound to a constant other than *c*. The activation of the *to1* node projects the inhibitory signal which blocks the *BPM* between the source node and the target argument nodes. Note the dashed link from *to1* to one black dot near to the bottom of the network, which is connected to two other black dots by a dashed line. This is to abbreviate representation of a full connection from *to1* to each back dot. On becoming active, any node connected to one of these black dots send the same inhibitory signal to the rest of dots.

The CCM_v, by contrast, only needs the *mto1* node, which is a multiphase τ-or element (Fig. 18.8b). Whenever the right element of the source node receives two different constant bindings, the *mto1* node will detect this and projects the inhibitory signal to stop the flow of the activation from the source node to the target argument node.

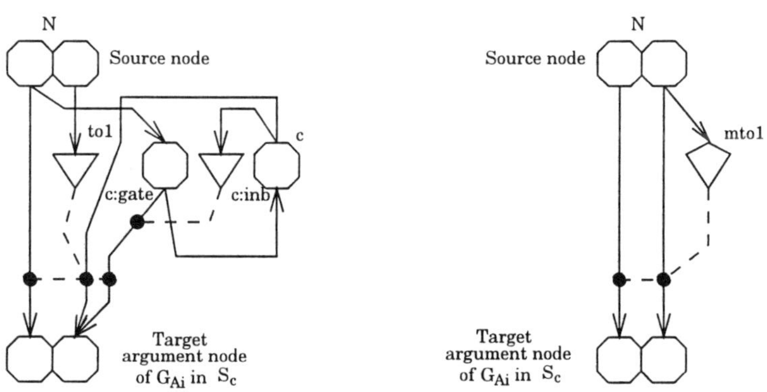

(a) A BPM for a constant UAG (b) A BPM for a variable UAG

Fig. 18.8. The structure of *CCMs*.

4.3.4. Binding Interaction Between UAGs. For any pair of UAGs in the antecedent, if either or both of them are constant UAGs or repeated variable UAGs, binding interaction between them and consistency checking after binding interaction is required to ensure proper propagation of bindings from the source predicate to the target predicate. There are three combinations in pairing all the different types of UAGs in the proposed inference architecture:

- a pair of a constant UAG and a variable UAG
- a pair of two variable UAGs
- a pair of two constant UAGs.

Binding Interaction Between Constant and Variable UAGs: For any two constant and variable UAGs, if the same variable filler is assigned to arguments belonging to them, the binding obtained between the variable filler and any arguments of the constant UAG must migrate to the arguments of the variable UAG. This situation can be seen when the fact, *p(U,U)*, is presented to the following rule:

$$p(c, X) \rightarrow q(c,X)$$

Presenting the fact first generates the bindings between the variable fillers (*U*'s) and the two arguments of the antecedent, which results in the set of bindings, {U/p:c, U/p:X}. Because the arguments *p:c* and *p:X* are bound to the same variable filler, binding interaction between these two arguments is required during inference to produce the desirable result *q(c, c)* from the consequent of the rule.

The submechanism that carries out this task is called a binding interaction submechanism between a constant and a variable UAG (BIM_{cv}). The pairs of UAGs requiring this submechanism are determined by the following condition:

$$BIM_{cv} = \{(G_{Ai}, G_{Aj}) \mid G_{Ai} \in S_a \wedge G_{Aj} \in S_a \wedge const(Ai) \wedge var(Aj)\}.$$

The structure of a BIM_{cv} is shown in Fig. 18.9a. The node *to1* is used to detect the situation where the same variable filler is assigned to the source node N_i of a constant UAG and the source node N_j of a variable UAG. Activation of the *to1* node projects the inhibitory signal which blocks direct binding propagation from the source nodes to the target argument node. The intermediate bindings generated as a result of binding interaction between two UAGs then will be represented on the binding node, *b2*. As inference continues, these bindings will propagate to the target argument node to complete inference. The *c:gate* is a node associated with the constant node *c*, and the *mto2* node is used for consistency checking after binding interaction.

Binding Interaction Between Variable UAGs: A binding interaction submechanism between variable UAGs (BIM_{vv}) is similar to the BIM_{cv} except the condition that at least one of UAGs should have repeated arguments rather than a single argument. This submechanism is not needed between any two UAGs that have a single variable argument because no consistency checking is required in this case. The example rule which requires a BIM_{vv} is

$p(X, X, Y) \rightarrow q(X, Y)$.

Presenting the fact, $p(a, U, U)$, to the antecedent of the rule generates the set of bindings, $\{a/p{:}X, U/p{:}X, U/p{:}Y\}$, which require binding interaction between the repeated argument $p{:}X$'s and the third argument Y during inference to produce the desirable result $q(a, a)$. Therefore, a submechanism is needed for binding interaction between these two groups of unifying arguments.

The pairs of UAGs requiring this submechanism are determined by the following condition:

$$BIM_{vv} = \{(G_{Ai}, G_{Aj}) \mid G_{Ai} \in S_a \wedge G_{Ai} \in S_a \wedge var(Ai) \wedge var(Aj) \\ \wedge Ai \cong Aj, size(G_{Ai}) > 1 \text{ or } size(G_{Aj}) > 1\}.$$

Figure 18.9b illustrates the structure of a BIM_{vv}.

Binding Interaction Between Constant UAGs: This refers to the situation where the same variable filler is assigned to two different constant argument nodes as exemplified with the following rule:

$$p(a, b) \rightarrow q(a, b).$$

Presenting the fact $p(U, U)$ should fail the matching between the presented fact and the antecedent of the rule because the same variable filler U is bound to two different constant arguments a and b. This indicates that for any two different constant UAGs in the antecedent, we need a binding interaction submechanism (BIM_{cc}) that detects this situation and prevents the rule from firing during inference. These pairs of UAGs can be determined by the following condition.

$$BIM_{cc} = \{(G_{Ai}, G_{Aj}) \mid G_{Ai} \in S_a \wedge G_{Aj} \in S_a \wedge const(Ai) \wedge const(Aj) \wedge Ai \cong Aj\}$$

Figure 18.9c depicts the structure of a BIM_{cc} between two source nodes, N_i and N_j, belonging to two different constant UAGs. Whenever the right elements of these source nodes become active in the same phase (i.e., if they are bound to the same variable filler) the *to1* node becomes active and projects an inhibitory signal to stop binding propagation from the source nodes to the target argument nodes.

4.4. A Rule Encoding Example

To demonstrate the entire rule encoding procedure, let us reconsider the following example rule:

$p(X, X, Y) \rightarrow q(X, Y)$.

Encoding the rule starts by constructing the two predicate assemblies corresponding the antecedent and the consequent of the rule as follows:

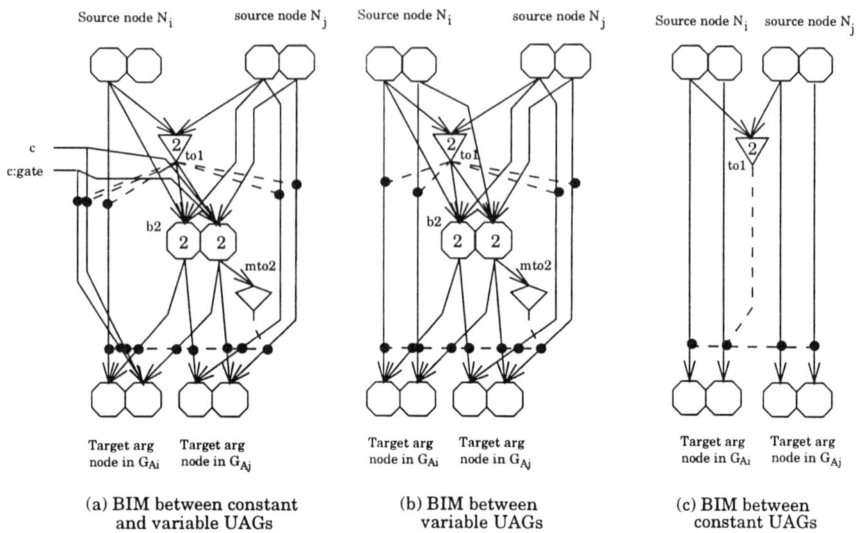

Fig. 18.9. The structure of binding interaction submechanisms.

$$p{:}\{X_1([0],[0]),X_2([0],[0]),Y([0],[0])\},$$
$$q{:}\{X([0],[0]),\ Y([0],[0])\}.$$

Then the intermediate mechanism is built between them, which involves the following procedure to determine the required submechanisms.

First of all, syntax of the rule is checked to obtain UAGs. From the example rule, we will get

$$S_a = \{G_X, G_Y\},\ \text{where}\ G_X = \{p{:}X_1,\ p{:}X_2\},\ G_Y = \{p{:}Y\},$$
$$S_c = \{G_X,\ G_Y\},\ \text{where}\ G_X = \{q{:}X\},\ G_Y = \{q{:}Y\}.$$

Second, the number of arguments of each UAG in S_a is examined. The antecedent of the example rule has two UAGs: G_X for the repeated variable arguments X's and G_Y for the single variable argument Y. Since $size(G_X) > 1$ and $size(G_Y) = 1$, only G_X requires the binding collection submechanism (*BCM*):

$$BCM = \{G_X\}.$$

Third, the matching between UAGs in S_a and those in S_c must be checked. This is carried out by examining each UAG in S_a which has the related UAG in S_c. Because both UAGs in S_a have related UAGs in S_c, binding propagation submechanisms (*BPM*s) are needed between the argument nodes of G_X in S_a and those of G_X in S_c as well as between the argument node of G_Y in S_a and that of G_Y in S_c. This is indicated by

$$BPM = \{G_X, G_Y\}.$$

In the next stage, in order to determine the consistency checking submechanisms, the type and size of UAGs in S_a are checked. In the case of the example rule, we only need CCM_v for the UAG, G_X, because it is a variable UAG and its size is greater than 1. This CCM_v ensures the consistency condition where all variable fillers bound to these repeated arguments of G_X should be the same constant filler or variable fillers. Thus we get

$$CCM_c = \{\}, CCM_v = \{G_X\}.$$

Finally, binding interaction submechanisms between UAGs will be accommodated. In the case of the example rule, a binding interaction submechanism between variable arguments (BIM_{vv}) is needed for the pair of UAGs, G_X and G_Y:

$$BIM_{cv} = \{\}, BIM_{vv} = \{(G_X, G_Y)\}, BIM_{cc} = \{\}.$$

Figure 18.10c shows the complete network generated for the example rule. Two base predicate assemblies are shown at the top and bottom of the network and between them are the *BCM*, the *BPM*, the CCM_v, and the BIM_{vv}. The binding node *b1* is used for the *BCM*, the *mto1* for the CCM_v, and the rest for the *BPM* and the BIM_{vv}. Although the complete network looks very complex, it is modularised. Figure 18.10a shows the network only with the *BCM* and the *BPM* and Fig. 18.10b with additional the CCM_v. As can be seen, the complexity of the network is mainly due to the binding interaction mechanisms between two UAGs. Rules not requiring this mechanism are encoded with a much simpler intermediate mechanism.

4.5. Performing Inference

Once a set of symbolic rules are encoded into corresponding SPNs, the inference architecture can perform forward chaining inference over the network. A step of inference is started by presenting a fact to the network. Presenting the fact involves specifying the argument bindings between the presented fact and the corresponding predicate assembly matched in the network. The SPN shown in Fig. 18.10c, for instance, presenting the predicate, *p(a, U, U)*, to the network will set up initial bindings, {a/p:X_1, U/p:X_2, U/p:Y}, by activating the filler nodes and their corresponding argument nodes in the following phases:

$$a[1], U[2], p{:}\{X_1([0],[1]), X_2([2],[0]), Y([2],[0])\},$$

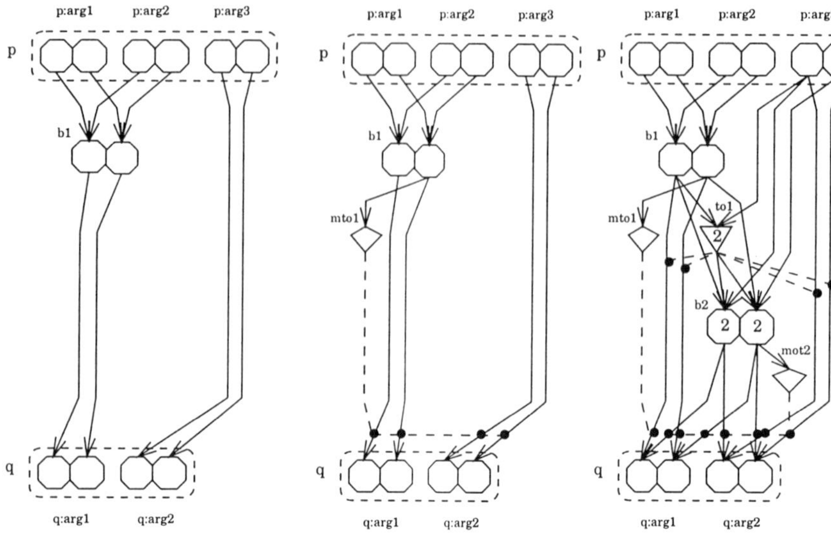

Fig. 18.10. Building the intermediate mechanism for the rule *p(X, X, Y)* → *q(X, Y)*.

where the numbers specify particular phases. As inference continues, these activations propagate to the *q* predicate assembly through the intermediate mechanism. This automatic binding propagation eventually activates the argument nodes of the *q* predicate assembly as follows:

$$q{:}\{X([2],[1]),\ Y([2],[1])\}.$$

The right elements of the argument nodes represent the constant bindings and the left elements the variable bindings. Consequently, the result of inference, *q(a, a)*, is obtained from the *q* predicate assembly as well as the result of unification produced during the inference, {a/U}.

5. COMPARISON WITH OTHER WORK

Because the proposed inference architecture is inspired by Shastri and Ajjanagadde's connectionist system SHRUTI, it is interesting to compare their system with ours. First, SHRUTI's binding mechanism only represents constant bindings explicitly. It represents variable bindings by inactivity of argument nodes during inference. It does not, therefore, differentiate one variable binding from others which is a basic, and fundamentally important, feature of symbolic inference. Second,

SHRUTI's rule encoding mechanism does not consider all the restrictions on variable binding that symbolic rules may impose. In particular, a submechanism for binding interaction between groups of unifying arguments is not considered in their system at all. However, our model can represent variable bindings because it uses an extended dynamic binding mechanism. Its rule encoding mechanism can encode rules that require binding interaction between groups of unifying arguments during inference.

Two other similar systems are described in Sun (1992) and Lange and Dyer (1989). Sun (1992) has proposed the network model, called CONSYDERR, for common sense reasoning. It consists of two subsystems one of which uses distributed representation, the other localist representation. The localist subsystem can deal with various knowledge representation issues such as consistency checking, unification, and so forth. The major difference between his localist subsystem and our network model lies in the functional requirements of nodes in a network. We use only one type of assembly which consists of entity nodes. The behaviour of the assembly is quite transparent because, apart from temporal behaviour, each element of the entity nodes in the assembly performs very simple processing (summing of weighted inputs and thresholding over temporal phases). Sun's subsystem, however, uses three different types of assemblies and unification, for example, is performed by what he calls a *complex assembly*. This complex assembly performs complex computations to support unification during inference (see Sun, 1992, p. 106). Although it does not use temporal phases, the need for high computational ability of assemblies adopted and the use of abstraction which hides network details is beyond simple summation with thresholding and so demands much more sophisticated neural elements than we require.

Lange and Dyer (1989) describe a connectionist system, ROBIN, capable of performing high level inferences over structured connections of nodes that encode world knowledge in semantic networks. It uses structured connections of nodes to encode a semantic knowledge base of related frames. When constructing a structured semantic network, a special node called a *signature node* is attached to each node representing a concept. During inference, ROBIN permanently allocates a unique numerical signature to each constant and represents dynamic argument-constant bindings by propagating the signature of the appropriate constant to the argument to which it is bound. Therefore, it can maintain large number of dynamic bindings and deals with rules having multiple variables. A problem with the use of signatures is that the signatures become high precision quantities if each entity has a unique signature. Thus, propagating bindings will require nodes to propagate and compare high precision analog values. Another limitation is that their model does not deal with consistency checking and unification issues.

6. CONCLUSION

Any connectionist architecture that aspires to replicate symbolic inference should be able to represent dynamic bindings and rules with embedded control mechanisms. Shastri and Ajjanagadde's SHRUTI is a step in this direction but it does not provide a connectionist equivalent of a naming system for unbound variables, which is a fundamental requirement in all of the standard symbolic reasoning systems. In addition, it does not consider all the binding restriction specified in symbolic rules when it encodes them. This limits the expressive power of their model.

The inference architecture proposed in this chapter shows how oscillation of neurons can efficiently be used to support constant and variable bindings using entity nodes with simple behaviours. This new rule encoding mechanism provides a way of representing not only a group of unifying arguments but also many groups of such arguments with appropriate consistency checking between groups. This extends the expressive power of the proposed inference architecture. Because of the space limitation, we do not deal with encoding facts into the corresponding SPNs. Although described here is a forward chaining style inference, the basic concept of the proposed connectionist architecture can be used to encode facts to support backward chaining inference with only slight adjustments (Park & Robertson, 1995).

The proposed inference architecture provides a mechanism that translates a significant subset of first-order Horn clause expressions into a connectionist representation which may be executed very efficiently. However, in order to have the full expressive power of Horn clause FOPL, we need to add the ability to represent structured terms as arguments of a predicate and recursion in rules. Currently, no connectionist system has provided a convincing solution to all these problems and to do so, in general, we would have to sacrifice one of the most attractive features of this class of system: its ability to guarantee an answer in finite time.

ACKNOWLEDGMENTS

This work was partly supported by the Ministry of Science & Technology, Korea, and the British Council under Grant SCOT/KOR/2923/37/A.

REFERENCES

Ajjanagadde, V., & Shastri, L. (1991). Rules and variables in neural nets. *Neural Computation*, *3*, 121-134.

Clossman, G. (1988). A model of categorisation and learning in a connectionist broadcast system. Unpublished doctoral dissertation, Department of Computer Science, Indiana University.

Eckhorn, R. (1993). Dynamic bindings by real neurons: Arguments from physiology, neural network models and information theory. Open peer commentary, *Behavioural and Brain Sciences*, *16*, 457-458.

Engel, A. K., König, P., Kreiter, A. K., Gray, C. M., & Singer, W. (1991). Temporal coding by coherent oscillations as a potential solution to the binding problem: Physiological evidence. In H. G. Schuster & W. Singer (Eds.), *Nonlinear Dynamics and Neural Networks*. Weinheim.

Fahlman, S. E. (1979). *NETL: A System for Representing Real-world Knowledge*. Cambridge, MA: MIT Press.

Fodor, J. A., & Pylyshyn, Z. W. (1988). Connectionism and cognitive architecture: a critical analysis. In S. Pinker & J. Mehler (Eds.), *Connection and Symbols* (pp. 3-71). Cambridge, MA: MIT Press.

Horn, D., Sagi, D., & Usher, M. (1991). Segmentation, binding, and illusory conjunctions. *Neural Computation*, *3*, 510-525.

Hummel, J. E., & Biederman, I. (1992). Dynamic Binding in a neural network for shape recognition. *Psychological Review*, *99*, 480-517.

Lange, T. E., & Dyer, M. G. (1989). High-level inferencing in a connectionist network. *Connection Science*, *1*, 181-271.

Luger, G. F. & Stubblefield, W. A. (1989). *Artificial Intelligence and the Design of Expert Systems*. Redwood City, CA: Benjamin/Cummings.

McCarty, J. (1988). Epistemological challenges for connectionism. Open peer commentary to "proper treatment of connectionism" by P. Smolensky. *Behavioral and Brain Sciences*, *11*, 44.

Park, N. S., & Robertson, D. (1995). A localist network architecture for logical inference based on temporal synchrony approach to dynamic variable binding. In R. Sun & F. Alexandre (Eds.), *The Working Notes of the IJCAI-95 workshop on Connectionist-Symbolic Integration*, pp. 63-68.

Park, N. S., Robertson, D., & Stenning, K. (1995). An extension of the temporal synchrony approach to dynamic variable binding in a connectionist inference system. *Knowledge-Based Systems*, *8*, 345-357.

Shastri, L., & Ajjanagadde, V. (1993). From simple associations to systematic reasoning: A connectionist representation of rules, variables, and dynamic bindings using temporal synchrony. *Behavioral and Brain Sciences*, *16*, 417-451.

Strong, G. W., & Whitehead, B. A. (1989). A solution to the tag-assignment problem for neural nets. *Behavioral and Brain Sciences*, *12*, 381-433.

Sun, R. (1992). On variable binding in connectionist networks. *Connection Science*, *4*, 93-124.

Wang, D. L., & Terman, D. (1995). Locally excitatory globally inhibitory oscillator networks. *IEEE Transactions on Neural Networks*, *6*, 283-286.

19

Oscillations in Discrete and Continuous Hopfield Networks

Arun Jagota
University of California at Santa Cruz

Xin Wang
University of Southern California

ABSTRACT

This chapter is crisply partitioned into two parts: one dealing with oscillations in discrete Hopfield networks and the other with oscillations in continuous Hopfield networks. The single theme spanning both parts is that of the Hopfield model and its energy function. The first part deals with *analyzing* oscillations in the discrete Hopfield network with symmetric weights, and speculating on possible uses of such behavior. By imposing certain restrictions on the weights, an exact characterization of the oscillatory behavior is obtained. Possible uses of this characterization are examined.

The second part deals with *injecting* chaotic or periodic oscillations into continuous Hopfield networks, for the purposes of solving optimization problems. When the continuous Hopfield model is used to solve an optimization problem, the results are often mediocre because of the convergent nature of its dynamical algorithm. To circumvent this limitation, we develop mechanisms for injecting controllable chaos or periodic oscillations into the Hopfield network. We allow chaotic or oscillatory behavior to be initiated and converted to convergent behavior at the turn of a "knob," in rough analogy with simulated annealing. The resulting algorithm, called *chaotic annealing*, is evaluated on instances of Maximum Clique — an NP-hard optimization problem on graphs — and shown to exhibit a significant improvement over the convergent Hopfield dynamics.

1. INTRODUCTION

This chapter is crisply partitioned into the following two parts:

- Analysis of oscillations in a discrete Hopfield network under synchronous updates and investigation of their possible uses.

- Synthesis of oscillations in a continuous Hopfield network for the purposes of solving optimization problems.

The single theme spanning both parts is that of the Hopfield model and its energy function.

The first part deals with analyzing oscillatory behavior in discrete Hopfield networks with symmetric weights. It is well known that under synchronous updates, such networks can oscillate between two states but higher order oscillations are not possible (Goles, Fogelman-Soulie, & Pellegrino, 1985). Such two-state oscillations are called *two-cycles*. Unfortunately, no useful characterization of the two-cycles themselves that holds for arbitrary networks is known. By imposing certain restrictions on the weights of the network, we obtain an exact characterization of the two-cycles. This characterization is obtained in terms of a certain graph underlying such a network instance. This characterization is shown to have the following possible uses. First, in small network instances of this kind, it becomes clear that all two-cycles can be easily found merely by inspecting their underlying graphs. Second, in network instances — small or large — whose graphs have certain structure, the two-cycles reveal themselves readily. We are especially interested in knowing when a network instance is devoid of two-cycles, for then synchronous updates always converge to fixed points. Third, these two-cycles are shown to have possible uses to associative memories, although our arguments in this regard remain quite speculative in nature.

The second part, somewhat more practical in intent, deals with injecting chaotic or periodic oscillations into continuous Hopfield networks for the purposes of solving optimization problems. The dynamical equations of the continuous Hopfield network with symmetric weights exhibit convergent behavior to fixed points (Hertz, Krogh, & Palmer, 1991; Hopfield, 1984). This is convenient for applying the continuous Hopfield model to solving optimization problems (Hertz, Krogh, & Palmer, 1991; Hopfield & Tank, 1985) by encoding feasible solutions of a mapped optimization problem into the fixed points of the network's dynamical equations. On the other hand, because this convergent behavior is gradient-descent in nature, it is also responsible, in part, for the often mediocre performance of the continuous Hopfield model on such problems. To remove this defect, we develop mechanisms that inject controllable chaos or periodic oscillations into the dynamical equations of the continuous Hopfield network. Our mechanisms allow chaotic or oscillatory behavior to be initiated and converted to convergent behavior at the turn of a "knob." This process, which we call *chaotic annealing*, is motivated by an analogy to simulated annealing in which the behavior is relatively random at high temperature and relatively convergent at low temperature. Just like lowering the temperature gradually allows simulated annealing to work better on optimization problems than gradient descent, it is hoped that turning the "knob" gradually, to go from chaotic to periodic to convergent behavior, will work better on optimization problems than the convergent dynamics of the Hopfield network. To demonstrate this, chaotic annealing is evaluated on instances of Maximum Clique — an NP-hard optimization problem on graphs — and shown to exhibit a measurable improvement over the convergent Hopfield dynamics.

2. OSCILLATIONS IN DISCRETE NETWORKS

The *Discrete Hopfield Network* (Hopfield, 1982) is composed of n units 1, ..., n, interconnected with symmetric weights $w_{ij} = w_{ji} \in \Re$ for all $i \neq j$ and with $w_{ii} \geq 0$ for all i. Each neuron I has a state $X_i \in \{0, 1\}$ and a time-invariant external input $I_i \in \Re$. The dynamical behavior of the network is governed by the following state update rule:

$$X_i(t+1) := \left\{ \begin{array}{ll} 1 & \textit{if } I_i + \sum_{j=1}^{n} w_{ij} X_j(t) \geq 0 \\ 0 & \textit{if } I_i + \sum_{j=1}^{n} w_{ij} X_j(t) < 0 \end{array} \right\}. \qquad (1)$$

We say that (1) is updated *asynchronously* if, in time step t, only *one* neuron I is picked to update its state according to (1). The picked neuron is assumed to be fairly chosen, in the sense that in any infinite sequence of updates according to (1), every neuron is picked to update its state infinitely-often. We say that (1) is updated *synchronously*, if, in time step t, *all* neurons update their states according to (1). If (1) is updated asynchronously, then the network eventually converges to a fixed point $\mathbf{X}(t+1) = \mathbf{X}(t)$ from any initial state vector $\mathbf{X}(0)$ (Hopfield, 1982). If (1) is updated synchronously, then the network eventually converges to either a fixed point $\mathbf{X}(t+1) = \mathbf{X}(t)$ or to an oscillation between two states: $\mathbf{X}(t)$ and $\mathbf{X}(t+1)$ (Goles et al., 1985). It is interesting that this result rules out cycles of period greater than two.

2.1. Computational Applications

Almost all known applications of the discrete Hopfield model crucially depend on its convergent behavior to fixed points under asynchronous updates. Information is typically stored in such fixed points and retrieved by the network's asynchronous dynamics. In the application area of *associative memories,* memories are stored in the fixed points. The initial state serves as the fragment, or cue, from which a memory is to be retrieved. The asynchronous dynamics performs the recall process from this initial state. In the application area of *optimization*, feasible solutions of an optimization problem are stored in the fixed points. A cost is associated with each fixed point, which is proportional to the energy of that fixed point (Hopfield, 1982). The objective is to find a fixed point of minimum cost. The asynchronous dynamics is used as a local search (hill-climbing) method to attempt to find a fixed point of small cost.

We are not aware of any application that exploits the two-cycles present in the discrete Hopfield network. The challenge — apparently not an easy one — is to characterize the two-cycles present in a network and find useful applications. Ours is preliminary work in this direction.

2.2. The Hopfield-Clique Network

The *Hopfield-clique Network* (HcN); (Jagota, 1994a) is a special case of the discrete Hopfield network in which, for all $i \neq j$, $w_{ij} = w_{ji} \in \{\rho, 1\}$ for $\rho < -n$, where n is the number of neurons in the network.

It is useful to define a graph $G_N = (V, E)$, underlying the network, as follows. The vertex-set $V = \{1, ..., n\}$ of the graph is the set of units of the network. A pair of vertices $\{i, j\}$ is an edge in the graph if and only if $w_{ij} = 1$ in the network.

For any vector $\mathbf{X} \in \{0, 1\}^n$, let $S_x = \{i \mid X_i = 1\}$ denote the set of vertices in V associated with $\mathbf{X}$. Conversely, for any set $U \subseteq V$, define $\mathbf{X}^u$ by

$$X_i^u = \begin{Bmatrix} 1 & \text{if } i \in U \\ 0 & \text{otherwise} \end{Bmatrix}.$$

We next describe the network state, using the vector or the set notation interchangeably.

In a graph G, two vertices are called *adjacent* if they are connected by an edge. A set of vertices S is called a *clique* if every pair of vertices in S is adjacent. A clique S is called *maximal* if no superset of S is a clique. The following result is in Jagota (1994a).

Theorem 19.1. In an HcN network N, a vector $\mathbf{X}$ is a fixed point of (1) if and only if S_x is a maximal clique in its underlying graph G_N.

Theorem 19.1 gives an exact characterization of the fixed points of the HcN in terms of a simple property in its underlying graph. This characterization is useful for the theory and application of the HcN (Jagota, 1990, 1994a).

Theorem 19.1 holds for asynchronous updates. What about synchronous updates? Can we obtain an exact characterization of the two-cycles in analogous fashion? Before proceeding further, why should we be interested?

- Curiosity.
- Might open up new applications.
- Remarkably, synchronous updates in the HcN converge in ≤ 3 iterations (Shrivistava, Dasgupta, & Reddy, 1990). In fixed-point applications, if an HcN instance could be shown to be devoid of two-cycles, synchronous updates could be used for efficient retrieval. In two-cycle applications, synchronous updates would have the added bonus of efficient convergence.

2.3. Characterization of Synchronous Updates in HcN

In this section, we characterize synchronous operation of (1) on the HcN. More precisely, we describe the next state as a function of the current state in terms of certain properties of the graph underlying the network. This characterization leads us to the characterization of two-cycles. This characterization will also be of independent interest in possible applications, as we speculate shortly.

The characterization will heavily use set-theoretic notation and it is helpful to review such notation here. A *set* is an unordered collection of distinct elements, explicitly represented as $A = \{,,...,\}$. The empty set is denoted by $\varnothing$. Given two sets A and B, $A \cup B$ denotes their *union* (the set of elements that are in A or in B or in both), $A \cap B$ denotes their *intersection* (the set of elements that are both in A and in B), $A \setminus B$ denotes *subtraction* (the set of elements that are in A but not in B), and $\bar{A}$ denotes the *complement* (the set of elements that are not in A but are in some prespecified superset of A called the universe).

In this section, we use $U \subseteq V$ as notation for a network state. Let $S(U)$ denote the state that follows the state U under synchronous updates. Let $N(U)$ denote the set of vertices v in $V \setminus U$ such that v is adjacent to every vertex in U. Define $N(\varnothing) = V$. The notation $N(U)$ generalizes the usual concept of the neighbor-set of a vertex v, denoted by $N(v)$. Let $A(U)$ denote the set of vertices v in U such that v is adjacent to all vertices in U. Define $A(\varnothing) = \varnothing$. Lemma 19.2 characterizes the next state under synchronous updates.

Lemma 19.2. $S(U) = N(U) \cup A(U)$.

Proof: The proof is easy and is omitted.

Figure 19.1 illustrates Lemma 19.2.

2.4. Examples and Applications of Synchronous Updates

In an earlier paper (Jagota, 1994b), several kinds of discrete structures arising in AI applications were encoded into the HcN, with knowledge items in these structures stored into the fixed points of the network. In this section, we reexamine several of these encodings, and speculate on how synchronous updates may be used to retrieve information different from that stored in the fixed points.

2.4.1. Emergent Rooms Schemata. The emergent rooms schemata is an example taken from McClelland and Rumelhart (1986, chap. 14, p. 22). In this example, microfeatures representing objects and features found in rooms are represented as neurons in a network whose interconnection weights are determined by which pairs of microfeatures are correlated, which are anticorrelated, and which are uncorrelated. In McClelland and Rumelhart (1986), this example was used to demonstrate that distributed schemata could emerge spontaneously from microfeatures represented as neurons and correlational associations between them represented as weights in a PDP network

A few years back we took this same example and encoded it, in slightly simplified form, into the HcN (Jagota, 1994b). Figure 19.2 shows the graph underlying the network after the encoding. At that time, as noted earlier, our interest was in fixed-point computations. Here our interest is in synchronous updates.

Consider the following questions:

Q1. List the microfeatures that are contained in every room.

Q2. List each of the microfeatures that appear in a room that contains the microfeatures *ceiling* and *walls*.

The answer to **Q1** is $S(V)$, which is computable in one synchronous update step from V. By Lemma 19.2, $S(V) = \{ceiling, walls\}$. The answer to **Q2** is $S(U)$, where $U = \{ceiling, walls\}$. Since $A(U) = \{\text{ceiling, walls}\}$ and $N(U) = \{bed, dresser, ..., fridge\}$, by Lemma 19.2, $S(U) = V$.

2.4.2. Stored Relations. Let $\alpha^n = \{(x_1, ..., x_n) \mid x_i \in \alpha \text{ for } I = 1, ..., n\}$ denote the set of all n-tuples on a finite set α called the alphabet. A subset R of α^n is called an *n-ary relation* on alphabet α. For example, $R = \{ (0,1,0), (1,1,0), (0,0,0)\}$ is a relation on the alphabet $\alpha = \{0, 1\}$ with $n = 3$. R is better known to some as a collection of three 0/1 vectors of length 3.

All of the following are special cases of n-ary relations.

- Some set of n-bit binary vectors with $\alpha = \{0, 1\}$.
- Some set of n-bit q-state vectors with $\alpha = \{0, 1, ..., q - 1\}$.

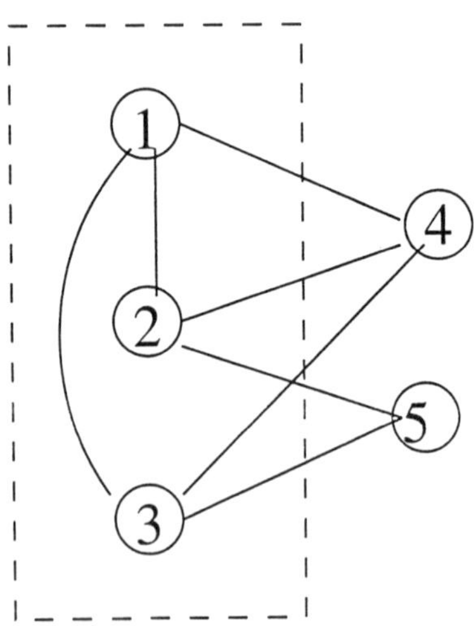

Fig. 19.1. $N(\{1, 2, 3\}) = \{4\}$. $A(\{1, 2, 3\}) = \{1\}$. Therefore, $S(\{1, 2, 3\}) = \{1, 4\}$.

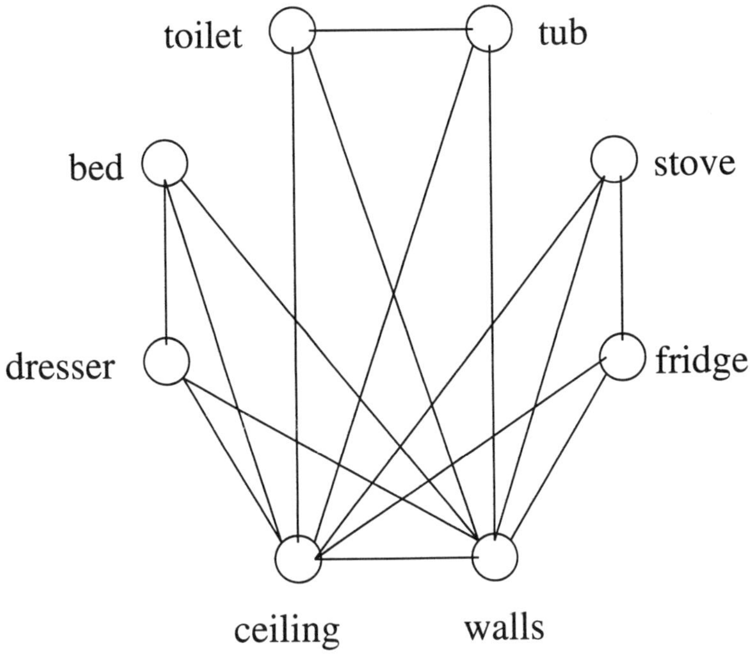

Fig. 19.2. A small version of the rooms schemata example.

- Some set of strings of length n on the English alphabet $\alpha = \{a, b, ..., z\} \cup \{A, B, ..., Z\}$.
- Some single relation in a relational database.

In earlier work (Jagota, 1994a), it was shown that any n-ary relation R could be encoded into an HcN instance employing $|\alpha| \times n$ neurons in such a way that every n-tuple of R was encoded into a fixed point of the HcN in an injective way (i.e., distinct n-tuples were encoded into distinct fixed points). We called this the *stable storage property* of the HcN. This result is in sharp contrast to the poor stable storage capacity of the Hopfield model under the Hebb storage rule (Hertz, Krogh, & Palmer, 1991).

Figures 19.3 and 19.4 give examples of relations encoded into the HcN. Similar examples are in Jagota (1991d). In the example of Fig. 19.3, we can see that each of the tuples is stored as a unique fixed point of the network; and likewise in the example of Fig. 19.4. Our interest here is not in the information stored in the fixed points, but in retrieving information via synchronous updates.

Consider the following questions:

Q1. Which courses did Jeff receive an "A" in?

Q2. Which letters fill the blank in ca_?

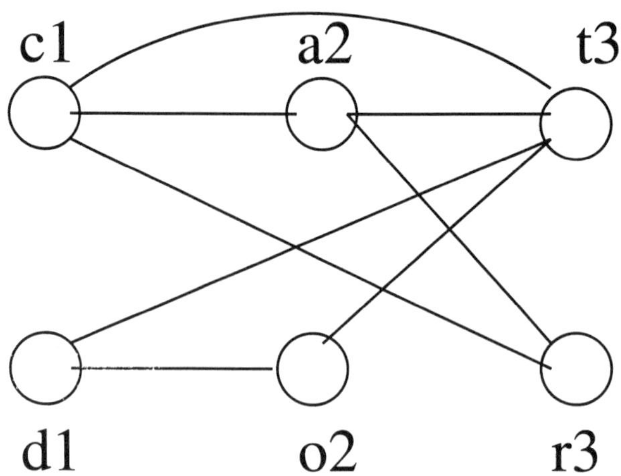

Fig. 19.3. The words *cat*, *car*, and *dot* stored into HcN using the representations {c1, a2, t3}, {c1, a2, r3}, and {d1, o2, t3} respectively.

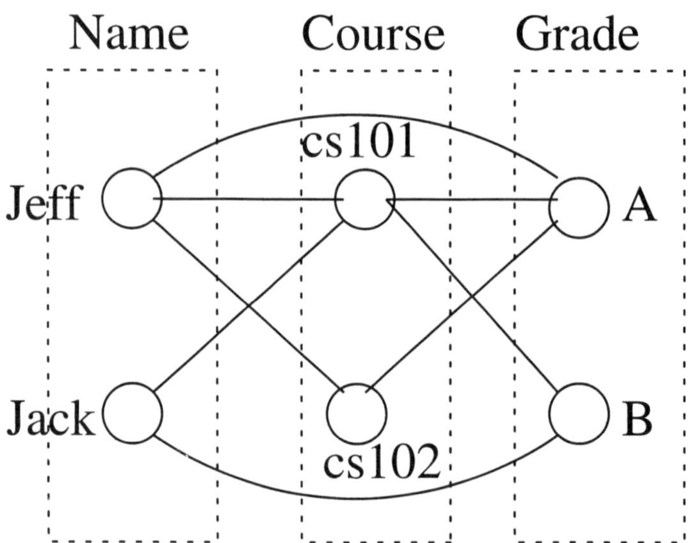

Fig. 19.4. The tuples {name = Jeff, course = cs101, grade = A}, {name = Jack, course = cs101, grade = B}, and {name = Jeff, course = cs102, grade = A} of a relation in a database, stored into HcN.

The answers to both **Q1** and **Q2** are $S(U) \setminus U$. For **Q1**, $U = \{\text{Jeff, A}\}$. Since $A(U) = U$ in this case, and $N(U) = \{\text{cs101, cs102}\}$, by Lemma 19.2, $S(U) \setminus U = \{\text{cs101, cs102}\}$. For **Q2**, $U = \{\text{c1, a2}\}$. Since in this case also $A(U) = U$, and $N(U) = \{\text{t3, r3}\}$, by Lemma 19.2, $S(U) \setminus U = \{\text{t3, r3}\}$.

Thus, both answers are obtainable in one synchronous step from the state U.

The main limitation of this scheme is that, although it gives the correct answer in these toy examples, the answer need not be correct on arbitrary relations encoded into HcN. The reason for this is that storing certain relations into HcN causes *spurious* fixed points to develop. Consider the set of strings $D = \{\text{car, con, for}\}$. Storage of D in HcN, in the manner exemplified in Fig. 19.3, creates a spurious fixed point, one associated with the string $\{cor\}$ which is not in D. Consider the question: *which letters fill the blank in c_r and form a word in D*? The expression $S(U) \setminus U$ — where $U = \{\text{c1, r3}\}$ — equals $\{\text{a2, o2}\}$, and contains a spurious element o2 which comes from the spurious fixed point associated with *cor*. Nevertheless, for this type of question, we can guarantee that $S(U) \setminus U$ is a superset of the correct answer.

A third example involves storing some collection of binary vectors. Such a collection, as we noted earlier, is an n-ary relation on the alphabet $\alpha = \{0, 1\}$. Suppose, for instance, that a set I of binary images is stored in HcN. Let U denote a subimage of some image in I. U is the set of indices of the black pixels in the subimage. Then $S(U) \setminus U$ equals $N(U)$, the set of indices of black pixels outside U, each of which is in a fixed point — an image or a spurious image — containing U. This might be of use in showing all completions of the subimage U.

2.5. Characterization of Two-Cycles in an HcN

Define $\bar{A}(U) = U \setminus A(U)$. The following characterization of two-cycles in an HcN was obtained jointly by the author and K. W. Regan, his Ph.D. advisor.

Proposition 19.3. The pair $<U, S(U)>$ is a fixed point or a two-cycle of an HcN if and only if both **C1** and **C2** hold:

C1. The set $A(N(U))$ equals the empty set Ø.

C2. The set $N(A(U) \cup N(U))$ equals the set $\bar{A}(U)$
The pair $<U, S(U)>$ is a two-cycle of an HcN if and only if both **C1** and **C2** hold but U is not a maximal clique, the condition for which event is:

C3. The set $N(U)$ equals the empty set ⌀ *and* the set $A(U)$ equals the set U.

The proof is omitted.

Figure 19.5 diagrams the important sets used in the statement of Proposition 19.3.

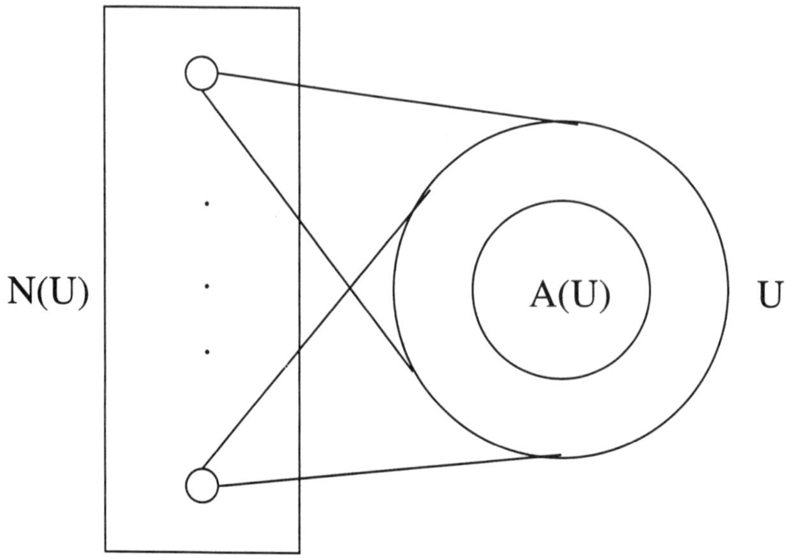

Fig. 19.5. The set U, its subset $A(U)$, and the set $N(U)$ are shown.

2.5.1. Examples Using This Characterization. We now describe, with the help of this characterization, the nature of the two-cycles in the HcN instances whose underlying graphs have very special structures. These are intended mainly as examples, because the graphs are too specialized to be of practical use (except, perhaps, the last one). Figure 19.6 diagrams all these graphs.

A graph is called a *matching* if no two of its edges share a common endpoint. A graph is called *complete* if between every pair of vertices there is an edge. A graph is called *bipartite* if its vertex-set V can be partitioned into two sets V_1, V_2 so that all edges cross the partition. A bipartite graph is called *complete* if all possible crossing edges are present. For an in-depth introduction, the reader is referred to Bondy and Murty (1976).

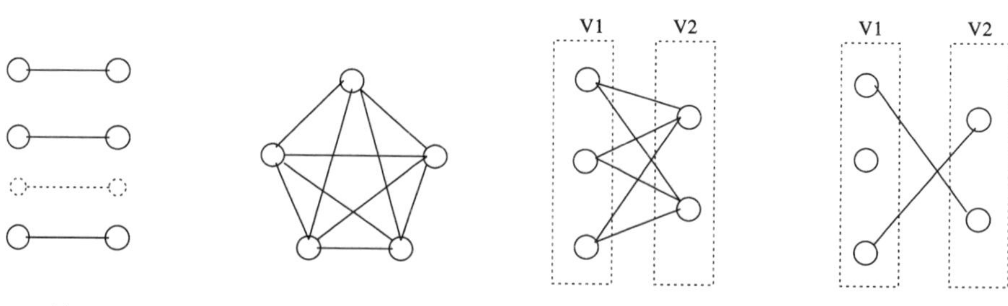

Fig. 19.6. (a) matching, (b) complete graph, (c) complete, bipartite graph, (d) bipartite graph.

- When G_N is a *matching*, <∅, V> is the only two-cycle.

- When G_N is the *complete* graph, there is no two-cycle.

- When $G_N = (V_1, V_2, E)$ is a *complete, bipartite* graph with $V_1| \geq 2$ and $V_2| \geq 2$, the following are the only two-cycles: (I) $<V_1, V_2>$, (ii) $<\emptyset, V>$, (iii) $<\{v_1\}, V_2 \setminus \{v_1\}\}>$ for all $v_1 \in V_1$, and (iv) $<\{v_2\}, V_1 \setminus \{v_2\}\}>$ for all $v_2 \in V_2$.

- When $G_N = (V_1, V_2, \text{E})$ is any *bipartite* graph with $|V_1| \geq 2$ and $|V_2| \geq 2$, the following are two-cycles: (I) if $|N(V_1)| \geq 2$ then $<V_1, N(V_1)>$, (ii) if $|N(V_2)| \geq 2$ then $<V_2, N(V_2)>$, (iii) if $N(V_1) = v_2$ then $<V_1 \cup \{v_2\}, \{v_2\}>$, and (iv) if $N(V_2) = v_1$ then $<V_2 \cup \{v_1\}, \{v_1\}>$.

We do not know if there are more two-cycles.

These examples suggest that when an HcN instance has a specialized structure, it may be feasible to determine its two-cycles analytically.

2.5.2. An Average-Case Result. Define a random HcN instance on n neurons as one in which each weight w_{ij}, $I \neq j$, is set to 1 or to ρ with equal probability one-half, independently of the other weights. This procedure samples a HcN instance *uniformly at random* from the sample space of all n-neuron HcN instances. It has been shown that the probability of the event "a random HcN instance on n neurons contains a two-cycle" approaches 1 as n approaches infinity (Jagota, 1993). Thus, almost every HcN instance contains a two-cycle.[1]

2.6. Conclusion to Part I

We conclude the first part of this chapter by itemizing the main points:

- Fixed points in the HcN were known to have a simple and useful characterization.

- Now synchronous updates also have a simple, and somewhat useful, characterization.

- Two-cycles in an HcN have an interesting but slightly more complicated characterization. So far, the usefulness of this characterization has been seen only in helping identify two-cycles in HcN instances possessing specialized structure. Other uses are not yet transparent.

---

[1] When the probability of some event E approaches 1 on a uniformly random element in a sample space S, it is reasonable to conclude that the event E occurs for *almost every element* of S (Bollob'as, 1985).

- Almost every HcN instance contains a two-cycle.

3. OSCILLATIONS IN CONTINUOUS NETWORKS

This part deals with injecting chaotic or periodic oscillations into continuous Hopfield networks for the purposes of solving optimization problems.

The *Continuous Hopfield Network* (Hopfield, 1984), like its discrete version, is composed of n units 1, ..., n, interconnected with symmetric weights $w_{ij} = w_{ji} \in \Re$ for all $I \neq j$. Each neuron has a constant external input $I_i \in \Re$. Unlike the discrete version, $w_{ii} \in \Re$ for all I, and each neuron I has a state $X_i \in [0,1]$. The dynamical behavior of the network is governed by the following system of coupled, nonlinear differential equations (Cohen & Grossberg, 1983; Hopfield, 1984):

$$\frac{d\boldsymbol{X}}{dt} = -\boldsymbol{X} + \boldsymbol{G}_\lambda(\boldsymbol{W}\boldsymbol{X} + \boldsymbol{I}) \tag{2}$$

where **X** is the network state vector, **I** the vector of external inputs, $g_\lambda(x) \equiv 1/(1+e^{-\lambda x})$ a sigmoid with gain λ, and $\boldsymbol{g}_\lambda$ a vector map in which g_λ is applied component-wise.

When the vector **I** is constant, every trajectory of (2) is guaranteed to converge asymptotically to some fixed point of (2) (Cohen & Grossberg, 1983; Hopfield, 1984). As λ is increased, the fixed points of (2) approach fixed points of the discrete network with the same W and I (Hopfield, 1984). On an HcN this means that, for a sufficiently large λ, the network eventually converges to a state vector from which a maximal clique in the graph underlying the network can be recovered. Thus (2) may be used as a local optimization method which finds a maximal clique in an encoded graph (any graph).

The evolution of (2), however, performs gradient-descent on an energy function (Cohen & Grossberg, 1983; Hopfield, 1984) and therefore finds only locally optimal solutions. How can this limitation be removed? One approach, called *mean field annealing* (Bilbro et al., 1989; Peterson & Anderson, 1988), involves varying λ sufficiently slowly as (2) is evolved. Mean field annealing is known to approximate simulated annealing in its performance (Bilbro et al., 1989; Hertz, Krogh, & Palmer, 1991), which explains why it often works well in practice (Bilbro et al., 1989; Jagota, 1995).

A second approach — the one we employ in this chapter — is to inject controllable chaotic or periodic oscillations into (2). These oscillations are injected into (2) through the external input **I**. Initially, chaotic oscillations are injected into **I**, which in turn induce oscillations in the evolution of (2). The oscillations injected into **I** are gradually changed to periodic ones by turning a "knob." Finally, constant input is fed into I, which makes the evolution of (2) undergo a phase transition to convergent behavior. We call this algorithm *chaotic annealing*. Chaotic annealing is motivated by analogy with simulated annealing (and also mean field annealing). Just as simulated annealing exhibits relatively random behavior at high temperature which transitions to convergent behavior at low temperature — which is what makes it usually work better than low fixed-temperature convergent dynamics — we expect that chaotic annealing — which makes (2) exhibit chaotic behavior initially, and convergent behavior eventually — will work better than convergent-only evolution of (2).

3.1. Related Work

There is some previous work along these lines (Vepralainen, 1991; Wells, 1992). In Vepralainen (1991), a chaotic annealing method is proposed and a theoretical result, establishing a connection between that method and simulated annealing, is obtained. Our method in this chapter is somewhat different. We also evaluate our method experimentally, on the Maximum Clique problem, whereas the results in Vepralainen (1991) are theoretical in nature.

During revisions on this chapter, we were informed of another approach to chaotic annealing for combinatorial optimization due to Chen and Aihara (1995) that is quite related to ours. (See Chen & Aihara, 1995, also for other related earlier work.) This approach, like ours and unlike stochastic simulated annealing, uses deterministic chaos. This approach, like ours, uses a network with continuous-valued sigmoidal neurons. This approach, like ours, starts the network in transient chaotic mode and uses a bifurcation parameter to transition the network dynamics to an eventually convergent one.

And now the differences. This approach, unlike ours, builds chaotic behavior into the dynamical rules governing the operation of the network itself. Our approach, in contrast, uses a standard continuous-state, continuous-time Hopfield network and injects chaotic signals from a two-neuron oscillator into this network via the external input to each neuron. This scheme, we feel, has the following benefits. First, it is *modular*, using the Hopfield model as a standard component. In particular, the Hopfield network has been widely used for solving a variety of combinatorial optimization problems (each use differs, in essence, only in the weights and biases used to encode some optimization problem). In principle, one may use our chaotic annealing scheme on any of these networks simply by coupling our two-neuron oscillator to such a network. Second, it is simpler to control and analyze the dynamical behavior of the two-neuron oscillator than it might be to control the non fixed-point behavior of an *n*-neuron network. In particular, for our two-neuron oscillator, we know exactly how to evolve the bifurcation parameter to generate chaotic signals, then transition to periodic signals, and then eventually to produce a constant output. And lastly, the approach in Chen and Aihara (1995) is tested on the TSP problem as well as on a maintenance scheduling problem. Our approach is tested on a different problem — the maximum clique problem.

3.2. Chaotic Annealing

Figure 19.7 shows the architecture of our chaotic annealing network. The network consists of two subnetworks coupled together: HcN and a two-neuron chaotic oscillator (Wang, 1991). A graph G, denoting an instance of the maximum clique problem, is encoded into the HcN network, as follows. The network weights are set so that the graph G_N underlying the network, described in Section $\Re$f{HcN}, equals G. When the HcN network is decoupled from the oscillator by setting $c = 0$, the network exhibits convergent behavior according to (2), and eventually settles to a maximal clique. When the oscillator is coupled to an HcN, it may be used to pump chaotic or periodic oscillations into the external input of each neuron of the HcN, which in turn induces oscillations in the evolution of the HcN network according to (2).

The two-neuron chaotic oscillator is taken from Wang (1991), and is illustrated in Fig. 19.7a. The network evolves according to:

$$\mathbf{Y}(t+1) = \mathbf{g}_{\mu}(\mathrm{V}\mathrm{Y}(t)) \qquad (3).$$

Here V is an arbitrary 2×2 matrix (i.e., not necessarily symmetric) and $\mathbf{Y} \in [0,1]^2$ is the network state vector. $\mathbf{g}_{\mu}$ is the sigmoid vector map defined following (2), with gain $\mu \in [0,\infty)$. Notice that (3) is a discrete-time variant of (2), but with the difference that the external bias vector $\mathbf{I}$ equals zero and V is not necessarily symmetric. We have the following theorem from Wang (1991).

Theorem 19.4. Consider the iterated map given by (3), with the weight matrix

$$\begin{pmatrix} a & -a \\ b & -b \end{pmatrix}.$$

If $b < a < 0$ and $d = b/a \geq 2$, or $a > b > 0$ and $d = b/a \leq ½$, then the family of iterated maps (3) is topologically (1, 0)-conjugate to a full family of S-unimodal maps on the interval [0,1] with $\mu \in (0, \infty)$.

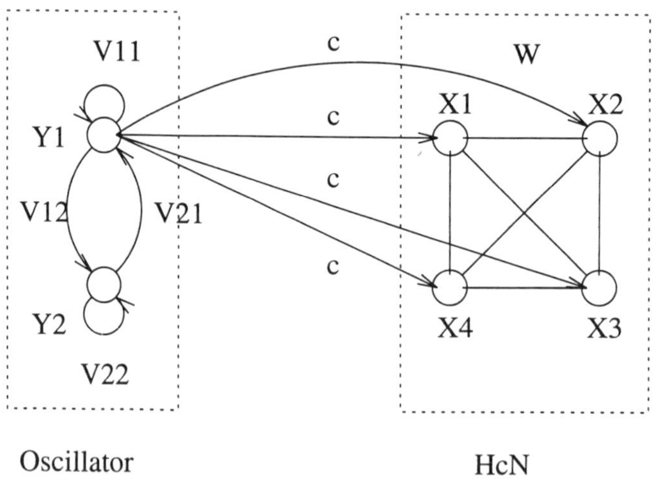

Fig. 19.7. The two-neuron oscillator coupled to a four-neuron HcN network.

According to properties of a full family of *S*-unimodal maps (Devaney, 1986), there exists mathematically a period-doubling route to chaos and possible strange attractors in this simple two-neuron network.

Our full chaotic annealing algorithm, CA(μ, c), in the form it was experimented with, is now described formally as follows:

ALGORITHM CA (μ, c)
INPUT: α, c
1 $\mathbf{X} := (0.5 \pm r)^n$
2 $\mu := 4$
3 while = $\mu \geq 0.1$ do
3a $\quad \mathbf{Y} := (0.35, 0.55)$
3b $\quad$ repeat five times
3b1 $\quad\quad \mathbf{Y} := \mathbf{g}_\mu(\mathrm{V}\,\mathbf{Y})$
3c $\quad$ repeat n times
3c1 $\quad\quad \mathbf{Y} := \mathbf{g}_\mu(\mathrm{V}\,\mathbf{Y})$
3c2 $\quad\quad \mathbf{I} := (|\rho|\ c\mathrm{Y}_1)$
3c3 $\quad\quad \mathbf{X} := \mathbf{X} + \gamma\,[-\mathbf{X} + \mathbf{g}_\lambda(\mathrm{W}\mathbf{X} + \mathbf{I})]$
3d $\quad \mu := \alpha\,\mu$
3e $\quad c := \alpha\,c$

The description is not complete without the following remarks:

- Both the oscillator gain μ and the oscillator-to-HcN coupling constant c are annealed geometrically, as shown in Steps 3d-e, at the same rate $\alpha \in (0,1)$. α and c are parameters to the algorithm. The extreme values of μ, $\mu = 4$ and $\mu = 0.1$, were chosen because at the former extreme (3) exhibits chaotic oscillations, and at the latter extreme (3) exhibits convergent behavior (Wang, 1991).

- In Step 1, r is a random number in (0, 0.05) and is used to break the symmetry of the initial HcN network state vector $\mathbf{X}$.

- The oscillator weight matrix V is chosen as

$$\begin{pmatrix} -5 & 5 \\ -25 & 25 \end{pmatrix}.$$

- Step 3b is employed to get the transients out of the evolution of (3).

- For each fixed μ, a choice was made to iterate the oscillator and the HcN network, in lock-step fashion, n times (Step 3c). In one iteration, first the oscillator was iterated once (Step 3c1), from which the external input **I** to HcN was constructed (Step 3c2), and then the HcN network was iterated once (Step 3c3). Notice that the external input vector **I** was constructed from only the first component Y_1 of the oscillator output vector **Y**. (Every component of **I** is given the same value, $|\rho|\,\mathbf{c}\mathbf{Y}_1$.) From Theorem 19.4, the iterated map (3) is topologically conjugate to a one-dimensional map. Indeed, just the first component Y_1 of **Y** exhibits the oscillations we desire.

- In Step 3c3, which is a discretized version of (2), the Euler step size γ was chosen to be 0.1 and the neuron gain λ to be 1. These settings were arrived at after experimentation. In the future, we hope to use results from Wang, Jagota, Botelho, and Garzon (1995), which mathematically analyzed the model of Step 3c3, to help choose a larger step size γ while guaranteeing convergence to a fixed point. This could speed up the CA(μ, c) algorithm. The effect of increasing γ on the clique size found would have to be determined experimentally.

- We also experimented with a variant of CA, called CA(μ), in which the coupling constant c was kept unchanged (i.e., Step 3e of algorithm CA(μ, c) was deleted).

It is useful to note that the number of annealing steps (i.e., the number of iterations of the while} loop in Step 3) is $\log_{1/a} 40$ which depends only on a. By contrast, the number of annealing steps in a geometrically annealed mean field annealing algorithm for the Maximum Clique algorithm evaluated earlier {Jagota, 1995} grew in proportion to $\log_{1/a} n^2$ because the initial temperature T_0 that was used had a value proportional to n^2 (Jagota, 1995). In subsequent work (Jagota, Sanchis, & Ganesan, 1995), an MFA schedule with only two annealing steps was employed. However this didn't work as well as the geometric-schedule-based MFA of Jagota (1995). To summarize then, our chaotic annealing algorithms — CA(μ, c) and CA(μ) — are more efficient than geometrically annealed MFA but less efficient than two-temperature MFA. We have no results on the quality of the solution found by CA(μ, c) or CA(μ), in comparison with the two versions of MFA.

3.2. Preliminary Experimental Results

Table 19.1 reports preliminary results of experiments to evaluate the algorithm CA(μ). Each row corresponds to a p-random n-vertex graph, that is, a graph on n vertices in which each of the $\binom{n}{2}$ edge-slots contains an edge with probability p, independent of the other edge-slots. For the CA(μ) algorithm, the choice of a was optimized and is not reported here; c was chosen equal to 1. The column labeled *Greedy* denotes the following greedy algorithm: I) start from the entire graph and delete, one by one, the lowest degree vertex from the graph until a clique C remains, (ii)extend this clique by adding vertices, one by one, until the result is a maximal clique. The discrete HcN can be made to emulate this algorithm; see the algorithm SD(V) described in Jagota (1995). The column labeled C-HcN denotes the continuous HcN network with constant external input **I**, evolved according to (2).

n	p	Greedy	C-HcN	CA'
30	0.5	5.73	5.66	5.6
100	0.5	8.0	7.73	7.93
100	0.909	29.8	28.66	29.4
400	0.909	47.13	43.73	44.0

Table 19.1. The size of the clique returned by the three algorithms, averaged over 15 graphs in each row.

From Table 19.1 we see that algorithm CA(μ) consistently finds a larger clique, on average, than does algorithm C-HcN. However, the greedy algorithm consistently finds significantly larger cliques, on average, than both. The size of the largest clique in a 0.5-random 100-vertex graph is 10 almost surely (Bollob'as, 1985; see Jagota, 1995, for more details.) The sample size of 15 random graphs in each row is sufficient to draw these conclusions because the variances of the sizes of the cliques found by these algorithms on random graphs are quite small, as demonstrated in some detail in Jagota (1995).

Table 19.2 reports preliminary results of experiments to evaluate the algorithm CA(μ, c). Each row corresponds to a p-random n-vertex graph. The column labeled C(0.1) denotes a nonannealing version of the CA(μ, c) algorithm, Steps 3a-3c3 only, operated with $\mu = 0.1$. At this fixed value of μ, the CA algorithm is expected to behave like the C-HcN algorithm, that is, one with constant external input. The value of the coupling constant c for CA(0.1) was set to 1. For the CA(μ, c) algorithm, described in column four, the initial value of c was set to $\bar{e}$, where $\bar{e}$ is the average degree of a vertex in the complement graph $\bar{G}$. This setting is explained in the next paragraph. For a p-random graph, $\bar{e} = (1 - \text{p}) \times (n - 1)$, which was the value used for the initial c. For the CA(μ, c) algorithm, the annealing rate α — the same rate for the annealing of μ as well as of c — was set to ½. For both C(0.1) and CA(μ, c), ρ was set to $-4n$.

The initial value of c requires some explanation. Neurons are not committed to 0 or 1 values in the initial stages of the CA(μ, c) algorithm, so it is reasonable to assume an activity of ½ on average of a neuron. Under this assumption, the incoming input to a neuron from other neurons is on average $(\frac{1}{2})\rho\bar{e}$. The desirable range, to allow the external input to a neuron to have a significant effect on the dynamics, is between 0 and $|\rho|\bar{e}$. Since $Y_1 \in [0,1]$ and, from step 3c2, $\mathbf{I} := (|\rho| c Y_1)$, we can achieve this desired range by setting the initial c to $\bar{e}$. In a later stage of the evolution of the CA(μ, c) algorithm, the neurons are likely to be more committed to 0 or 1 values and, since the size of the largest clique in a random graph is very small, the average activity of a neuron is expected to be much smaller than ½. The corresponding decrease in the range of **I** is achieved by decreasing (annealing) c, as shown in step 3e of the CA(μ, c) algorithm.

n	p	CA(0.1)	CA
30	0.5	2.4	5.86
100	0.5	7.3	8.31
100	0.909	29.0	30.53

Table 19.2. The size of the clique returned by two algorithms, averaged over thirteen graphs in the second row, and fifteen graphs in the first and third rows.

From Table 19.2, we see that algorithm CA(μ, c) consistently finds a significantly larger clique, on average, than does algorithm C(0.1). Of the thirteen 0.5-random 100-vertex graphs, C(0.1) found a larger clique than CA(μ, c) on just one graph, an equal-size clique on two graphs, and a smaller clique on ten graphs. Of the fifteen 0.909-random 100-vertex graphs, C(0.1) found a larger clique than CA(μ, c) on two graphs, an equal-size clique on two graphs, and a smaller clique on eleven graphs.

Although the graphs in Tables 19.1 and 19.2 were not identical, their statistical parameters were the same, allowing indirect comparisons. Such comparisons indicate that the algorithm CA(μ, c) probably works slightly better than even the greedy algorithm SD(V). Further comparisons with Jagota (1995, Table 1) support this tentative conclusion and, furthermore, also indicate that algorithm CA(μ, c) approaches competitiveness with geometrically annealed MFA.

3.3. Conclusion to Part II

This part dealt with injecting oscillations into a continuous Hopfield network, for solving a mapped optimization problem. The continuous Hopfield algorithm to solve an optimization problem is gradient-descent in nature. To circumvent this limitation, a mechanism was developed for injecting controllable chaos or periodic oscillations into the Hopfield network. Chaotic or oscillatory behavior was initiated, and converted to convergent behavior at the turn of a "knob," in analogy with simulated annealing. The resulting algorithm, called chaotic annealing, was evaluated on instances of the Maximum Clique optimization problem on graphs. The chaotic annealing algorithm exhibited a significant improvement over the convergent Hopfield dynamics. One version of the chaotic annealing algorithm appears to also be competitive with some other approaches that work better than the convergent Hopfield dynamics.

ACKNOWLEDGMENTS

The authors thank Tim Shirey for formatting and style comments, and David DeMaris for suggesting better names for the chaotic annealing algorithms and for pointing us to the closely related chaotic annealing work of Chen and Aihara (1995).

REFERENCES

Bilbro, G., Mann, R., Miller, T. K., Snyder, W. E., van den Bout, B. E., & White, M. (1989). Optimization by mean field annealing. In D. S. Touretzky (Ed.), *Advances in Neural Information Processing Systems 1* (pp. 91-98). San Mateo, CA: Morgan Kaufmann.

Bollob'as, B. (1985). *Random Graphs*. New York: Academic Press.

Bondy, J. M., & Murty, U. S. R. (1976). *Graph Theory with Applications*. New York: North-Holland.

Chen, L., & Aihara, K. (1995). Chaotic simulated annealing by a neural network model with transient chaos. *Neural Networks*, *8*, 915-930.

Cohen, M. A., & Grossberg, S. (1983). Absolute stability of global pattern formation and parallel memory storage by competitive neural networks. *IEEE Transactions on Systems, Man, and Cybernetics*, *13*, 815-826.

Devaney, R. L. (1986). *An Introduction to Chaotic Dynamical Systems*. Menlo Park, CA: Benjamin/Cummings.

Goles, E., Fogelman-Soulie, F., & Pellegrin, D. (1985). Decreasing energy functions as a tool for studying threshold networks. *Discrete Applied Mathematics*, *12*, 261-277.

Hertz, J., Krogh, A., & Palmer, R. G. (1991). *Introduction to the Theory of Neural Computation*. Reading, MA: Addison-Wesley.

Hopfield, J. J. (1982). Neural networks and physical systems with emergent collective computational abilities. *Proceedings of the National Academy of Sciences*, *79*, 2554-2558.

Hopfield, J. J. (1984). Neurons with graded responses have collective computational properties like those of two-state neurons. *Proceedings of the National Academy of Sciences*, *81*, 3088-3092.

Hopfield, J. J., & Tank, D. W. (1985). "Neural" computation of decisions in optimization problems. *Biological Cybernetics*, *52*, 141-152.

Jagota, A. (1990, April). Applying a Hopfield-style network to degraded printed text restoration. *Conference on Neural Networks and PDP, Indiana-Purdue* (pp. 20-30). Fort Wayne, IN: Purdue Research Foundation.

Jagota, A. (1993b). *The Hopfield-clique Network, Associative Memories, and Combinatorial Optimization*. Unpublished doctoral dissertation, State University of New York at Buffalo, Department of Computer Science, 224 Bell Hall, Amherst, NY 14260, 1993. Also available as Tech. Rep. TR 93-12 from above address.

Jagota, A. (1994a). A Hopfield-style network with a graph-theoretic characterization. *Journal of Artificial Neural Networks*, *1*, 145-166.

Jagota, A. (1994b). Representing discrete structures in a Hopfield-style network. In D. S. Levine and M. Aparicio, IV (Eds.), *Neural Networks for Knowledge Representation and Inference* (pp. 123-142). Hillsdale, NJ: Lawrence Erlbaum Associates.

Jagota, A. (1995). Approximating maximum clique in a Hopfield-style network. *IEEE Transactions on Neural Networks*, *6*, 724-735.

Jagota, A., Sanchis, L., & Ganesan, R. (1995). Approximating maximum clique using neural network and related heuristics. In D. S. Johnson & M. Trick (Eds.), *DIMACS Series: Second DIMACS Challenge*. Providence, RI: American Mathematical Society Press.

McClelland, J. L., Rumelhart, D. E., & the PDP Research Group (1986). *Parallel Distributed Processing: Explorations in the Microstructure of Cognition* (Vol. 2). Cambridge, MA: MIT Press.

Peterson, C., & Anderson, J. R. (1988). Neural networks and NP-complete optimization problems; a performance study on the graph bisection problem. *Complex Systems, 2*, 59-89.

Shrivistava, Y., Dasgupta, S., & Reddy, S. M. (1990). Neural network solutions to a graph theoretic problem. *Proceedings of IEEE International Symposium on Circuits and Systems* (pp. 2528-2531). New York: IEEE.

Vepralainen, A. M. (1991). Annealing with chaotic neurons in "artificial neural networks." In T. Kohonen, O. Simula, K. Makisara, & J. Kangas (Eds.), *International Conference on Artificial Neural Networks* (Vol. 1, pp. 181-186). Amsterdam: North-Holland.

Wang, X. (1991). Period-doublings to chaos in a simple neural network: An analytic proof. *Complex Systems, 5*, 425-441.

Wang, X., Jagota, A., Botelho, F., & Garzon, M. (1995). Absence of cycles in symmetric neural networks. In D. S. Touretzky, M. C. Mozer, & M. E. Hasselmo (Eds.), *Proceedings of Ninth Neural Information Processing Systems Conference* (pp. 372-378). Cambridge, MA: MIT Press.

Wells, D. M. (1992). Solving degenerate optimization problems using networks of neural oscillators. *Neural Networks, 5*, 949-959.

20

Modeling Neural Oscillations Using VLSI-Based Neuromimes

Seth Wolpert

Pennsylvania State University at Harrisburg

ABSTRACT

As a prelude to a VLSI implementation of a live locomotory control network, the phenomena of reciprocal inhibition and recurrent cyclic inhibition were recreated and subjected to parametric tests of their oscillatory range and stability. Networks were constructed from comprehensive VLSI-based artificial neurons, or neuromimes, which are efficient and convenient, yet configurable and comprehensive, allowing a variety of cellular transient and steady-state characteristics to be precisely and continuously varied. In initial tests, both oscillator types were found to operate over a broad range of cellular and network frequencies. In those tests, it was noted that oscillation by reciprocal inhibition between two neurons requires that each possess some measure of synaptic dynamics, while neurons in the cyclically inhibited networks did not. This suggests that the two oscillators utilized different temporal mechanisms. In circuit tests, individual cells self-oscillated over a wide range of frequencies in response to cell threshold, refractory period, and postsynaptic inhibition. In subsequent network tests, the cyclic networks were found to be sensitive to cellular threshold, yet insensitive to refractory period duration. Conversely, the reciprocal networks were found to be sensitive to refractory period duration, yet immune to cellular threshold. This complementary relationship suggests an advantage for biological oscillatory networks that incorporate both types.

1. INTRODUCTION

Neuronal oscillators have been documented as Central Pattern Generators (CPGs) of efferent signals that elicit rhythmic motor responses in a variety of organisms. As a result, CPGs have been the object of a large amount of neuroscientific investigation. Swimming motion has been studied in mollusks by Satterlie and Spencer (1985), in tritonia by Getting (1989), in medicinal leeches by Friesen (1989), and in sea lampreys by Grillner, Waller, Brodin, and Lanser (1991). Pyloric oscillations have been studied in the lobster by Selverston (1985), locomotion has been studied in locusts by Robertson and Pearson (1985), and repetitive aspects of snail feeding have been studied by Elliott and Benjamin (1985). From observations of morphological data, intracellular signal patterns, and outward behavior, the structure and interconnectivity of these and other CPGs have been postulated on a neuron-by-neuron, synapse-by-synapse basis. That level of detail makes CPGs excellent candidates for recreation in electronic hardware. In the past, such endeavors would have necessitated an extremely elaborate circuit based on discrete devices, such as the model of avian retina by Runge et al. (1968). With the advent of broad access to custom VLSI technology, arbitrary configurations of nerve cells may now be recreated efficiently and accurately in electronic hardware using a comprehensive IC-based artificial nerve cell, or neuromime.

Neuromimes have historically been pursued within the limitations of available electronic technology. Crane (1962) devised the Neuristor, a device that processes pulse trains through either trigger or refractory junctions, and propagates them along a simulated axon. Set forth as a platform on which to investigate neural computation, the Neuristor captured mathematical, if not aesthetic characteristics of biological neurons. Hiltz (1965) made extensive use of silicon devices in an artificial neuron that replicates many behavioral aspects of neuronal function, including threshold, action potential generation, accommodation, refractoriness, burst firing, adaptation, and strength-latency correspondence. In the succeeding years, many new models of neuronal behavior were devised. Jenik (1962), Fitzhugh (1966), Lewis (1968a, 1968b), Johnson and Hanna (1969), French and Stein (1970), Roy (1972), Pottala (1973), MacGregor and Oliver (1973), Brockman (1979), Mitchell and Friesen (1981), and more recently, in VLSI form by Mahowald and Douglas (1991), Elias and Northmore (1995), DeYong, Findley, and Fields (1992), and Linares-Barranco, Sanchez-Sinencio, Rodriguez-Vazquez, and Huertas (1991) all devised neuromorphic circuits that improved on the accuracy or versatility of some aspect of neuronal behavior. Organization of these circuits has tended to follow two approaches, the Fitzhugh-Nagumo models, which simulate membrane ionic currents from simplifications of the Hodgkin-Huxley equations, and the "integrate-and-fire" models, which generate electrical signals corresponding to membrane potential and threshold potential and arbitrate output activity based on an analog comparison of the two signals. Notable among the integrate-and-fire models is the implementation by French and Stein (1970), which featured an organization that is not only highly cohesive to outward neuronal response, but is also composed of subcircuits that are appropriate for implementation in analog CMOS VLSI.

The neuromime designed by French and Stein is organized around an analog voltage comparator that continuously monitors the transient signals that represent cell membrane potential and threshold potential, and initiates the synthesis of an output impulse, or action potential whenever the threshold is exceeded. This organization is shown in Fig. 20.1, and was modified to form the basis for the VLSI prototype. This configuration offers tremendous flexibility in modeling the behavior of an arbitrary biological neuron. It is capable of assimilating a virtually unlimited quantity of input and output signals, both excitatory and inhibitory. It allows independent, continuous, and precise control over the time constant and resting level of the cell's dendritic or postsynaptic membrane potential, threshold potential, and axonal, or presynaptic membrane potential. With minor modification, it can assign uniquely addressable synaptic weights to each sensory input. This model also offers control of the resting level, shape, amplitude, and duration of the neuronal output pulse, or action potential. With threshold potential continuously accessible, control over the strength and duration of the refractory period is possible, and threshold-related phenomena, such as fatigue, facilitation, and accommodation are also easily accomplished.

The VLSI-based neuromime, as implemented in this study, is organized as shown in Fig. 20.2. Steady-state resting levels and time constants for membrane and threshold potentials are maintained off-chip by R-C networks, with transients controlled by active devices on-chip. All synaptic inputs to the cell are assimilated through CMOS buffers, which provide extremely high input impedance and low input capacitance. Once buffered, synaptic stimuli are standardized with respect to duration, amplitude, and offset by truncation into fixed-width pulses. This is performed by monostables with nominal output pulse widths of approximately 20 microseconds. These brief excitatory and inhibitory pulses are then assimilated into postsynaptic membrane potential, V_{post} via a push-pull stage consisting of MOSFETs M_1 and M_2. Excitatory stimuli activate M_1, which deflects V_{post} upward to represent depolarization of the neuron's cell membrane. Inhibitory stimuli activate M_2, which deflects V_{post} downward, representing further polarization of the cell membrane.

Threshold transients for refractory period, fatigue, and facilitation are controlled on-chip by the threshold generator, and may be further augmented by supplemental active components off-chip. The voltage comparator senses Vm_{post} and threshold, and triggers the action potential generator (APG) whenever threshold is exceeded. The APG synthesizes an action potential waveform upon the presynaptic membrane potential node, V_{pre}. The output buffer converts action potential impulses on V_{pre} to binary impulses able to drive a large number of other neuromime inputs or standard CMOS and TTL digital logic. Input and output buffers may also be adapted to sense and generate biologically compatible signals in parallel, affording the facility to translate impulses from digital to biological levels and vice versa. The comprehensiveness of this model however, is based on the off-chip accessibility of the R-C networks for threshold and membrane potentials. As such, the time constants and resting levels for each are independently, continuously, and precisely controllable.

The use of artificial neurons to recreate cellular oscillators has been notably accomplished in a study published by Friesen and Stent (1977). There, discrete neuromimes as designed by Lewis (1968b) were employed to realize ringlike cellular

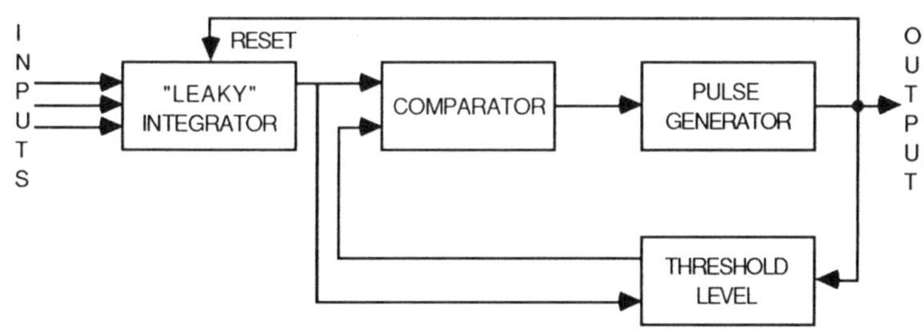

Fig. 20.1. Organization of the integrate-and-fire neuromime model described by French and Stein (1970).

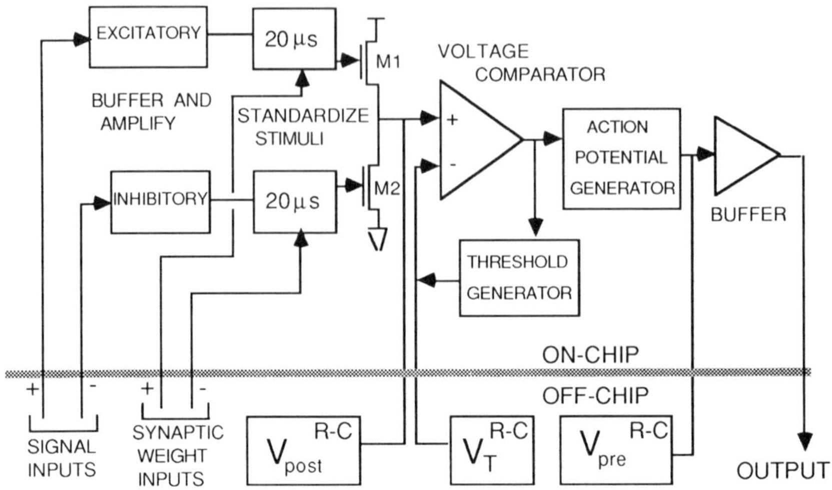

Fig. 20.2. Organization of the VLSI-based neuromime, as published by Wolpert and Tzanakou (1986).

networks that oscillate by the principle of recurrent cyclic inhibition (RCI). After building and characterizing ring networks composed of three, four, and five cells, they proceed to embed a five-cell network into an electronic model of a small segment of the CPG, as mapped out in the leech in earlier studies by Friesen (1989). Interconnecting the eight neuromime circuits they had available and driving any significant outside inputs with artificial signals analogous to those emanating from other parts of the network, they reconstructed a neuron-by-neuron mockup of a segment of the oscillator network, and found its period and duty cycle to approximately agree with physiological data. This is a remarkable achievement in light of the fact that the leech CPG is a phase-locked network distributed over 21 body segments and composed of hundreds of neurons, some of which have 10 synaptic inputs or more. The extent of this interconnectivity is belied by an observation by Friesen and Stent (1977) that signals from a minimum of six intact ganglia are necessary to obtain oscillatory behavior in physiological studies. This fact also relates the complexity of the task of identifying the location and extent of the CPG network throughout 42 ganglia, and consisting of tens of thousands of neurons.

In morphological studies, many topologies have been observed as bases for cellular oscillator networks. Two commonly observed configurations are reciprocally inhibitory pairs of cells and cyclically inhibitory rings of three or more cells. Reciprocal oscillators are characterized as consisting of two cells, each of which exhibits tonic activity and inhibits its counterpart with some mechanism of fatigue, in either the cell's own excitability or its counterpart's responsiveness to inhibition. The latter mechanism of fatigue is the more commonly observed in biological networks, and is phenomenologically known as *postinhibitory rebound* (PIR). Such networks exhibit alternating bursts of impulses, where the impulse frequency within each burst is approximately the tonic output frequency of each individual neuron, and the frequency of the bursts themselves depends primarily on the latency of cellular rebound from sustained inhibition. This topology and its signal patterns are given in Fig. 20.3.

Alternately, cyclic oscillators are characterized by arrangement of an odd number, N, of constituent cells in a ring configuration, with each cell exhibiting tonic activity and inhibiting an adjoining cell in one direction. Bursts of impulses then propagate around the ring in the opposite direction. The number of bursts present in the ring at any one time is $(N-1)/2$, and the period of the oscillator is $2*N*T_R/(N-1)$, where T_R is to the time it takes for a cell to recover from sustained inhibition. The interconnectivity described holds for rings with any odd number of cells, and at any given time, one cell in the ring is in the process of recovery from inhibition, while all remaining cells assume an alternating sequence of active and inhibited states. This arrangement of cells and the signal patterns that result in the case of a five-celled ring are illustrated in Fig. 20.4. Note that the duty cycle in this type of oscillator is 40%, rather than 20%, as two cells are active at any time. It should also be mentioned that rings containing an even number of cells may also be implemented in symmetrically interconnected ring structures, but more elaborate inhibitory interconnectivity schemes must be employed in order for cyclic oscillation to occur.

One long-term objective of this research is to implement an electronic model of the CPG for swimming motion in *hirudo medicinalis,* the medicinal leech from morphological data and electrophysiological recordings. In order to be applicable to the task, the VLSI-based neuromime must be able to assume the transient characteristics of tonic excitation, as well as both of the oscillatory modalities described earlier, as all three phenomena have been observed in the structure of the *hirudo* network. It is the short-term objective of this study to demonstrate the suitability of the VLSI-based neuromime to this task by implementing both oscillator types and characterizing oscillatory response to a simulated variation in a number of environmental parameters. If their behavior is consistent with physiological data, then the way is clear to a number of long-term objectives relative to this procedure.

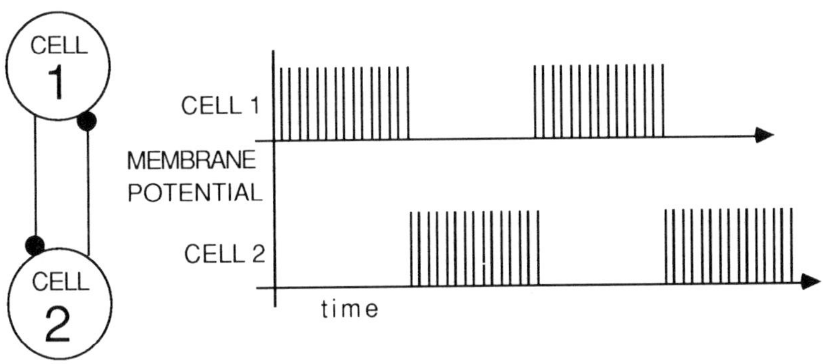

Fig. 20.3. Topology and signals in a mutually inhibitory network.

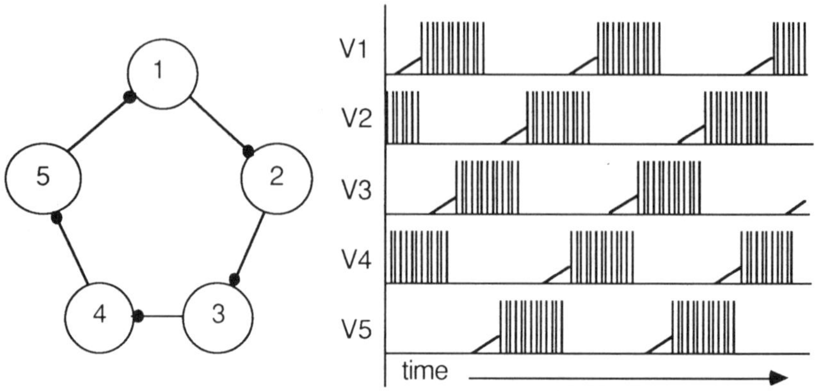

Fig. 20.4. Structure and signal patterns of a five-cell RCI network

The first such objectives will be to evaluate the completeness and correctness of the existing *hirudo* swim CPG model. Once implemented, the VLSI model may then be used as a platform to extend the model by evaluating additional connections that have been postulated, but never confirmed. Subsequent objectives will be to examine the singularity of the relationship between neuronal "hardware" and its associated "software." This will attempt to address the issue "Do the structure and connectivity of a neuronal network dictate the signal patterns that reside within it? Conversely, is a neural network like a digital computer, able to run different programs on the same physical platform?" The third objective of this project is to formalize a methodology for recreating neuronal circuits from biological sources for application to contemporary tasks in computation, control, image processing, and pattern recognition.

2. THE NEURONAL MODEL

The IC-based neuromime was first described by Wolpert and Tzanakou (1986), and is based on the organizational shown in Fig. 20.2. Organizationally simple, it is closely based on the outward function of a generic neuron. It is also flexible and can therefore assume specific characteristics of a wide variety of neurons from both biological and mathematical sources. The model is organized around three critical circuit nodes: namely postsynaptic membrane potential (V_{post}), which corresponds to the neuronal membrane potential in the soma and dendritic segments of the cell; presynaptic membrane potential (V_{pre}), which corresponds to the neuronal membrane potential in the axon of the cell; and threshold potential (V_T), which is the magnitude of V_{post} required to elicit an action potential on V_{pre}. Each of these nodes is biased by an off-chip R-C network, and as such, their resting levels and time constants are externally controllable.

Varying the resting level of V_{post} allows for the individual and relative magnitudes of the cell's responsiveness to excitatory and inhibitory stimuli to be closely and continuously controlled. Varying the time constant of V_{post} allows for the magnitude and temporal persistence of synaptic stimuli to be closely and continuously controlled. This also provides control over temporal summation of excitatory and inhibitory stimuli to be controlled. Varying the resting level of threshold allows for the excitatory threshold of the cell (the number of excitatory stimuli required to drive the cell to excitation) to be controlled. Varying the time constant of threshold potential allows for the refractory period duration to be controlled. Varying the resting level and time constant of V_{pre} allows for its temporal duration and waveshape in terms of peak, slope, and after-potential to be matched to specific biologically aesthetic action potentials.

Waveforms resident in the artificial nerve cell are depicted in Fig. 20.5. Note that the depolarizing "blip" on V_{post} exactly coincides with the 20 microsecond pulse emerging from the monostable. Also, note that, for clarity, the initiation of the action potential was slightly delayed after the rising edge of the voltage comparator output. Although delay is a feature built into the neuromime circuit, normal cell operation would be characterized by the action potential waveform commencing on the rising edge of the comparator output signal.

The model, as depicted in Fig. 20.2, has been specifically configured for the cellular oscillators in this study, having only one each of the excitatory and inhibitory input pathways. Even so, its input capacity may be easily expanded by combining all stimuli of a given polarity into composite spike trains by a simple logical OR operation. This provides a good approximation of temporal summation as long as the frequency of incident excitatory or inhibitory stimuli does not approach levels that will cause temporal overlap of the waveforms. If more accuracy in temporal summation is warranted, additional input buffers can easily be incorporated into the on-chip circuitry. This facility allows stimuli from each source to have separate pathways to the postsynaptic membrane potential node, each with a synaptic weight that is independently and continuously controllable.

Also noteworthy in the model is the observation that the neuromime nominally standardizes all excitatory inputs and all inhibitory inputs to a fixed duration, and hence, synaptic weight. This design decision was made because the offset, waveshape, and duration of a given stimulus should not dictate its synaptic weight. Instead, other methods, some as simple as digital divide-by-n counters may be used to modulate synaptic weight from off-chip. Another option available is to alter the 20 microsecond duration to which each stimulus is truncated by means of a separate control input. Thisfacility was also implemented in the neuromime with independent control inputs for each input pathway, excitatory or inhibitory, and in a way that lets the 20 microsecond duration be either lengthened or shortened to any duration desired. With this circuit organization, the duration of this pulse is linearly proportional to the voltage deflection that results in V_{post}. This provides an accurate mechanism for modulating synaptic weight in a manner that may be implemented under both static and dynamic conditions.

In order to realize the oscillator networks in this project, the neuromime will be required to exhibit tonic activity, that is, generate a continuous and constant stream of

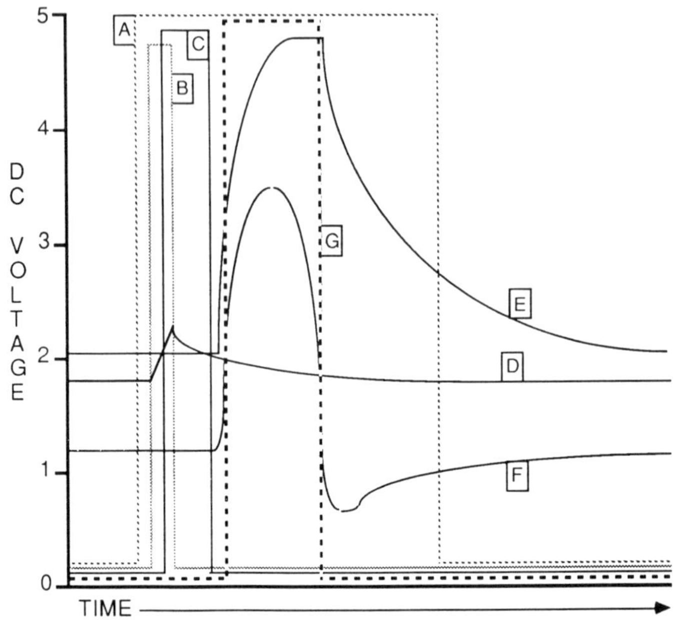

Fig. 20.5. Waveforms resident in the IC-based neuromime including an excitatory input (A), the 20 microsecond pulse to which it is truncated (B), the voltage comparator output (C), V_{post} (D), threshold (E), V_{pre} (F), and the binary level output impulse (G).

action potentials in the absence of any external excitatory stimuli. The structure of this model makes this phenomenon easily accomplished. If the nominal resting level of V_{post} is set to be greater than that of threshold potential, the voltage comparator will attempt to trigger action potentials on a continuous basis. With the advent of the first action potential, the threshold potential will be pulled up to it supply voltage (V_{DD}) to simulate the absolute refractory period. As soon as threshold exceeds V_{post}, the voltage comparator output will return to a low, inactive state. After the action potential has elapsed, threshold will decay back to its resting level to simulate the relative refractory period. Once it has decayed to a level below that of V_{post}, the comparator output will return to its active state, initiating synthesis of another action potential by the APG. In this way, a constant stream of action potentials is generated, with an interpulse interval equal to the duration of the relative refractory period. Waveforms associated with this chain of events are depicted in Fig. 20.6. Not only does the organization of the neuromime support this mode of operation, but it affords control over the frequency of tonic excitation via three different mechanisms. The interpulse interval may be controlled by the time constant of the threshold potential node, which varies the duration of the relative refractory period. The interval may also be controlled by varying the magnitude of the voltage gap between V_{Mpost} and the threshold potential. Finally, the level of tonic excitation may be reduced by the introduction of inhibitory stimuli of various frequency and synaptic weight from off-chip. Conversely, it may be increased by the introduction of excitatory stimuli of varying frequency and synaptic weight. In realizing the oscillators described in this study, it will be necessary to invoke all of the features of the model mentioned in this section.

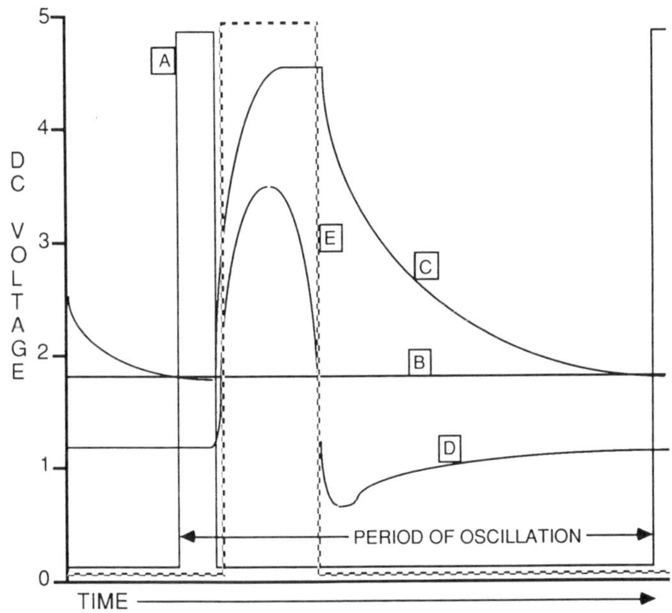

Fig. 20.6. Waveforms resident in the IC-based neuromime undergoing tonic excitation, including the comparator output (A), V_{post} (B), Threshold (C), V_{pre} (D), and the binary output pulse (E).

3. CIRCUIT DESCRIPTION

Circuitry for the IC-based neuromimes used in this study was simulated using SPICE3 and physical design was carried out using MAGIC6. Both processes were carried out using DECstation 2100 work stations. The integrated circuits were fabricated using a 2-micron double-level metal technology. Finished ICs contained three complete neuromimes, and were packaged in 600-mil 40 pin dual inline ceramic housings for easy handling and testing. Each neuromime circuit occupies approximately 0.6 square millimeters of chip area. Electrically, the circuit is powered by a single-ended 5 to 10 volt DC supply, and being CMOS, it dissipates minimal power on-chip.

The majority of the subcircuits in the neuromime are standard analog CMOS VLSI, and are described in detail elsewhere (Wolpert & Tzanakou, 1986). Only the circuit for standardizing all stimuli into 20 microsecond pulses is presented here, as it is the site for synaptic learning. This circuit is a monostable, logically organized as shown in Fig. 20.7. In this scheme, the rising edge of each stimulus propagates quickly through the circuit to bring about the leading of the output pulse. This same rising edge is also delayed by 20 microseconds through an R-C network. Its eventual arrival at the output of the monostable then brings about the trailing edge of the output pulse. The circuit node at the juncture of the resistor and capacitor of the R-C network is also bonded out off-chip. There, supplemental capacitance may be added in order to extend the R-C time constant to any duration desired. As the time constant is extended, the pulse emerging from the monostable extends as well, and the push or pull MOSFET that drives V_{post} effects a greater polarization of that node.

In order to establish references for waveforms to be presented later, actual waveforms of the neuromime's response to one supraliminal stimulus were digitally sampled, and are shown in Fig. 20.8. Figure 20.8 shows an excitatory stimulus, along with the response of V_{pre}, the threshold potential node, and the binary output. All of the oscillator networks described in this chapter require that the neuromime be adjusted to undergo tonic excitation. The resting levels of V_{post} and threshold were transposed, and

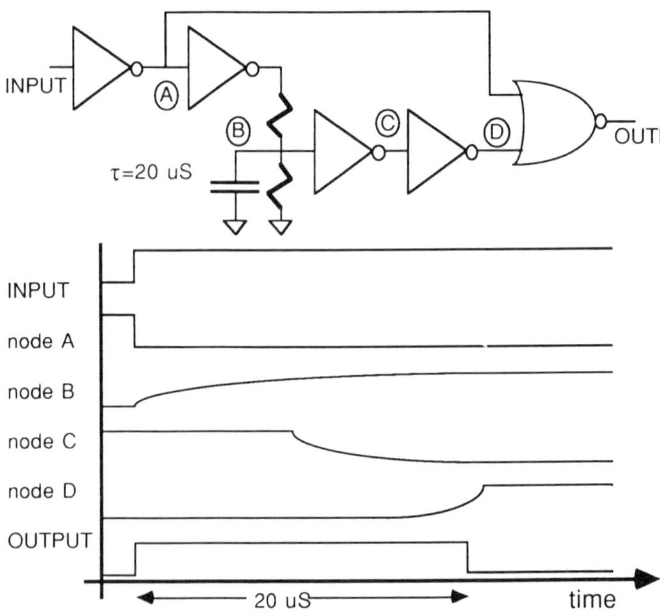

Fig. 20.7. Logical organization of the monostable used to standardize all stimuli to 20 microseconds and waveforms resident in that circuit.

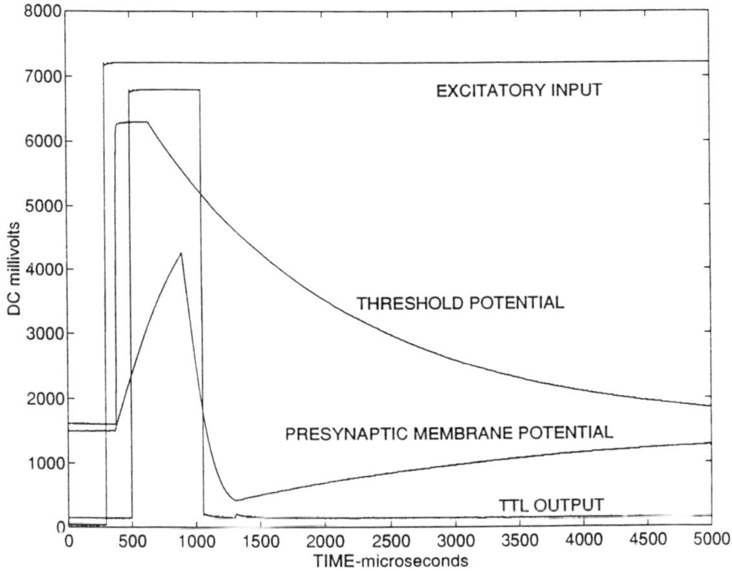

Fig. 20.8. Digitally sampled waveforms resident in the neuromime during the acquisition of a supraliminal excitatory stimulus. Waveforms shown are the excitatory stimulus (A), threshold potential (B), presynaptic membrane potential (C), and the TTL level output (D).

the digitally sampled waveforms that occurred as a result are shown in Fig. 20.9, including signals on V_{post}, threshold, the voltage comparator output, and V_{pre}. With this organization, the IC-based neuromime can not only exhibit continuous tonic activity without supplemental circuitry, but can do so over a wide range of output frequencies. This provides excellent flexibility in characterizing the relationship between the output frequency of an oscillator network and the output frequencies of the cells that comprise it.

Oscillatory behavior, as observed in biological systems, has been attributed to a number of neurodynamic mechanisms. Two such processes are particularly prominent-reciprocal inhibition and recurrent cyclic inhibition. Reciprocal or mutual inhibition occurs between a pair of tonically active cells, each of which possess some mechanism of fatigue in its own activity level or in its responsiveness to outward inhibition. The latter mechanism is known as postinhibitory rebound (PIR), and has been described by Perkel and Mulloney (1974). Recurrent cyclic inhibition occurs in a circular arrangement of tonically active neurons, as described by Szekely (1965). In order to accurately replicate the activity in the biological oscillator in this study, it would be necessary for the neuromime to replicate both of these oscillatory modalities.

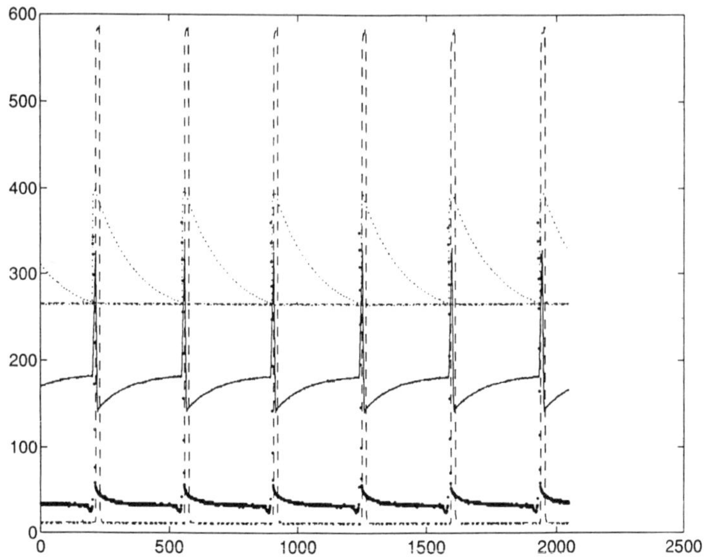

Fig. 20.9. Digitally sampled waveforms resident in a neuromime undergoing tonic excitation. Shown are waveforms of a binary output pulse (A), threshold potential (B), postsynaptic membrane potential (C), presynaptic membrane potential (D), and the voltage comparator output (E).

3.1. The Cyclically Inhibitory Networks

A ring containing an odd number of three or more tonically active neurons, each with an inhibitory connection to its neighbor in the clockwise direction will produce cyclic bursts of impulses that propagate counterclockwise. All neurons in the ring are behaviorally similar, and additional synaptic delay may be introduced at any point or points in the ring. Kling and Szekely (1968) analyzed such networks, and found that any ring with an odd number of cells interconnected in this way will oscillate with a period equal to the number of cells in the ring multiplied by the time required for each cell to recover from sustained inhibition to its nominally active state. Rings with even numbers of cells interconnected in this way exhibit bistable behavior, but may be made to oscillate if additional inhibitory interconnections are added. The majority of circuit testing in this study was conducted with a five-celled ring, but rings of three cells and seven cells were also demonstrated to function in accordance with Szekely's observations.

The five-celled ring network shown in Fig. 20.4 was the first to be assembled. Each neuromime was set to the following parameters: V_{DD} = 7.0 volts DC, V_{post} rests at 2.7 volts DC with a time constant of 116 milliseconds, V_{pre} rests at 1.9 volts DC with a time constant of 7.0 milliseconds, and threshold rests at 2.4 volts DC, with a time constant of 1.4 milliseconds. With these settings, each neuromime was observed to generate impulses at a frequency of 100 Hz in the absence of external inhibition, and exhibit total inhibition when a 100-Hz inhibitory signal is introduced. When five neuromimes were assembled into a ring, the circuit exhibited oscillatory behavior according to Szekely's observations, and did so without requiring transient modifications to any circuit nodes. Multiprobe tests revealed that, at any one time, two cells were found to be active, two inhibited, and the remaining cell in the process of recovering from inhibition. Digitally sampled waveforms from two nodes of this circuit are shown in Fig. 20.10. From this point onward, a number of parametric tests were conducted on this network to assess its stability with respect to a number of simulated chemical and electrical variations in neuronal operating conditions. Results from these tests are presented in the next section.

3.2. The Mutually Inhibitory Networks

The two-phase mutually inhibitory oscillator was implemented using a pair of identical neuromime circuits whose outputs cross-connect to an inhibitory input of their counterpart cell, as shown in Fig. 20.3. Each neuromime was configured with the same

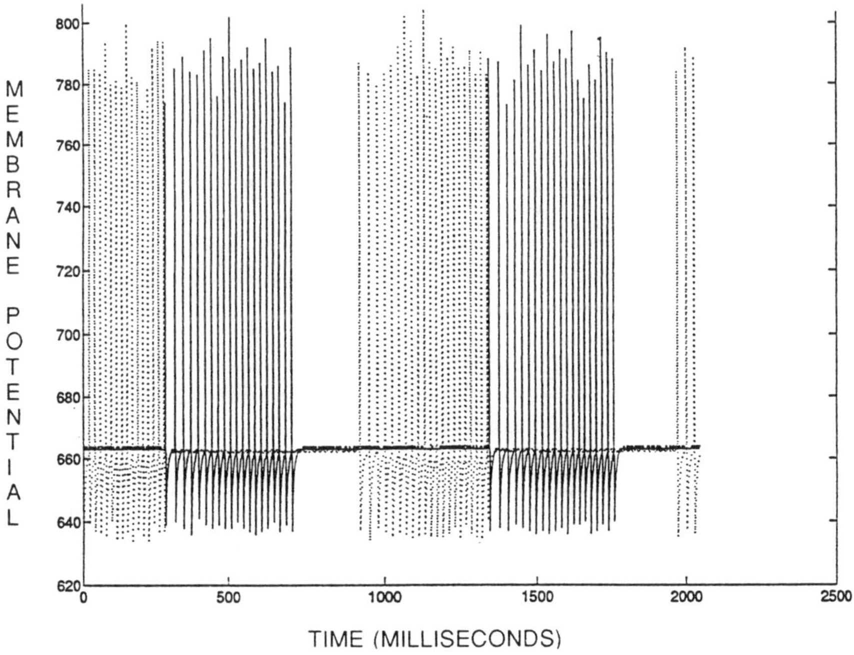

Fig. 20.10. Digitally sampled waveforms of V_{pre} from two adjoining cells of the five-celled cyclic inhibitory ring network.

V_{DD}, resting levels, and time constants as used in the cyclic oscillators. As such, it was confirmed to tonically excite at a rate of 100 Hz and exhibit zero output activity with a 100-Hz inhibitory stimulus. Interconnecting a pair of neuromimes configured in this way, however, failed to produce the expected behavior. Instead, the network was observed to exhibit one of two possible responses: Either one cell would remain active and inhibit its counterpart indefinitely, or the pair of cells would both oscillate at some intermediate frequency, simultaneously and partially emitting impulses and inhibiting their counterparts. With this observation, it became clear that function of a network in this configuration depends on how tonic excitation is inhibited, not only at the active and inhibited frequencies, but all points in between. Although the neuromime does not support variation of the linearity of the synaptic weight, this effect may be approximated by manipulating the temporal course of it inhibitory synaptic weight. The result of this change was that the same two behaviors were observed but, in the case of both cells being partially active, that frequency would be reduced. Because the neuromime's temporal summation response to a single input is consistent with biological models, the solution to this problem then had to be in the incorporation of transient responses. This was the avenue pursued in order to reproduce PIR.

The key to implementing PIR lies in the plasticity of the synaptic inhibitory input. Empirically, PIR may be described as a neuron possessing a high innate sensitivity to inhibition and, as more inhibitory stimulation is incurred, that sensitivity drops to a level not normally sufficient to suppress tonic excitation. The neuron then rebounds to some reduced level of output activity, and generates action potentials that will inhibit its counterpart. Once the inhibition received from its counterpart has ceased, the neuron immediately reverts to its nominal output frequency and its synaptic sensitivity returns to its nominal high value a short time later. This sequence of events was achievable through both implicit and explicit mechanisms of synaptic weight modification.

Implicit synaptic weight reduction was accomplished with the introduction of an additional capacitance to the node onto which V_{post} is discharged with each inhibitory stimulus. This circuitry is illustrated in Fig. 20.11, which shows this capacitor C_F, as well as the MOSFETs that charge and discharge it, M2A and M2B, respectively. Each inhibitory stimulus discharges C_{MEM} into C_F, elevating the voltage on C_F from ground toward V_{post}. As this voltage increases, the net polarization of V_{post} that occurs with each inhibitory stimulus is diminished, and the effects of synaptic weight reduction are manifest. Eventually, inhibitory stimuli become unable to hinder the target cell's own tonic excitation, and the cell rebounds to its spontaneously active state.

Implementing this circuit revealed that several adjustments and conditions had yet to be considered. First, the inhibitory stimuli to one cell originate from the other cell that is just emerging from an inhibited state. Such cells do not rebound to the same frequency at which they tonically excite. Therefore, the neuromimes must be adjusted so that they are completely inhibited at frequencies significantly less than 100 Hz. Furthermore, in order to replicate the behavior of biological PIR oscillators, the onset of inhibitory stimuli must bring about an immediate end to neuronal activity. This means that the very first pulse alone is enough to shut down the target cell. As a result, the nominal inhibitory sensitivity must be far greater than had first been anticipated. This is an adjustment that is made outside of the learning circuit. With the innate inhibitory sensitivity always so high, the neuromime was found to have more difficulty in rebounding from inhibition. This restriction necessitated an extra measure of circuit tuning in the inhibitory synaptic weight, but finally yielded two-phase PIR oscillatory behavior. Digitally sampled waveforms from the mutually inhibited PIR oscillator are shown in Fig. 20.12.

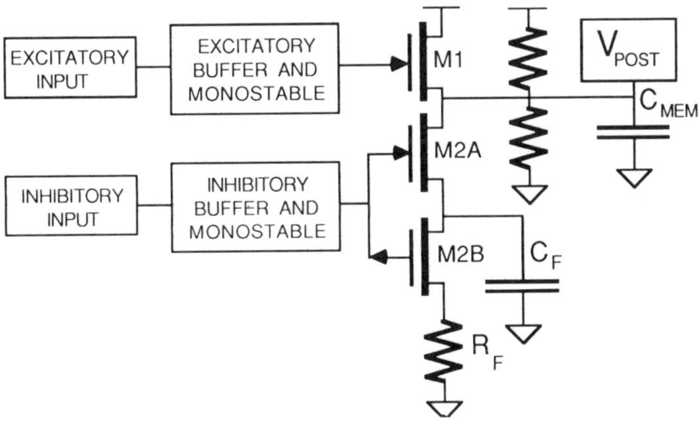

Fig. 20.11. Supplementary circuitry used to implement synaptic weight modification for postinhibitory rebound.

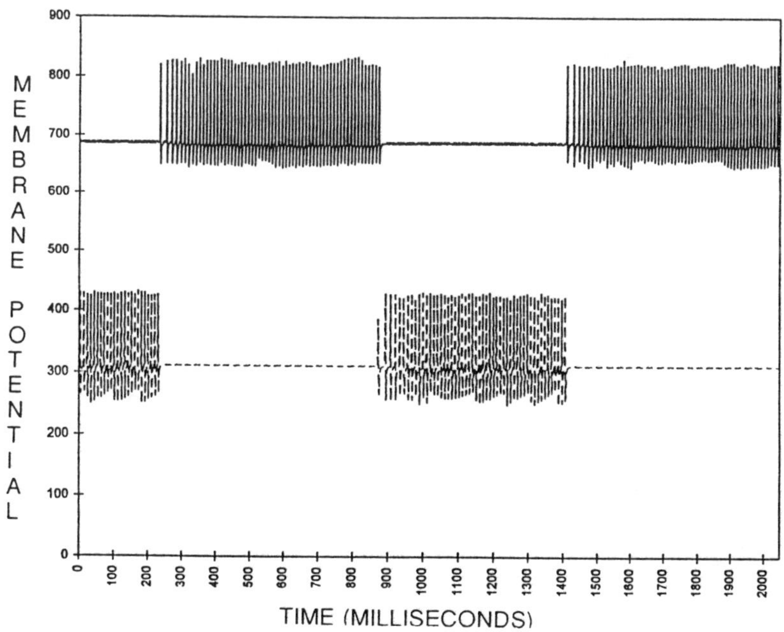

Fig. 20.12. Digitally sampled waveforms of presynaptic membrane potential from the mutually inhibitory two-phase oscillator network with explicit synaptic weight modification.

4. RESULTS

Bench tests performed on neuronally-based oscillators were conducted in two phases. The first phase involved characterizing the frequency of tonic excitation in individual neurons as a response to variation in environmentally derived parameters, such as resting membrane potential, threshold potential, threshold time constant, and incident inhibitory stimuli. The second phase encompassed characterizing the frequency of the network's reciprocal and cyclic oscillation in response to variation in the frequency of self-excitation of its component neurons. The objective of these tests is to evaluate the stability of the oscillator in response to a variety of parametric variations. Results will help to assess the validity of the neural reconstruction methodology to be developed later in this study. All of the parameters in this study are easily and precisely controllable due to the flexible organization of the component neuromimes, and form analogs to environmental variations such as ambient temperature and the concentration of various ionic species, such as sodium, potassium, and chloride.

4.1. Characterization of Individual Nerve Cells

In the first phase, each of the five neuromimes was configured as described earlier, with a V_{DD} of 7.0 volts DC, V_{post} resting at 2.7 volts DC, and threshold potential resting at 2.4 volts DC. This biasing arrangement leaves V_{post} resting 0.3 volts DC above threshold, causing the neuron to tonically excite at 100 Hz. In the course of this test, the resting level of V_{post} for each cell was varied upward so that it nominally exceeded the threshold potential by from 0.1 to 1.1 volts DC. This test was conducted for the nominal threshold time constant of 1.4 milliseconds, and repeated for time constants of 0.4 and 14 milliseconds. Results of these tests are given in Fig. 20.13. Some of the flexibility of the neuromime design is borne out in this test, as the frequency of cellular tonic excitation is seen to vary smoothly from under 10 Hz to over 600 Hz without any additional circuit modifications.

From the disparities of these three curves, it is apparent that the level of tonic activity is also highly dependent on the duration of the relative refractory period, which is controlled in the neuromime by the capacitor placed on the threshold potential node. By dictating the rate of decay of threshold from its absolute maximal value back to its resting level, this capacitor allows another mechanism for continuous and precise control over the frequency of tonic excitation. In the second phase of testing, this relationship was examined. Capacitors of varying values were placed on the threshold potential node for all five neurons in the ring, and results are shown in the log-log graph of Fig. 20.14. Once again, the frequency of tonic activity is seen to be widely and smoothly controllable over the range from 0.1 to over 600 Hz with no other modifications made to the circuit.

Finally, the rate of tonic excitation may be modulated by means of applying tonic inhibitory stimuli from an independent source. The effect of such inhibition on a cell that nominally excites at 100 Hz is shown in Fig. 20.15. In the course of circuit tests,

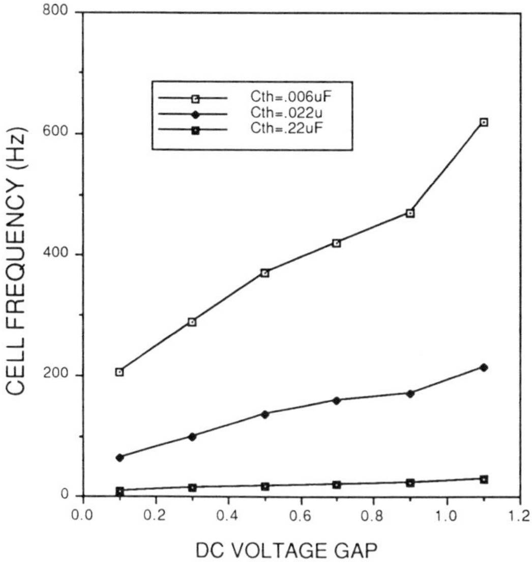

Fig. 20.13. The effect on cellular tonic excitatory frequency seen by varying the cellular threshold, as defined by the voltage gap between V_{post} and threshold potential for relative refractory period durations of 0.4 milliseconds (top), 1.4 milliseconds (center), and 14 milliseconds (bottom) curve, as simulated by different capacitance values on the threshold potential node.

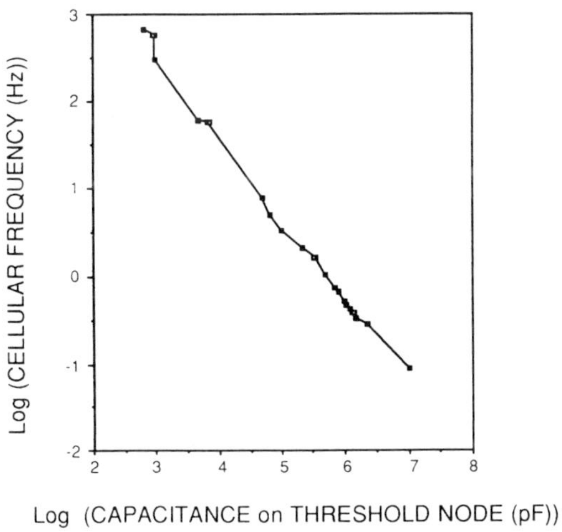

Fig. 20.14.. The effect on cellular frequency seen by varying the time constant on the threshold potential node.

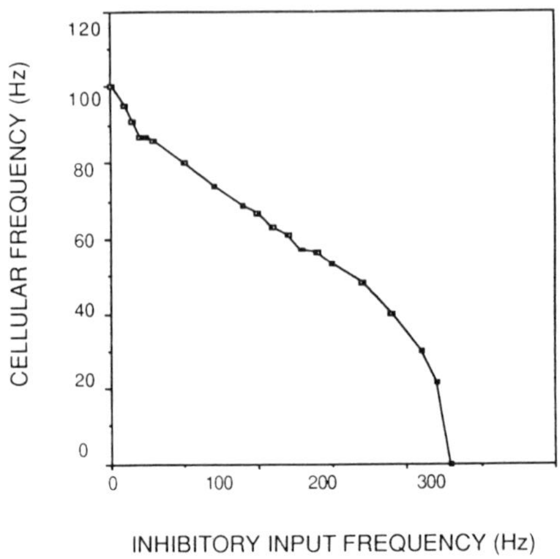

Fig. 20.15. The effect on tonic excitation frequency seen by varying the intensity of an external inhibitory stimulus.

this relationship exhibited an appreciable amount of variability, not only in response to the inhibitory frequency, but also with respect to synaptic weight and transient synchronization of off-chip stimuli with on-chip events. This facility, along with the two previously mentioned, and an independent and continuous control over all synaptic weights offers a tremendous flexibility in simulating a number of transient characteristics in individual nerve cells and circuits they comprise.

4.2. The Cyclically Inhibited Networks

In the second phase of testing, the overall response of cyclically inhibited networks to variation of the parameters that so dramatically affect tonic activity level was evaluated. Whereas the synaptic weight and input stimulus frequency of the inhibitory signal path are constrained to ranges that enable the circuit to support tonic activity, the other two parameters under investigation, (I) voltage gap between V_{post} and threshold and the (II) threshold time constant were varied, and the impact on cyclic output frequency assessed in two circuit tests. In the first test, the voltage difference between V_{post} and threshold was varied, and the overall ring operating frequency recorded. Results of this test are shown in Fig. 20.16. In the second test, the duration of the refractory period for

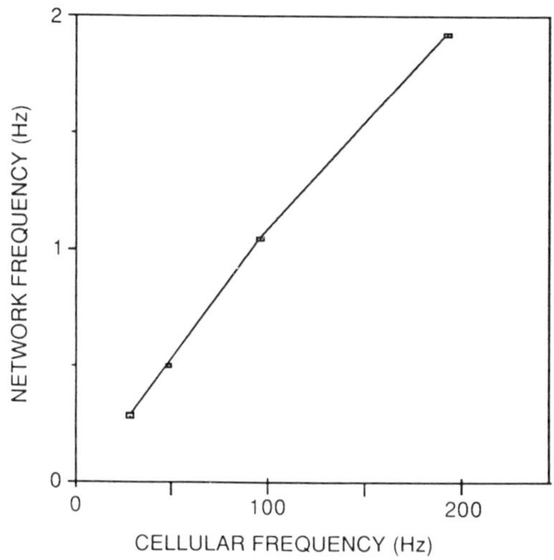

Fig. 20.16. Relationship between frequency of the five-cell cyclic oscillator and the tonic cellular frequency, as varied by altering the gap between resting levels of V_{post} and threshold potential.

all five cells was varied, and the ring output frequency recorded. Data from this test are presented in Fig. 20.17.

Data from the graph of Fig. 20.17 indicate that the frequency of cyclic oscillation is roughly proportional to the frequency of tonic excitation over the range of cyclic frequency from 0.3 to 2.0 Hz when tonic excitation is varied by means of the gap between V_{post} and the resting threshold potential. With this arrangement, the number of individual impulses in each burst would be relatively constant. In tests, this was observed, with 38 to 41 pulses observed in each burst. Data from the graph of Fig. 20.17b indicate that the frequency of cyclic oscillation is relatively insensitive to variation in cellular frequency when cell frequency is modulated by varying the duration of the refractory period. This observation was especially pronounced for higher levels of the voltage gap between V_{post} and threshold, and held over the range of cellular frequencies from near zero to over 600 Hz, as shown in Fig. 20.17a. These results, along with those of Fig. 20.16 suggest that the output frequency of cyclic oscillators are sensitive to cellular parameters affecting threshold, and immune to cellular parameters affecting refractory period.

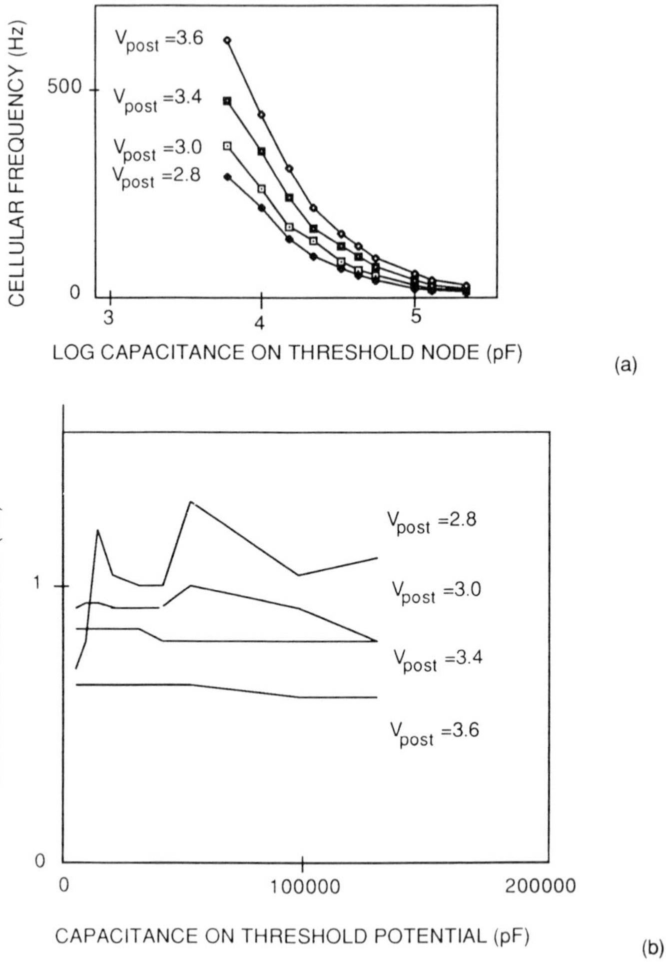

Fig. 20.17. Variation in cellular frequency, as induced by altering the duration of the relative refractory period (A, above) and response of the five-cell ring to that variation (B, below). These measurements are repeated for four different values of resting level of V_{post} from 2.8 to 3.6 volts DC.

4.3. The Reciprocally Inhibitory Networks

Tests of the Reciprocally Inhibitory networks were also carried out in two phases. The resistor and capacitor labeled R_F and C_F of Fig. 20.11 were used to determine the magnitude and latency of synaptic fatigue for each artificial nerve cell. In a series of tests, the value of C_F was varied and its effect on reciprocally inhibitory behavior recorded. In those tests, the network demonstrated smoothly variable and stable oscillations over the range of cellular frequency from 15 to 450 Hz, over the range of network output frequency from 0.1 to 18 Hz, and from six to several thousand impulses per burst.

Network response to the value of C_F for constituent cellular frequencies of 130, 200, and 300 Hz were all found to be smoothly and continuously variable, as illustrated in the log-log graphs of Fig. 20.18. Once it was confirmed that C_F, which controls the latency of onset of synaptic weight modification, coherently affected the network frequency, the effect of cellular threshold on overall network frequency was then assessed.

In the final series of tests, the cellular threshold, as manifest by the value of V_{post}, was varied over a wide segment of its operating range and the effect on cellular and network frequency observed. Results from this test are given in Fig. 20.19. There, it was observed that the cellular frequency varied in a manner consistent with the data of Fig. 20.14, whereas the overall network remained relatively close to its nominal operating frequency of approximately 1 Hz.

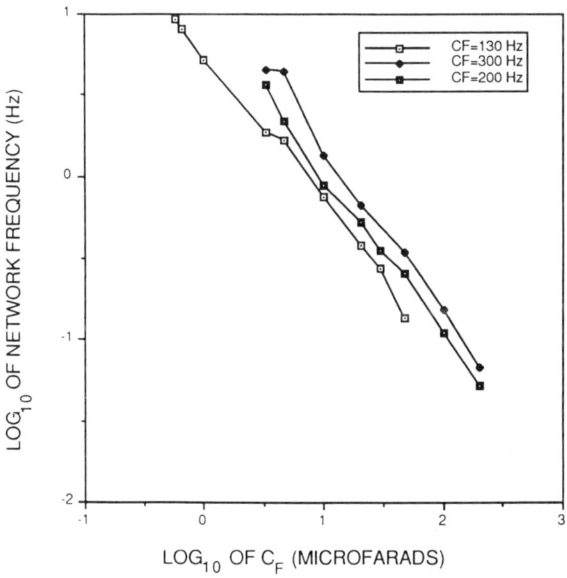

Fig. 20.18. Oscillatory frequency of the reciprocally inhibitory network as a function of the value of C_F. The network uses implicit synaptic modification and the cells of the network tonically excite at cellular frequencies (CF) of 130 Hz (leftmost curve), 200 Hz (center curve), and 300 Hz (rightmost curve).

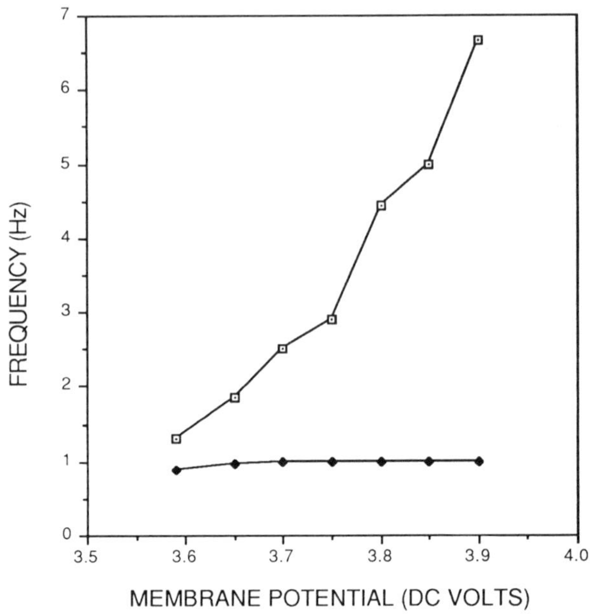

Fig. 20.19. Response of constituent cells (upper curve) and the mutually inhibitory network (lower curve) to variation in cellular threshold, as controlled by the resting level of V_{post}. For reasons of scaling, note that the cellular frequency is normalized to its minimal value of 137 Hz.

5. DISCUSSION

For any living organism, the likelihood and efficiency of day-to-day survival are most assured if the neuronal elements that control its sensation, motion, and information processing maintain their rhythm in the face of transient variation in environmental conditions such as temperature, ionic concentrations, and the availability of various nutrients. Parametric tests of such oscillator networks will allow us to draw several conclusions about the networks and their design. Circuit tests showed, for example, that reciprocally inhibiting two-phase networks and cyclically inhibited five-phase ring networks demonstrated operation over a wide range of cellular and network frequencies, and tolerated variation in cellular parameters that would have seriously disrupted the operation of tonically active single cells. In addition, these network configurations showed parametric sensitivities that complemented one another, providing maximal stability to any oscillator network that employs combinations of both types. This relationship also suggests that such networks possess time constants that transcend those of their elemental cells, and that they may be made highly immune to parameters that are expected to vary widely day-to-day.

It is well known that the function of a single nerve cell varies dramatically with respect to variation in outward and inward environmental conditions in terms of its innate excitatory and inhibitory responsiveness, resting membrane potential, and the very shape, duration, and amplitude of the action potential through which it communicates with other nerves and effectors. As is the case with artificial systems, the overall response of a system can be made to maintain its operational state in spite of the parametric sensitivities of the components from which it is composed. This is the phenomenon observed in the mockup of the five-cell ring oscillator.

It was expected that the frequency at which the cyclic inhibitory network oscillates be closely dependent on the frequency at which its component neurons oscillate. For a network to follow this trend, the number of impulses in each burst would remain relatively constant. This tendency was observed in three-celled ring networks by Friesen and Stent (1977), and confirmed in five-celled rings, as shown by the data of Fig. 20.18. By changing the mechanism that limits the self-excitation frequency, however, it was also shown that the frequency of network oscillation can be largely independent of the frequency at which the component neurons oscillate. Data from Fig. 20.19 indicate that, for larger gaps between threshold and V_{post}, the overall frequency of cyclic oscillation is very consistent, even though the frequency of tonic excitation of the individual cells varies over two orders of magnitude. Networks following these conditions would exhibit the number of impulses per burst varying dramatically. In such networks, the time constant that dictates the duration of these bursts is dependent on some other temporal mechanism other than the refractory period.

Although these data agree with those obtained by Friesen and Stent (1977), there are also stark contrasts between this study and theirs. In their study, most tests were conducted with the intensity of tonic excitation being the input to the system. This parameter corresponds to the systemic enabling of the oscillator while its own internal parameters were held relatively constant. In the current study, the response of the internal parameters was examined, while the systemic gating or enabling of the system was held constant. The other contrast apparent between these studies is that the Friesen and Stent model relied on frequency-invariant intersegmental temporal delays for system stability, while the VLSI-based models demonstrate that such stability may be brought about by a mechanism innate to the structure of the network. In the next phase of this project, the VLSI-based five-celled ring will be incorporated into a more precisely configured and interconnected model of the leech swimming network, as recently detailed by Friesen (1989). With the low cost, convenience and circuit density afforded by VLSI technology, such a task is far more attainable today than in the time the original models were constructed.

The improved comprehensiveness afforded by the VLSI-based neuromime has already yielded insights to neuronal function not disclosed in studies using discrete circuits or software simulation. This facility will be used in future studies to construct comprehensive neuron-by-neuron, synapse-by-synapse mockups based on morphological data and cell-cell interactions. Signal patterns resident in such networks will be compared with those of electrophysiological data and outward behavioral observations in order to evaluate the completeness and accuracy of the biological model. Once a methodology for this practice is developed, it will be applied to other biological neural systems, in order to provide new insights into neural mechanisms of motion, signal processing, and pattern recognition.

ACKNOWLEDGMENTS

Developmental work on the IC-based Neuromime and neural oscillator networks was supported by NSF grants MIP-9210945 and EID-920039. The author wishes to thank Andrew J. Laffely and Alifya E. Chinwalla[1] for their assistance in designing and testing VLSI prototypes.

REFERENCES

Brockman, W. H. (1979). A simple electronic neuron model incorporating both active and passive responses. *IEEE Transactions on Biomedical Engineering*, *26*, 635-639.

Crane, H. D. (1962). Neuristor — A novel device and system concept. *Proceedings of the IRE*, *50*, 2048-2060.

DeYong, M. R., Findley, R. L. & Fields, C. (1992). The design, fabrication, and test of a new VLSI hybrid analog-digital neural processing element. *IEEE Transactions on Neural Networks*, *3*, 363-374.

Elias, J. G., & Northmore, D. P. (1995). Switched-capacitor neuromorphs with wide-range variable dynamics. *IEEE Transactions on Neural Networks*, *6*, 1542-1548.

Elliott, C. J., & Benjamin, P. R. (1985). Interactions of pattern-generating interneurons controlling feeding in *Lymnaea Stagnalis*. *Journal of Neurophysiology*, *54*, 1396-1411.

Fitzhugh, R. (1966). An electronic model of the nerve membrane for demonstration purposes. *Journal of Applied Physiology*, *21*, 305-308.

French, A. S., & Stein, R. B. (1970). A flexible neuronal analog using integrated circuits. *IEEE Transactions on Biomedical Engineering*, *17*, 248-253.

Friesen, W. O. (1989). Neuronal control of leech swimming Movements. In J. W. Jacklet (Ed.), *Neuronal and Cellular Oscillators* (pp. 269-316). New York: Marcel Dekker.

Friesen, W. O., & Stent, G. S. (1977). Generation of a locomotory rhythm by a neural network with recurrent cyclic inhibition. *Biological Cybernetics*, *28*, 27-40.

Getting, P. (1989). A network oscillator underlying swimming in tritonia. In J. W. Jacklet (Ed.), *Neuronal and Cellular Oscillators* (pp. 215-236). New York: Marcel Dekker.

Grillner, S., Wallen, P., Brodin, L., & Lansner, A. (1991). Neuronal network generating locomotor behavior in lamprey: Circuitry, transmitters, membrane properties, and simulation. *Annual Review of Neuroscience*, *14*, 169-199.

Hiltz, F. F. (1963). Artificial neuron. *Kybernetik*, *1*, 231-236.

Jenik, F. (1962). Electronic neuron models as an aid to neurophysiological research. *Ergebnisse Biologie*, *25*, 206-245.

Johnson, R. N., & Hanna, G. R. (1969). Membrane model: A single transistor analog of excitable membrane. *Journal of Theoretical Biology*, *22*, 401-411.

Kling, V. & Szekely, G. (1968). Simulation of rhythmic nervous activities I — Action of networks with cyclic inhibitions. *Kybernetik*, *5*, 89-103.

---

[1] NSF-REU participant, 1992-93.

Lewis, E. R. (1968a). An electronic model of the neuroelectric point process. *Kybernetik, 5*, 30-46.

Lewis, E. R. (1968b). Using electronic circuits to model simple neuroelectric interactions. *Proceedings of the IEEE, 56*, 931-949.

Linares-Barranco, B., Sanchez-Sinencio, E., Rodriguez-Vazquez, A., & Huertas, J. L., (1991). A CMOS implementation of Fitzhugh-Nagumo model. *IEEE Journal of Solid-State Circuits, 26*, 956-965.

MacGregor, R. J., & Oliver, R. M. (1973). A general purpose electronic model for arbitrary configurations of neurons. *Journal of Theoretical Biology, 38*, 527-538.

Mahowald, M., & Douglas, R. (1991). A silicon neuron. *Nature, 354*, 515-518.

Mitchell, C. E., & Friesen, W. O. (1981). A neuromime system for neural circuit analysis. *Biological Cybernetics, 40*, 127-137.

Perkel, D. H., & Mulloney, B. (1974). Motor pattern production in reciprocally inhibitory neurons exhibiting postinhibitory rebound. *Science, 185*, 181-183.

Pottala, E. W., Colburn, T. R., & Humphrey, D. R. (1973). A dendritic compartment model neuron. *IEEE Transactions on Biomedical Engineering, 20*, 132-139.

Robertson, R. M., & Pearson, K. G. (1985). Neural circuits in the flight system of the locust. *Journal of Neurophysiology, 53*, 110-128.

Roy, G. (1972). Simple electronic analog of the squid axon membrane: The NeuroFET. *IEEE Transactions on Biomedical Engineering, 18*, 60-63.

Runge, R. G., Uemura, M., & Viglione, S. S. (1968). Electronic synthesis of the avian retina. *IEEE Transactions on Biomedical Engineering, 15*, 138-151.

Satterlie, R. A., & Spencer, A. N. (1985). Swimming in the pteropod mollusc *Clione Limacina* II. *Journal of Experimental Physiology, 116*, 205-222.

Selverston, A. I. (1985). *Model Neural Networks and Behavior*. New York, Plenum Press.

Szekely, G. (1965). Logical network for controlling limb movement in *Urodela*. *Acta Physiologica of the Academy of Sciences of Hungary, 27*, 285-289

Wolpert, S., & Tzanakou, E. (1986). An integrated circuit realization of a neuronal model. In S. C. Orphanoudakis (Ed.), *Proceedings of the IEEE 12th Annual Northeast Bioengineering Conference*, Yale University, New Haven, CT, March 13-14, 1986.

Author Index

Italics denote pages on which complete references appear.

C

L

Y

Z

Subject Index

M

N

O

P